Praise for *Healthy Teens, Body and Soul*

"For parents who are struggling with their teen's health, this book is vital."
—Lynn E. Ponton, M.D., author of *The Romance of Risk:
Why Teenagers Do the Things They Do* and *The Sex Lives of Teenagers:
Revealing the Secret World of Adolescent Boys and Girls*

"This book is a model for helping parents and young people become partners to support thriving in adolescence, rather than merely surviving it."
—Karen Hein, M.D., President, William T. Grant Foundation

"*Healthy Teens, Body and Soul* brings a new and refreshing perspective. . . . I highly recommend this book for all parents seeking to help guide their children through adolescence."
—Arthur Elster, M.D., Director, Medicine and Public Health,
American Medical Association

"*Healthy Teens, Body and Soul* will help parents as they advise their sons and daughters how to stay healthy in the second decade of life. Marks and Rothbart have made a valuable contribution to the popular health literature by clarifying the health issues in a positive manner."
—Charles E. Irwin, Jr., M.D., Director, Division of Adolescent Medicine,
University of California, San Francisco Children's Medical Center

"Parents of teens: This is it. This is the book to put parents in-the-know so they can help their teens toward a healthy independence. Marks and Rothbart have given parents not just a roadmap, but a comprehensive field guide for sharing their teen's journey through adolescence toward adulthood."
—Marlin S. Potash, Ed.D., and Laura Potash Fruitman,
mother-daughter coauthors of *Am I Weird or Is This Normal?*

Healthy Teens, Body
AND
Soul

A Parent's Complete Guide
to Adolescent Health

Andrea Marks, M.D.

Betty Rothbart, M.S.W.

A Skylight Press Book

A FIRESIDE BOOK
Published by Simon & Schuster
New York   London   Toronto   Sydney   Singapore

FIRESIDE
Rockefeller Center
1230 Avenue of the Americas
New York, NY 10020

A Skylight Press Book

For information about special discounts for bulk purchases,
please contact Simon & Schuster Special Sales:
1-800-456-6798 or business@simonandschuster.com

Designed by Christine Weathersbee

Manufactured in the United States of America

10 9 8 7 6 5 4 3 2 1

Library of Congress Cataloging-in-Publication Data

Marks, Andrea, M.D.
  Healthy teens, body and soul : a parent's complete guide / Andrea Marks, Betty Rothbart.
    p. cm.
  Includes index.
  1. Teenagers—Health and hygiene. 2. Teenagers—Psychology. I. Rothbart, Betty.
II. Title.

  RA777.M267 2003
  613'0433—dc21   2002190999

ISBN 0-7432-2561-9

Permissions appear on page 359.

Dedicated with love to my partners in life . . .
my parents, Ruth and Stanley Marks;
my children, Gillian and Jordana Warmflash;
my husband, David Warmflash.
—Andrea Marks, M.D.

Dedicated with love to my parents,
David and Dorothy Rothbart, who gave me life
and showed me how to live it,
and to my children, Lila and Jacob Smith,
who keep the love flowing.
—Betty Rothbart, M.S.W.

Acknowledgments

Andrea Marks, M.D.

Healthy Teens, Body and Soul is based on the research and teachings of specialists in the field of adolescent medicine. A relatively new medical specialty, adolescent medicine was founded in 1951 by Dr. J. Roswell Gallagher, who, believing that adolescents are different and require a distinct kind of health care, established the first adolescent clinic in the United States at Children's Hospital of Boston. Twenty-three years later, I had the privilege of doing my training in adolescent medicine at Boston Children's with Dr. Gallagher's successor, Dr. Robert Masland, an inspiring and thoughtful teacher, and my exceptional colleagues, Drs. Jean Emans and Norman Spack.

A second learning spurt occurred in my first "real job" in the Division of Adolescent Medicine at Montefiore Medical Center in the Bronx, New York. Dr. Michael I. Cohen, mentor extraordinaire, and my colleagues, Drs. Ken Schonberg, Iris Litt, and Karen Hein, were (and, as national leaders in the field, continue to be) models of commitment and academic rigor.

My training complete, a few years later I accepted the offer of Dr. Mervin Silverberg to establish the new Division of Adolescent Medicine at North Shore University Hospital in Manhasset, New York. With the undaunted support of Dr. Silverberg and the perseverance of terrific colleagues, most especially Dr. Martin Fisher, we built a program to take care of teens, train pediatricians and aspiring specialists in adolescent medicine, and conduct research in adolescent health.

Years later, I felt a tug to put all I had learned in academia into practice in the "real world" and in 1990 opened a private practice for adolescents and young adults (ages 9 to 30) in New York City. No surprise, my learning curve escalated even more steeply, and I thank our wonderful patients and their parents for their intelligence, openness, and trust. They have taught me important lessons in adolescent medicine, most especially about the complexities and subtleties of caring for teens within the context of family. I thank my dedicated associate, Dr. Karen Rosewater, and my devoted office manager, Harriet Rasch, for their wisdom and spirit.

The Society for Adolescent Medicine (SAM) was founded by the pioneers in our field in 1968 and has grown into a multidisciplinary, international organization of health professionals committed to improving the health and well-being of adolescents. To have served the Society as director of scientific programs and a member of the board of directors has been among the most enriching experiences of my career. To have been selected to be the President of SAM in 2004 is a great honor. My numerous friends in SAM are professionals I am extremely lucky and proud to know.

Healthy Teens, Body and Soul is a synthesis of thirty years of thinking about and caring for teens. Writing this book with Betty Rothbart has been a magnificent journey, and I thank her deeply for the experience. Thank you, Lynn Sonberg of Skylight Press, for introducing us and for your guidance, and Caroline Sutton, our editor at Simon and Schuster, for your enthusiastic support.

Finally, what teens and families are all about . . . I thank my parents, Ruth and Stanley Marks, and my sister, Marjorie Marks, for the happiness and security I felt during my own adolescence. I thank my daughters, Gillian and Jordana Warmflash, for the sheer joy I have experienced raising such loving and honest young adults. I thank my husband, David Warmflash, for being a model parent to our children and an unwavering support to me in all aspects of our lives.

Betty Rothbart, M.S.W.

Perhaps my work on this book really began many years ago, on the day my father hauled scrap lumber into the house and built five mailboxes, one for each member of the family. The mailboxes didn't particularly coordinate with the living room decor, but they certainly made *living* easier. My sisters and I were teenagers then, so emotional that my father found it hard to have an orderly conversation with us, and my mother was worn out trying. My dad figured that if we couldn't talk together, we might as well *write*. And so we did.

Letters flew in and out of those mailboxes. I penned passionate pleas for later curfews, shorter skirts, and permission to turn the garage into a dance studio. My father typed his replies on yellow paper, balancing the typewriter on his knees as he sat in his armchair, while my concise, ever-frugal mother scribbled responses on scrap paper and the backs of envelopes.

Of course, we often spoke, too! But when discussions got too heated, we'd shift the conversation to paper. All that back-and-forth taught me a lesson that is reflected in this book: *Communication between parents and teens isn't always easy, but keeping it going even when it's tough is a sign of love.* Now I am committed to communicating with my own teenagers—and, through writing, to encouraging other parents to do so, too.

First, therefore, I thank my parents, David and Dorothy Rothbart, for their ongoing inspiration and support, and my children for theirs. My daughter,

Lila, and my son, Jacob, delight and teach me, and I am proud to be their mother. Thanks to their devoted dad, Stuart Smith, for raising our healthy teens with me.

For their loving encouragement and words of wisdom, my thanks to Gloria Cohen, Karen Curlee, Eleanor Rothbart Goldman, Judith Rothbart Kline, Dexter Lane, Ruth Rothbart Mayer, Irv Rothbart, Harriet Sirof, Alice Soloway, Ken Wampler, and my "Ivy Street family."

For their wonderful tales of adolescent health, many thanks to John, Michael, and Julia Chelen; Alexandra DeMeglio; Josh Ross; and the many other parents and adolescents I spoke with for this book.

Andrea Marks has become a friend as well as a co-author, and working with her has been a warm, harmonious, and rewarding experience.

Lynn Sonberg of Skylight Press has been an enthusiastic guiding spirit whose excellent suggestions have strengthened this book.

Thanks go to our editor at Simon & Schuster, Caroline Sutton, for her insightful guidance and appreciative support, and to her assistant, Nicole Diamond, for her kindness and attention to detail. Thanks also to Chris Lloreda, Deputy Publisher, and Marcia Burch, Vice President for Publicity, for their warm support.

Over the years I have treasured friendships and collaborations with fellow social workers, as well as with colleagues at Planned Parenthood Federation of America, SIECUS, and Bank Street College of Education. Currently, through the New York City Department of Education, I am privileged to work with intelligent, dedicated administrators, teachers, parents, and students on such projects as writing curriculum, creating health and literacy programs, leading teacher and parent workshops, and exploring new ways to expand health knowledge and improve health care access within New York's vibrant, culturally diverse communities.

I am also fortunate to work with wonderful colleagues from the New York State Department of Education, the Mayor's Office of Health Insurance Access, the New York City Department of Health and Mental Hygiene, the New York Academy of Medicine, and other health, mental health, and arts organizations.

Finally, thanks to the American Society of Journalists and Authors, an incomparable source of camaraderie and professional development.

Contents

Introduction

We chose the title *Healthy Teens, Body and Soul* because we feel optimistic and upbeat about adolescence as a time of great energy, resilience, and potential. Yet many health professionals, educators, and above all parents anticipate adolescence with trepidation, fearful that communication and camaraderie, contentment and safety will be difficult to sustain. Indeed, for some adolescents, the teen years are fraught with high levels of stress, unhealthy behaviors, and a decline in overall well-being. But for the great majority of young people, adolescence is a stage of remarkable positive growth in both body and soul.

In a mere ten flash-by years our young children become adults. Through their teen years they must build the knowledge and wisdom and strength to face the world independently. We believe that there are many significant ways their parents can help them thrive. We challenge the cliché that adolescence is a time when teens and parents inevitably must part company—going their separate, even antagonistic, ways. The parent-child relationship certainly *changes*, but teens still want and need their parents' love and involvement. Indeed, adolescents who feel connected to their families and their schools participate in fewer health risk behaviors and feel happier and more secure.

OUR EXPERIENCES HAVE TAUGHT US

Each of us brings to this book both a professional and a personal perspective.

Andrea Marks: As a doctor specializing in adolescent medicine for the past thirty years, directing hospital-based academic programs and in private practice, and the mother of daughters, now ages 18 and 20, I spend a great deal of time talking with teens. I have learned from listening to my patients and my own children how vital to them are the adults, especially parents, in their lives. While fully respecting adolescent patients' rights to privacy and confidentiality, I welcome their parents' involvement in their care. I have learned that it is far easier for parents to step back and let their children relate independently with me when they feel recognized, not marginalized. In fact, most adolescents are relieved and pleased that their parents get to know me. Maintaining that delicate balance between moving in and moving out is the art of adolescent medicine and the art of adolescent parenting. Mutual respect and trust among the members of the "health care team"—the teen, the doctor, the parent—are key to a successful outcome.

Betty Rothbart: As the mother of a daughter, 20, and a son, 16, and with more than twenty-five years' experience as a psychiatric social worker, educator, consultant to health organizations, and author of books on health and parenting, I have had various windows into adolescents' health needs, as well as their family, peer, and school experiences. Whether counseling teenage girls in a group home, training teachers in health and sexuality education, or teaching parent-adolescent communication workshops, time and again I have found a common thread. Adolescents yearn to be close with their parents (even though they might not show it), and parents want to be close with their adolescents (even though they aren't confident that they understand their children's world). The push-pull of adolescent-parent relationships is nothing new, of course. But in our fast-changing world, complicated by forces as varied as technological advances and terrorist threats, I observe that the role of parents as a stable source of love and guidance is more important than ever.

A HEALTH-PARTNERING APPROACH

Healthy Teens, Body and Soul gives you the facts about adolescent health, along with strategies for communicating with your teen. Our goal is to promote adolescent health, family closeness, and support during and beyond the teen years.

Parents can most successfully influence their adolescents' health by becoming their *health partners*. This means that over the course of adolescence, parents adapt their guidance and level of involvement to reflect and respond to their adolescents' evolving maturity and desire for independence. Throughout the book, you will find health-partnering tips that suggest large and small ways to support your adolescents' health and deliver or reinforce health messages.

How do adolescents grow and change? Chapter 1, "The Stages and Tasks of Adolescent Development," shows how their development can be understood as a series of three stages: early, middle, and late adolescence. At each stage, they grapple with the three tasks of adolescence: to gain independence, to clarify sexual identity, and to explore their self-image and their role in society. This chapter presents some fundamental ways that you can strengthen your relationship and communication throughout the adolescent years.

Chapter 2, "A Doctor of Their Own," introduces a key member of your adolescent's support team: a doctor or other health care provider who understands adolescents' needs. We discuss how to select the right doctor for your adolescent's ongoing care and what to expect from a health visit, especially the annual checkup.

Chapter 3, "The Basics: Nutrition, Exercise, and Sleep," addresses a crucial trio of core health practices that can support your adolescent's daily and long-term well-being.

In chapter 4, "Common Health Problems of Boys and Girls," we discuss a wide range of health problems of which all parents of adolescents should be aware. Chapter 5, "Health Issues for Your Daughter," and chapter 6, "Health Issues for Your Son," focus on gender-specific concerns.

Chapter 7, "Coping with Chronic Health Problems," addresses the coping skills needed by adolescents who do not have the luxury of taking their health for granted. Even as they must keep their special health needs in mind, these young people face the same tasks of adolescence as their peers.

Central concerns for all parents of adolescents are addressed in the next three chapters. Chapter 8, "Risks and Realities of Teen Sexuality," explores sexual health and decision making. In chapter 9, "No Teen Is Immune: Substance Use and Abuse," we discuss the dangers of tobacco, alcohol, and other drugs. Chapter 10, "Panic at the Mirror: Teens and Eating Disorders," helps you understand the "disordered eating" that can lead to anorexia, bulimia, obesity, and binge-eating disorder.

Chapter 11, "Your Teen's Mental Health," covers a broad spectrum of concerns ranging from common stresses associated with family life, school, and peers, to mental illnesses and how to get help for your child.

We conclude with chapter 12, "Preventing Accidents and Injuries," on how to help keep your teen safe on the athletic field, at an after-school job, on the road, and elsewhere.

Appendices provide you with books to read, organizations to contact, hot lines to call, and websites to consult. There is also a list of health-related fiction and nonfiction books that your adolescent can enjoy reading, learning from, and sharing with friends. Read these books yourself, too, so you can talk about them with your child and perhaps increase your awareness of adolescent life.

TAKE CARE, TAKE PRIDE

As parents of adolescents ourselves, we know how much fun—and how challenging—the experience can be. Children are never predictable. We can never chart a course for their lives and expect that they'll follow our hopeful plans. Every child is unique; what works with one might fail miserably with another. To help a child succeed, we must tune in to the individuality of his or her temperament, abilities, and hurdles. We must empathically teach our children to take responsibility and problem-solve in ways that work for them. Figuring out each child's subtle needs is a vital skill that makes parenting more gratifying.

As our children mature, we continue to support them in making their own plans and shaping their own lives. We take pride in their accomplishments, competence, and growth. We must never forget that the health decisions adolescents make along the way will affect their futures as much as—perhaps even more than—the other choices they make.

ONE: The Stages and Tasks of Adolescent Development

The best advice for parents of adolescents is the same as that for parents of newborns: *Enjoy your child.*

Adolescence—like infancy—is a time of transformation and discovery for both children and parents. Despite the challenges, the unsung fact is that most adolescents not only thrive and survive the teen years, they also manage to maintain a healthy and loving relationship with their parents.

It's just that the relationship changes. Adolescents gradually demand more independence; parents must gradually grant it to them. And yet, teenagers who continue to feel a connectedness to their parents as they grow up are *least likely* to partake in risky behaviors and more likely to emerge from the process healthier and more secure.

Nowhere is this more meaningful than in the area of health. Together, parents and adolescents navigate a social landscape strewn with health hazards and health opportunities. At some point, adolescents must take the lead. Increasingly on their own, they make choice after choice about opportunities to pursue, risks to take, hazards to sidestep. As adults, they will live with the legacy of the choices they made.

In Shakespeare's *The Winter's Tale*, an old shepherd laments that everyone would be better off if the trouble-prone adolescent years simply did not exist:

> *I would there was no age between ten and three-and-twenty; or that youth would sleep out the rest: for there is nothing in the between but getting wenches with child, wronging the ancientry, stealing, fighting.*

The problems the shepherd cites—teen pregnancy, disrespecting adults, getting into trouble with the law, violence—remain today's concerns, too. Like the shepherd, many parents probably wish that teens could magically leapfrog from childhood to adulthood, bypassing the perilous adolescent years. But both parents and children would be missing one of the most vibrant, interesting times of life, as magical in its way as the transformation from a newborn to a walking, talking, playing child.

WHAT TO DO ABOUT THE FEARS

Adolescence seems unpredictable. Can a child make the passage safely? And will parents be allowed to help? Parents often fear that when puberty strikes, their sweet child will transmogrify into a sullen, thorny creature, unknowable behind a thick bedroom door. As parents' sense of control diminishes, their concern for their child's physical and mental health escalates.

How can they continue to protect their child?

It might help to realize that most adolescents don't want to disappear or lose touch. Even as adolescents pursue independence and depend more on peer approval, they still want to stay connected with Mom and Dad. They need to feel they have a safe home base that will be there for them when they need it. But they also want to be given increasing privileges befitting adults-to-be.

Parents remain the most important adults in adolescents' lives, and adolescents crave their parents' love, respect, dependability, and guidance. Parents have countless opportunities to health-partner with their adolescent—to help guide their child toward becoming a physically, mentally, and emotionally healthy adult.

The art of health-partnering with adolescents is to give them a solid foundation in the basics of health, to keep communication open, and to guide them to take increasing responsibility for their own physical and mental health.

DEFINING ADOLESCENCE

Until the eighteenth century, adolescence was confused with childhood . . . The first typical adolescent of modern times was Wagner's *Siegfried* . . . that combination of (provisional) purity, physical strength, naturism, spontaneity, and joie de vivre which was to make the adolescent the hero of our twentieth century, the century of adolescence . . .

[Our] society has passed from a period which was ignorant of adolescence to a period in which adolescence is the favourite age. We now want to come to it early and linger in it as long as possible.

—Philippe Aries, *Centuries of Childhood:*
A Social History of Family Life[1]

Adolescence is the bridge from childhood to adulthood, spanning more than a decade. It begins at around age 10 and ends at around age 21, when former teens become young adults.

The onset of adolescence is easier to pinpoint because it is tied to a physio-logic event, the onset of puberty. The endpoint is more murky and debatable (some say adolescence lasts forever). At about age 21 young adults graduate from college or have progressed in jobs or the military. They have reached the legal age for drinking in most states and, solidly out of their teens, probably think of themselves as adults. Then again, some teens take on adult roles and responsibilities even before 21 (such as becoming parents themselves). And many teens still feel unsettled well beyond their twenty-first birthday. Certainly most parents are still very much involved in their children's lives beyond age 21, then gradually less so through their twenties.

Adolescence may be viewed as having three stages:

1. *Early adolescence:* the middle school and junior high school years, approximately ages 10 to 14.
2. *Middle adolescence:* the high school years, approximately ages 15 to 18.
3. *Late adolescence:* the few years after high school, approximately ages 18 to 21.

Take a moment to imagine a skating rink, then envision these three groups at play.

Early adolescents cling to their parents' hands or to the wall as they grope their way awkwardly along the ice, trying to stay upright.

Middle adolescents let go and skate with their friends.

And late adolescents are the dazzlers in the center, spinning, jumping, and trying ever more complicated moves.

THE TASKS OF ADOLESCENCE

Each stage of adolescence brings new challenges to face, new skills to master. These are the "tasks" of adolescence, the gauntlet of trials and triumphs that can ultimately propel adolescents to greater maturity, confidence, and sense of purpose. These tasks are:

- *To gain independence:* to feel capable of approaching life's challenges, based on a personal belief system of values and priorities.
- *To clarify sexual identity:* to feel comfortable in a mature body and in establishing close and intimate relationships.
- *To explore societal role and self-image:* to feel clarity of direction to assume mature roles based on interests, talents, and opportunities.

Following are portraits of how these tasks play out during the three phases of adolescence.

EARLY ADOLESCENCE

Ages 10 to 14—the Middle School/Junior High Years

The hallmark of early adolescence is puberty. For girls, puberty usually begins and ends in early adolescence. Boys usually enter puberty during early adolescence but continue to grow and develop well into middle adolescence. The girls look a lot older than the boys during this stage, making for some comical scenes, and undoubtedly some stress for the later-developing boys.

Early adolescents can't decide if they are children or adults. One minute they complain that their parents can't do anything right; the next minute they cuddle up like 5-year-olds. They are very excited about new bodily changes, and begin to dress like teen idols and people pictured in magazines. They become intensely involved with their own bodies and same-sex peers, while developing a new fascination with the opposite sex. They begin to collect CDs and listen to popular music. School becomes more challenging, too much so for those who had just gotten by in elementary school. Early adolescence is a time of heightened emotion and dramatic moments, as these early teens try to get everything right in the midst of physical and emotional changes they can't control.

This is a time for parents to enjoy and to empathize with, to be there and to stay away, to help their early adolescents manage but not try to control their lives. It is a time to offer kids options within the limits you set. Let them feel in control while you set the ground rules.

Although early adolescence is exciting, it is also an anxiety-producing time for both adolescents and their parents. Adolescents need their space and privacy, which are relatively easy to provide, and they also demand independence and freedom, which are harder for parents to feel comfortable with. Young teens want to travel alone, stay out later, and hang out with kids their parents might not know. Much of their life, at school and at play, becomes private, never discussed—except at rare moments when their guard is down . . . such as late at night when the lights are out and there is *no* eye contact.

The shyer or more reserved early adolescent might not feel ready for much independence or be all that interested in the fast-paced social life that begins to emerge among peers. For some adolescents, that social life includes coupling, along with various levels of sexual activity, from kissing, to "kissing with tongue," to touching clothed or unclothed, to oral sex or intercourse. Some early adolescents choose to "hook up," engaging in sexual play just for the fun of it, typically in "one-night stands." This is also the stage when adolescents begin drinking and smoking.

For quieter teens, this can be a difficult time, as they are not able or willing to participate and begin to feel marginalized.

Health-Partnering in Early Adolescence

During this stage, most parents are probably still making medical and dental appointments, continuing to be in charge but encouraging adolescents to take more responsibility.

This is a good time to assess whether to stay with the adolescent's current health provider (pediatrician, clinic) or to seek out a specialist in adolescent medicine (see chapter 2).

With puberty, some new discussions need to happen: about body changes, hygiene, mood fluctuations that accompany hormonal shifts. Whether your child is maturing slowly, quickly, or not yet at all, point out that there is a very wide range of normal.

If you haven't already talked with your adolescent about sexuality, smoking, alcohol, and other drugs, it is time to start. Chances are, if adolescents haven't already been exposed to them, they will be soon. At this point, adolescents are still very concrete thinkers, not able to project into the future the impact of their current health behaviors. So talk with them about the immediate ramifications. For example, rather than focusing on smoking's far-away consequences like lung cancer, talk about how smoking makes kids' breath and clothes smell bad and turns people off, causes coughing, and reduces stamina.

Help your adolescent explore talents and interests. Adolescents who are busy with constructive activities are more likely to envision a promising future and less likely to get in trouble with risk behaviors. Developing skills—whether in athletics, the arts, or entrepreneurial activities like baby-sitting, snow shoveling, and tutoring younger children—promotes a healthy self-image. Engaged adolescents have a place of their own, a role that matters to themselves and others.

MIDDLE ADOLESCENCE

Ages 15 to 18—the High School Years

Most girls in middle adolescence have completed their pubertal development, but boys at this stage are still growing and changing, especially in early high school. But now there is a more level playing field between the boys and girls, and they are beginning to notice each other more than in middle school—and in a more intense and serious way. Sexual feelings begin to surge, and relationships become more committed. "Hooking up" as a game is less likely among these more sophisticated teens. They are more likely to have strongly felt relationships with the opposite—or same—sex. Some high school romances last forever.

Serious sex, with planning ahead and birth control and talking with one's partner, is part of many of these relationships. Many teens, however, abstain from intercourse and explore other ways to express affection and desire. Although romance and true love can happen, most of these relationships are relatively brief, maybe a few months. But teens invariably describe them as "longtime" relationships.

Sometimes these relationships end because they take up too much precious time. High school kids have a lot on their plates. They have demanding schoolwork, passions to pursue (sports, music, the school play), friendships with same-sex peers and opposite-sex friends, family obligations, perhaps part-time jobs. Commitment to a partner is still not of prime importance at this stage of fickle alliances and conflicting demands. Many relationships fizzle.

During high school, adolescents are getting serious about their interests, their passions, and their time. They are learning that life requires choices. They are thinking more intently about who they are, what they love, and what their priorities are. The skills they began to develop during early adolescence become more finely honed—or outgrown, with new interests taking their place.

The future (college, the military, work) is not quite here yet, but it's not that far off, either. Teens are aware that decisions will soon have to be made and that how they perform now will have an impact on future opportunities. High school *counts*, as many kids say.

Family remains important. As teens become more independent—able to travel alone (car, subway, bus, taxi, pickup truck, bike), able to cook or sew or shop, able to hold a job—parents become more like friends and advisers. Increasingly parents are people to talk and debate with, to play tennis with as equals, to go with to a serious play or movie.

The push-pull of the middle school years is often gentler now, especially during the latter part of high school. That doesn't mean things have lulled into a Zen-like peace. Teens still slam doors, are intensely private, and give one-syllable answers. But most teens are beginning to feel more comfortable with themselves, and therefore also with their parents, at this stage.

Health-Partnering in Middle Adolescence

The stakes are higher now. In some areas parents need to move in even more than they did in early adolescence. Finding the right doctor might be critical. Teens might have sexuality-related needs, such as birth control, disease prevention, questions about their sexual orientation. There might be a need to seek professional help for any emotional and psychiatric difficulties, serious alcohol or drug problems, chain smoking. These problems, if left alone, are not likely to resolve by themselves or be outgrown.

Parents can have a critical role in helping teens make decisions about the future as long as they don't try to make the decisions for them. Practical guidance—how to fill out a college application, find a job, compare financial aid packages, drive a car—can be a great "meeting ground" for parents and teens. Parents become resources to the teen, rather than dictating how things are going to be.

LATE ADOLESCENCE

Ages 18 to 21—the Years After High School

It's a confusing age. Able to vote at 18 but not drink until 21. Neither a child nor an adult. Nor even a teen. For most late adolescents, this is a time to leave home in a new way. Their room or bed remains at home but they spend most of their time away. They are forced to become independent, like it or not. If they manage the transition successfully, their clothes will be relatively clean, nutrition reasonable, work habits in order, judgment good. But so suddenly are these skills demanded that it can all come as a shock.

The first year of college is the hardest, not academically for most, but for learning to organize and carry out their own life, on their own. Parents are not there to wake them up, remind them, serve them, help them, cuddle them. There's E-mail, phone calls . . . but parents are *not there.*

They have no idea where I am at four A.M. Am I up to this?

The change of location means making all new friends. Old high school friendships might strengthen, but most fade away. New friendships take time to develop, to feel safe, to feel real. This can be a lonely time.

It's not the same cozy school or familiar town anymore. It's a new world, maybe far away and surely very different. It's exciting and exhilarating and challenging and new . . . but there's that loneliness, at least at first. If friends have gone away and the teen has stayed home, there's that loneliness, too. The social landscape is full of holes.

Maybe one solution would be falling in love. But the stakes become higher now, and no one seems to date much anymore. They have one-night stands or exclusive and serious commitments involving intimacy and regular sex. The alternatives? Hanging out, getting drunk, not even sure quite what happened last night or with whom.

Late adolescents are likely to be clearer about their sexual orientation, or might experiment with new sexual behaviors. Sexually transmitted diseases are more of a threat than ever, and caution is essential. Older partners mean more serious risk. Alcohol is everywhere, and there are no parents around to help put on the brakes. Roommates don't check their breath when they come in at night, or worry about whether they are in their bed or not the next morning.

And the future is now, not next year. *What am I going to be when I grow up?* Probably not an actress or a baseball player, a fireman or policeman. Or maybe yes. *But most likely I need to find something practical so I can earn a living, eventually support a family . . .*

How frightening . . .

I won't think about this for a while. I will call home and chat with my parents instead. I just feel so young and overwhelmed.

Health-Partnering in Late Adolescence

Late adolescents may be on their own, but they still need their parents. Not to tell them what to do, but to be present—maybe not in person, but in spirit. These adolescents need to know that although they are away, they are not forgotten. E-mail is great, but snail mail gives them something they can touch and hold, solid evidence that you're thinking about them. They may not always return phone calls, but it matters that you've left a message. It could be, in fact, that one of these days you'll call at just the moment when your adolescent really needs to hear from you. You'll hear the hoarseness over the phone, find out that your kid is really run-down. And it will be at your urging that your adolescent will actually trek down the hill to the health center to get checked out.

Because health care is likely to shift locales, parents are less likely to meet the provider or even know who it is. But they can encourage their adolescent to use health facilities, even provide guidance in how to describe ailments to a doctor. As more abstract thinkers now, these older adolescents are better able to understand the long-term implications of the health decisions they make.

As adulthood gets ever closer, be sensitive to your adolescent's need to clarify what he or she will do or be in the coming years. Summer jobs, internships, volunteering, or travel can help expand your adolescent's world and open up new opportunities. Some adolescents research or come up with (and finance) these opportunities on their own, but many benefit from their parents' encouragement, collaboration, and contacts in identifying possibilities and making plans. As is the case during the earlier years, late adolescents who are occupied in meaningful activities are less likely to engage in risk behaviors that could compromise their future.

HEALTH-PARTNERING TIPS FOR PARENTS
• *Make your love the rock* your adolescent can always depend on—*no matter what.* Express your belief that your child can achieve his or her dreams. Spend time together and be available to listen.

FIVE KEYS TO RAISING TEENS*

1. Love and Connect.

   Key message: "Most things about their world is changing. Don't let your love be one of them."

2. Monitor and Observe.

   Key message: "Monitor your teen's activities. You still can, and it still counts."

3. Guide and Limit.

   Key message: "Loosen up, but don't let go."

4. Model and Consult.

   Key message: "The teen years: Parents still matter; teens still care."

5. Provide and Advocate.

   Key message: "You can't control their world, but you can add to and subtract from it."

- *Acknowledge what is going well.* Adolescents are more likely to address their shortcomings if they feel appreciated in other ways. You can always find something: *Thanks for doing the dishes without my asking. . . . Your little sister was happy that you read to her. . . . It was nice of you to shovel the neighbor's sidewalk. . . . Thank you for calling to let me know you'd be late. . . . You've been doing much better about getting to school on time.*
- *Avoid characterizing your adolescent as a problem.* When things are rough, express confidence that the problem can be overcome.

*Excerpted from *Raising Teens: A Synthesis of Research and a Foundation for Action*, a Harvard School of Public Health review of studies on adolescents.†

---

†A. Rae Simpson, *Raising Teens: A Synthesis of Research and a Foundation for Action.* Center for Health Communication, Harvard School of Public Health, 2001; accessed February 2, 2002.

- *Do not compare your adolescent with anybody else.* Mark Twain said, "Few things are harder to put up with than the annoyance of a good example." Comparisons only frustrate and shortchange your child.
- *Involve your adolescent in family responsibilities* to strengthen his or her sense of identity and self-worth. Doing household chores and running errands are also ways you can spend time together.
- *Be aware of your teen's whereabouts. Where are you going? What will you do? When will you be home?* Your teen might protest—but needs that attention and knows it shows that you care.
- *Get involved with your child's school.* Attendance at parent association meetings is generally highest in elementary school, then drops off dramatically in middle and high school. If anything, it is even *more* important during adolescence. You can network with other parents and learn of events and issues that your adolescent might not know or communicate—from academic and safety concerns to school trips, scholarships and contests, tutoring and enrichment opportunities, extracurricular activities, community involvement, and more.
- *Learn more about today's youth culture.* Read magazines targeted to adolescents. Listen to youth market radio stations. See teen films. Whether or not you like what you see, you will better understand your child's world.
- *Set few, fair, and consistent rules.* Focus on what really matters: respect, safety, school performance, health. Link actions to positive or negative consequences. Avoid physical or excessively harsh punishment.
- *Involve your teen in decision making.* The more teens are given a say about what happens, the more likely they are to cooperate.
- *Model how to cope with a mistake.* You do not have to be a saint. But when you apologize and try to make amends, your teen will learn to do so, too.
- *Emphasize education, creativity, and spirituality.* Encourage reading, limit TV. Go as a family to museums, plays, and spiritual or religious observances.
- *Help your adolescent discover positive community resources* that will help him or her fulfill talents, develop interests, and link up with positive peers. Volunteering for community service relieves teens of their self-focus, opens their eyes to others' situations, and affirms that they can make a positive difference in the world.

TWO: A Doctor of Their Own

What is the single most important trait doctors must have in order to work well with adolescents?

They have to like adolescents.

Not everybody does, you know. Some pediatricians are unfazed by screaming babies, charmed by truculent toddlers, and amused by back-talking 8-year-olds—but oh, how they dread adolescents. That don't-wanna-talk act tries their patience. And when teens do talk—well, how exactly do you handle a kid's telling you about his sexual experimentation without spilling the beans to his parents and urging them to ground him? There's too much tiptoeing around with adolescents, playing that delicate game of protecting their confidentiality while the parents worry in the waiting room. Better to stick with the little kids.

But other doctors would rather work with adolescents than with any other age group. For them, treating adolescents is the most exciting, dynamic, and rewarding field of medicine, despite the frustrations and challenges that inevitably come with the territory.

This doctor-patient relationship is unlike any other. The patient evolves from being a child who still relies on Mom or Dad to keep track of medicine to a grown-up medical consumer who makes independent decisions. The doctor guides the patient and parents on how to make healthy choices—and on the lifelong impact those choices may have.

A UNIQUE SET OF HEALTH RISKS

Dr. Adele Dellenbaugh Hoffman, a founder of the Society for Adolescent Medicine, recognized that adolescents constitute a distinctive constituency: "What we're talking about is a decade, an age of human growth and development that has tremendously unique things happening emotionally and biologically."[1]

Although many people believe teens are the healthiest age group, in fact they have many special needs and concerns. They benefit from seeing doctors or other health professionals who are trained to understand that social and psychological issues affect adolescents' physical health, and vice versa. This book refers to an adolescent's primary care provider as the "doctor," but some adolescents see a nurse practitioner or physician's assistant who has been specially trained in adolescent health care.

Adolescents' health problems may be:

- Unique to their age group (delayed puberty, scoliosis) or common to all age groups (colds, constipation, seasonal allergies).
- Behavior-driven (sexuality, substance use, accidents, and injuries).
- Related to body image (skin problems, eating disorders, piercing, tattoos).
- Symptomatic of emotional struggles, especially depression or stress (fatigue, headaches).
- Related to difficulties within the adolescent's world at home, in school, or with peers (abuse, learning disabilities, bullying).
- Chronic or handicapping conditions (asthma, migraines, cerebral palsy).

The adolescent's doctor must be able to consider the complex interplay between biologic health and disease and emotional well-being, helping teens and parents differentiate between normal and problematic changes and behaviors.

BUILDING TRUST

Central to the success of the relationship is a doctor's ability to establish rapport. Some adolescents are open, easy to talk with, eager to ask questions. Others resist, refuse to disclose what's really going on, and must be won over. Doctors need to find ways to let patients know they are on their side. To keep communication flowing doctors avoid asking yes-or-no questions and perfect the art of asking open-ended questions:

Tell me more about what it has been like starting a new school in eleventh grade.

How does the injury affect your ability to do things you want to do?

What do you think about the fact that some kids in your grade get drunk on Saturday night?

The goal is to convey interest in the adolescent's life and to appear nonjudgmental so the adolescent will feel comfortable describing life as it is, not as he or she thinks an adult believes it should be. The patient should come to regard the doctor as more of a resource than an authority figure. Over time, as the doctor gains the adolescent's trust, they can work together as a team to steer the healthiest route to adulthood.

The doctor must also develop trust with the parents. This can be achieved in several ways: including parents in office visits as appropriate, discussing straight medical matters with them, answering their phone calls promptly, and calling family meetings when needed.

TALKING ABOUT VALUES

"Family values" has become a heavily laden term in our society, almost synonymous with "conservative." But every family has—and should have—values, beliefs about the best ways to live. Adolescents need to know how their parents feel about such matters as sexual activity, drug use, and ethical relationships with others. It makes sense for parents to share their beliefs with their child's doctor and ask that they be respected. Sometimes such a discussion presents an opportunity for the doctor and parents to explore an issue together and determine the best approach for the adolescent.

For example, let's say that parents tell a doctor they expect their daughter to abstain from having sexual intercourse. They ask the doctor to limit discussions of sexual behavior to abstinence. The doctor might agree that abstinence is by far the healthiest, most appropriate choice for an adolescent—but points out that if she inquires about safer sex measures, it is the doctor's responsibility to provide correct information. Indeed, what the parents might not have considered is that learning about the risks of sexual activity (contraceptive failure, pregnancy, sexually transmitted diseases, emotional upheaval) might in fact help fortify their daughter's decision to abstain.

On the other hand, if she is determined to have sex, surely the parents would not want her to be vulnerable to those risks. If she is not informed about precautions, she will be more likely to get pregnant or contract a sexually transmitted disease.

In this discussion, parents might come to see the ramifications of their original request in a new way. The doctor might take extra care to talk with the girl about abstinence. The doctor would not only honor the family's values but also be sensitive to the emotional conflict the girl might have if she pursues a sexual relationship. Is it causing her increased stress? Does her ambivalence make her inconsistent in practicing safer sex—and therefore increase her risks? Is she caught between a boyfriend's desires and her parents' wishes? Is she aware that she has the right to stop having sex? Would she like the doctor to help her discuss the matter with her parents?

Throughout, the doctor must maintain the adolescent's confidentiality—unless she is behaving in ways that will cause harm to herself and others. (See "Privacy and Confidentiality," page 23.) But the doctor can incorporate the parents' views into the discussion.

An independent relationship with the adolescent does not usually require complete exclusion of the parent, nor do most adolescents want or prefer that. So the doctor has a balancing act to perform of being faithful to the adolescent's trust and confidence while maintaining communication with the parents so that they are comfortable entrusting their child's health care to that "doctor of their own."

A NEW ROLE FOR PARENTS

I like going to the doctor by myself. When it's only me, I just get in and get out. My mom asks too many irrelevant questions.

—Joseph, age 14

Parents are part of the health care team. But as a child gets older—perhaps with more secrets, more issues, more need for privacy—parents must increasingly accept a subsidiary role. Throughout childhood, the parents were right there in the examining room with their child. They described how their child felt while the child just sat there, rarely needing to chime in. And they got the doctor's impressions and instructions firsthand.

In early adolescence, when children are 9, 10, or 11 years old, parents begin to step back a little. But as time goes on, they must step back a lot, and eventually completely, to allow their teens to truly have a doctor of their own. Adolescents must learn to describe symptoms, answer the doctor's questions, weigh the options, and make and follow through on decisions.

Not only must the adolescent trust this person, the parents also must trust the doctor to care for their child, often without the parents' intimate (or any) involvement or knowledge of all the details, especially pertaining to "private" matters.

Even if parents intellectually understand this, their emotions might be a step behind. Relegated to the waiting room, they might feel demoted, distanced. It's unnerving to think that adolescents might have questions they don't want parents to hear, or that doctors might have answers parents won't get to hear.

YOUR TEEN IN THE DRIVER'S SEAT

Allowing a teen a more independent, grown-up relationship with a doctor acknowledges the child's passage to a new stage in life. It is also a pragmatic approach. If adolescents are not allowed that confidentiality, they might not seek or receive help they urgently need, such as contraception, treatment of a sexually transmitted disease, or pointers on how to quit smoking.

The process of giving adolescents greater responsibility for their health is comparable to teaching them to drive. Parents are used to being in the driver's seat. When a teen gets behind the wheel, parents get a whole new view from the passenger seat. At stop signs, they can't help stepping on the brake, but of course it's just an imaginary brake. The real one is underneath the improbably large sneaker of that impossibly big teen next to them. The car won't stop until the new young driver tells it to—and will go wherever the young driver steers it.

STAY WITH THE PEDIATRICIAN OR FIND A NEW DOCTOR?

Adolescents may stay with the pediatrician they already know, who might even have known them all their lives. This might provide continuity, reassurance, and comfort.

Or adolescents might prefer to switch to a new pediatrician or to a family doctor, internist, gynecologist, or specialist in adolescent medicine. Sometimes they want to go to a doctor recommended by a friend. Parents can network with other parents and teens, check with local hospitals or medical societies, or ask the Society for Adolescent Medicine for a referral to private doctors or to hospital, community, or school-based adolescent clinics. (Contact the society by phone, 816-224-8010; fax, 816-224-8009; E-mail—sam@adolescenthealth. org, or go to its website: www.adolescenthealth.org.)

Ask your child if the doctor's gender matters. One study found that a significantly higher percentage, 50 percent, of adolescent males preferred a female physician for a general physical exam compared with 40 percent who preferred a male physician. In the same study, almost as many males preferred a female physician for a genital exam. One researcher theorized that boys might expect greater "sensitivity" from a female doctor.[2]

Of course, not all families have the luxury of choosing a doctor. A health maintenance organization (HMO) or public clinic might assign a physician, although it might grant an adolescent's or parent's request for a different one if necessary. Some parents have found it helpful to ask the HMO receptionist about which doctors work best with adolescents.

Learn as much as you can about your health maintenance organization's policies and programs. You might find it helpful to read a book such as *Don't Let Your HMO Kill You: How to Wake Up Your Doctor, Take Control of Your Health, and Make Managed Care Work for You*, by Jason Theodosakis, M.D., and David T. Feinberg, M.D.[3]

Find out about school health programs. Some schools have school-based clinics where your adolescent can get a variety of services (medical and social services) that are low-cost (or free) and convenient (right in the school building, so they don't have to miss school).

AN OFFICE WITH TEEN APPEAL

Many adolescents like their pediatrician, but the office decor offends their dignity. They hate feeling like giants among the baby toys and picture books and yellow-ducky wallpaper. To retain adolescent patients, some pediatricians set up a separate reception area and make this waiting room a learning room, stocking it with teen magazines, brochures, and books on topics they want teens to talk about—body changes, smoking, sexually transmitted diseases, stress.

Doctors also decorate one or more examining rooms with teens in mind. They position the examination table for privacy, so the teen can't be seen when the door opens, and stock the room with plenty of examination gowns.

Ideally the doctor has an office (consultation room) for meeting privately with the teen before or after an exam. Teen care is often as much about talk as about a physical exam, as much about anticipating and preventing problems as about treating them. This room should be large enough to accommodate a family meeting, too. With the doctor preferably sitting beside, not behind, the desk, the family can gather to discuss medical care, social and family issues, and next steps.

If your child likes the pediatrician but not the setting, speak up. The doctor might use your feedback to make some much-needed changes, and will appreciate the opportunity to retain a patient.

THE FIRST VISIT
Information Parents Provide

The first visit with a new adolescent patient (under age 18) works out best if the doctor schedules time to meet separately and together with the parents and the child. This format takes at least an hour. Subsequent visits, depending on the reason for the visit, will take less time, generally from fifteen to thirty minutes.

It is nearly always best for the doctor and parents to meet alone first. This gives parents a private opportunity to express any concerns and their reasons for this visit. They can provide the child's medical history and the family medical history (significant health problems in immediate family members). They can also provide an overview of how the adolescent is doing at home, at school, and with peers.

The doctor should ask parents to review the child's medical history, including:

- *Pregnancy and birth:* Was the child full-term? Were there any problems during the pregnancy, delivery, or infancy? Where was the child born?
- *Adoption:* If the child was adopted, have the parents told him? How does he feel about it? What information do the parents have about the birth parents' medical history?

- *Major developmental milestones:* At what age did the child walk and talk?
- *Health history:* Has the child had any serious acute or chronic medical illnesses, accidents, injuries, hospitalizations, or operations? Any allergies (medications, food, seasonal, environmental)? Does the child take any medications? Nutritional or herbal supplements?
- *Health basics:* Describe the child's diet, sleep patterns, and fitness activities.
- *Environmental factors:* Are there pets in the home? Does the family live near a factory or waste disposal site?
- *Immunizations:* Is the child up-to-date on all immunizations required by the school? The parents should provide an immunization record. (See immunization section, later in this chapter.)
- *Mental health:* Parents should try to "paint a picture" for the doctor of the child's temperament, state of mind (mood), stress level, family interactions and activities, school performance and behavior, and relationships with peers.
- *Risk factors:* Do the parents have any concerns about the use of tobacco, alcohol, or other drugs? Sexual activity? Gang involvement? Unsafe driving or other reckless behavior? Do parents keep firearms in the home? If so, are they kept unloaded, locked, and safely stored?
- *Life changes:* Have there been any significant life changes recently, such as moving, a new school, the birth of a sibling, the illness or death of a family member or friend, a separation or divorce, a parent's loss of a job?
- *Religion:* What is the family's religion? Is the family observant? Do the parents and child practice their religion in the same way? Does the family follow any religious practices that might affect a child's diet or medical treatment?

Throughout this discussion, the doctor is listening not only to the information but also to the tone. Do the parents seem comfortable with their child's health and development? Are they excessively tense and worried, or surprisingly unconcerned? Do the parents seem to be aware of what is going on in their child's life?

Meeting the Teen

Next is the teen's turn to meet alone with the new doctor. This takes place in the doctor's office with the patient fully dressed, not in the exam room and not in an awkward exam gown, sure to inhibit and discomfort the teen.

The doctor immediately explains that meeting with parents first was not intended to exclude the adolescent, but rather to give the adolescent priority and to safeguard confidentiality. That way, if the adolescent shares any private or confidential information with the doctor, it will be after the interview with parents. Unless the confidential information is of a very serious nature, the doctor need not discuss it with the parents. If it is serious, the patient and doctor can first discuss how to inform them. But this is never done behind the adolescent's back or without the adolescent's knowledge.

This little introduction sets a welcoming and reassuring tone, which is important for most adolescents. For preteen or very young adolescents, this kind of introduction may be skipped in order not to overwhelm them. (See "Privacy and Confidentiality," on page 23.)

The Doctor-Teen Dialogue

A perceptive fly on the wall might be surprised that the conversation at first might have nothing to do with medicine. The doctor and the teen are talking about . . . whatever. School. Sports. Movies. Summer plans. The teen essentially sets the agenda. The doctor goes with the flow to give them a chance to get to know each other.

Gradually questions become more specific, starting with the patient's perspective on the reason for today's visit. The doctor proceeds to ask routine first-visit questions, starting with general inquiries about the adolescent's health:

Do you participate in sports or other exercise?

How many meals and snacks do you have each day and what do you eat?

Do you have any difficulty falling or staying asleep?

How is your energy level compared to other kids your age?

Does any part of your body hurt or bother you? For example, do you get headaches or belly pain?

Girls are also asked questions about their menstrual periods.

When did you get your first period?

How often do you get a period?

How many days does your period last? How heavy is the flow?

Any cramps, headaches, other associated problems?

Finally the doctor moves into more sensitive topics. The teen's relationship with parents. Feelings about school. Grades. Friendships. Whether the teen smokes, drinks alcohol, uses pot or other drugs. Involvement in any intimate (sexual) relationships.

The doctor also asks how the teen's mood is most of the time, any experiences with abuse, or serious accidents that have occurred. Of course, questions are asked in a way appropriate to the child's age, maturity, and reported behaviors. The doctor might ask preteens what they think about the use of substances or having sex in high school, rather than direct questions about themselves. Always the doctor remains sensitive to the patient's interest and comfort with the interview, and modifies questions accordingly.

Additionally, the doctor might ask:

How would you describe yourself?

What traits are most important to you about yourself?

Tell me about your interests, activities, values, what's easy for you and what's hard . . . whatever comes to mind.

A complete physical exam alone with the adolescent comes next (see page 25). Then the doctor asks if the adolescent has any questions, or if there is anything else that he or she might want to discuss before having the parents rejoin them.

Bringing the Full Team Together

Finally the parents are invited to join the conversation back in the doctor's office. This is the doctor's first opportunity to participate in a conversation with the family all together, observe their interactions, share impressions of the patient's health, and answer any questions. This very comprehensive first visit is designed to initiate a relationship with the parents and above all with the patient. The hope is that the visit will end with the adolescent and parents feeling satisfied and trustful that an important new relationship has begun.

PRIVACY AND CONFIDENTIALITY

Personal privacy and the confidentiality of their health care are very important to most adolescents. At the first visit the doctor must discuss both the need for and the limits of confidentiality. The topic might come up several times: in the meeting with parents alone, with the adolescent alone, and ideally also with them all together at the end of the first visit.

The doctor explains that most of what the adolescent shares remains confidential, but that there are limits to confidentiality. Serious health matters, or worrisome health risk behaviors involving drug or alcohol use, unsafe sexual practices, or very low mood that might include suicidal thoughts or actions, must be shared with parents for adolescents' well-being, especially since they will need their parents' help and support to tackle these issues. Before disclosing such matters to parents, however, the doctor will discuss them with the adolescent so that they may strategize together just how to inform and involve the parents. A cardinal rule is that the doctor never talks with parents behind the adolescent's back, a betrayal that almost guarantees that the doctor will lose the teen's trust, and thereby the opportunity to be helpful.

Of course, such matters are developmentally driven. Both the doctor and the parents will have a lower threshold for limiting confidentiality with a younger, immature, irresponsible, impulsive, or troubled teen. In such situations the behavior or problem might be more serious and there will be a more urgent need for parents to step in and help. The older, more mature, responsible, and thoughtful teen is in a better position to handle a situation with the doctor alone.

Often teens simply need some help from their doctor to inform their parents of something they themselves want to share. Other times teens may need just a little convincing from the doctor that they will feel much better about a situation if their parents know about it. It is very rare that a doctor will agree with an adolescent that withholding serious information from parents is in fact safer because the parent might react in a violent or destructive way. In such a situation, the doctor and adolescent must identify another adult (such as an aunt, uncle, or older sibling) who should be consulted instead. There are no hard-and-fast rules about this. Much depends on the doctor's judgment of the individual patient's situation, taking into account the seriousness of the matter, the patient's reliability and responsibility, and whether there are compelling reasons not to tell the parents.

FREQUENCY AND SCOPE OF VISITS

Adolescent medicine has a dual goal of prevention and treatment; doctors are both educators and practitioners. Just like general pediatricians, adolescent medicine specialists provide "anticipatory guidance." They give parents and teens a "heads up" about developmental changes they can expect—and the risk behaviors with which the teen might be confronted. By initiating these conversations, doctors give teens and their families an opportunity to discuss how they'll cross those bridges when they come to them.

The American Medical Association's *Guidelines for Adolescent Preventive Services* (*GAPS*)[4] recommends an annual health visit (the yearly checkup) from ages 11 to 21 to assess the adolescent's physical and psychosocial health.

It is a time to talk about the adolescent's development, safety practices (such as use of seat belts and bike helmets), diet, fitness, relationships, school, and any risk-taking behaviors such as smoking, drinking, taking drugs, having unsafe sex, or possession or use of weapons. The doctor also explores how the adolescent is coping with conflict and stress and whether there are any disturbances in mood. A physical examination is always done, and laboratory tests and immunizations are updated.

It is important for parents to feel that the doctor supports their role as their child's health partner and involves them in communicating positive health messages, both verbally and by example. Talking with parents helps the doctor know more about the adolescent and better understand the family. *GAPS* advises doctors to meet with parents at least once during early adolescence (ages 10 to 14) and middle adolescence (15 to 18). At these visits parents share information and receive guidance. A visit with parents during late adolescence (18 to 21) is recommended but optional.

THE ADOLESCENT CHECKUP

A year is a long time in the life of an adolescent. At the annual checkup the adolescent and doctor become reacquainted, and review ongoing health concerns as well as any health problems that might have occurred during the past year that the doctor didn't know about (for example, a fracture while skiing). They review the areas covered in the initial visit, including exercise, nutrition, sleep, energy, mood, menstruation, relationships with parents and peers, schoolwork, and health-risk behaviors (smoking, alcohol, drugs, sex, violence).

The annual checkup is above all a time to continue building a meaningful and more familiar relationship. It might also be the only time each year that the doctor does a complete physical examination and reviews whether any laboratory tests or immunizations are due. This comprehensive visit generally takes about half an hour. If important matters come up that require more time to address fully, a follow-up visit within the next week or two is scheduled.

Many adolescents long for a doctor who can read their minds. Although doctors are trained to look for health clues and to ask strategic questions, they must count on the adolescent to trust them enough to disclose what's really going on. Parents can help by reminding their adolescent that the doctor has experience treating a wide variety of problems. Whatever the adolescent's problem, the doctor has probably seen it before. One nice thing about the annual checkup is that the adolescent and doctor have met at least once previously, and the setting and routines are familiar. The adolescent should be less anxious than at the initial visit, and able to have a relaxed discussion that will prove informative and therapeutic.

The Physical Examination

After the checkup discussion, the adolescent moves from the doctor's office to the examination room and changes into a gown.

The exam is not a silent time. The doctor explains each step (*Your blood pressure is normal*), asks questions (*Have you been noticing any change in your vision?*), and discusses anything the adolescent is worrying or wondering about (*Why do my breasts feel tender before my period?*).

During the examination the doctor:

- Measures the adolescent's height, weight, blood pressure, and pulse.
- Examines the adolescent thoroughly, including skin, eyes, ears, nose, mouth, throat, lymph nodes, thyroid gland, lungs, heart, breasts, abdomen, and external genitalia.
- Examines the adolescent's spine for signs of scoliosis, a lateral deviation from a straight line of vertebrae down the back, which usually begins during early adolescence and can progress rapidly during growth in height (see chapter 4).
- Assesses the adolescent's overall development in accordance with the Tanner "sexual maturity ratings." This system evaluates adolescents' progress through five phases of development, based on a female's breast and pubic hair growth, and a male's genitalia and pubic hair growth. The five phases are useful for indicating slow or accelerated growth, both of which might indicate other problems. (See "Tanner Stages for Girls," chapter 5, and "Tanner Stages for Boys," chapter 6.)

A complete gynecologic examination might not be done at the annual checkup. For girls requiring one—those who have had sex, have a gynecologic problem, or simply request such an exam when over 18—a separate visit may be scheduled to ensure sufficient time for the exam and related discussion. However, if there are indications that a girl could be pregnant, has a sexually transmitted disease, is having unsafe sex, or would not return soon, then the gynecologic exam should be done during the checkup. (See chapter 5.)

Laboratory Tests

Routine laboratory testing at the initial visit or a checkup is very simple for most adolescents. Such testing is called *screening* when the adolescent feels okay (offers no complaints of any symptoms). The testing is done solely to uncover a possible unknown problem.

- *Urine:* An annual urine analysis is an easy and inexpensive screen for a variety of possible health problems, such as a urinary tract or sexually transmitted infection (white blood cells in urine), diabetes (sugar in urine), or kidney disorder (protein and/or blood in urine).

- *Blood:* A blood sample taken from a vein (a learning experience for many adolescents is that this procedure is neither painful nor scary) may be tested for a complete blood count (CBC). This is done primarily to check for a possible anemia (low count of red blood cells). The CBC also checks the white cell count and platelet count. On the same blood sample a chemical screen may be done. This includes many tests for organ function (liver, kidneys) as well as a cholesterol profile. Blood tests may be done every few years in a well adolescent.

- *Vision and hearing:* These screens are done periodically. An adolescent who falls outside the normal range of findings for hearing should be referred for further evaluation by an audiologist or otolaryngologist. By age 16 or 17, and certainly before graduating from high school, an adolescent should have a full eye exam by an ophthalmologist or optometrist. The eye exam should occur earlier, of course, if an adolescent has difficulty reading or seeing the chalkboard in school, fails an eye test when applying for a driver's license, or has headaches that may be related to eyestrain. Developing myopia (nearsightedness) is not uncommon during early or middle adolescence.

- *Intradermal Mantoux PPD (test for asymptomatic tuberculosis [TB] infection):* This test might be done if the adolescent lives in a community where TB exposure is a risk.

All other laboratory testing will depend on whether the adolescent reports certain symptoms (such as fatigue) or health concerns (such as very irregular periods) or risk behaviors (such as sexual activity or drug use).

Immunizations

Most adolescents should receive several immunizations between the ages of 10 and 21.

- *Tetanus-diphtheria (Td):* A 10- or 11-year-old often is due for a tetanus-diphtheria booster (given five years after completion of the primary series, which is usually completed around age 5 or 6); thereafter, a booster of Td is recommended every ten years.

- *Measles, mumps, rubella (MMR):* Adolescents should have received two doses of measles and at least one dose (preferably two) of mumps and rubella vaccines during early childhood. If this has not occurred, an MMR (measles, mumps, and rubella in one shot) booster is recommended.

- *Hepatitis B:* The hepatitis B vaccine (three-dose series) has been recommended for all newborns since 1991. Many states now require that all adolescents not previously immunized receive this vaccine series.
- *Varicella:* The varicella vaccine (two-dose series if over age 13) protects against chicken pox and is recommended for adolescents not previously immunized or who have not had chicken pox. A blood test may be done first to check immunity status of those teens uncertain whether they had the disease.
- *Hepatitis A:* The hepatitis A vaccine (two-dose series) is recommended in states and regions with a high prevalence of hepatitis A infection and for those adolescents traveling to high-risk areas or living in high-risk conditions.
- *Influenza:* The "flu shot" is recommended to be administered annually to adolescents with chronic illnesses such as asthma, diabetes, sickle cell disease, HIV, and heart disease, and may be administered to others desiring immunity for the season.
- *Pneumococcal:* The pneumococcal vaccine is recommended for adolescents with chronic illnesses similar to those listed above (see "Influenza").
- *Meningococcal:* The meningococcal vaccine is recommended for adolescents entering college and for others who live in close quarters such as dormitories. It protects against the most serious and sometimes fatal form of meningitis, caused by the bacteria *Neisseria meningitidis.*

Both the Centers for Disease Control and Prevention and the American Academy of Pediatrics publish recommendations for immunizations.

ADOLESCENTS AS MEDICAL CONSUMERS

Just as parents try to help their teens become smart shoppers (check quality, compare prices, wait for sales, seek good service), they also need to teach them how to be savvy medical consumers. It's not such an easy task, since many adolescents are intimidated by doctors or perceive other barriers to treatment.

Overcoming Barriers

According to one study, nearly one in five adolescents does not seek health care when he or she feels a need.[5] Whether rich or poor, teens cited the same reasons. Some of these reasons are not unique to teens:

The problem will go away.

I am afraid of what the doctor might find or do.

I can't pay.

I am having trouble making an appointment.

Other barriers to seeking needed care were more adolescent-specific:

I'm worried about confidentiality.

I can't get my parent or guardian to go with me.

Another major reason teens give for not seeking care for certain types of problems (overweight, sadness, fatigue, contraception, cigarette smoking) is that they do not think the doctor is knowledgeable or experienced in dealing with such issues and therefore will not be able to help them. Some teens have already had the experience of not being helped by their doctor with such problems.[6]

Following are some suggestions for how parents can respond when teens give these reasons for not seeking health care.

The problem will go away.

It is common and often reasonable for teens to wait and see if symptoms disappear before they see a doctor. Most colds go away within a few days. Some injuries, aches, and pains heal almost as quickly as they began. Home remedies or over-the-counter treatments take care of the occasional headache, indigestion, or cold sore.

But waiting to see a doctor can also be dangerous. Some symptoms signal the need to see a doctor immediately. Make sure your child knows to see a doctor *promptly* when experiencing one or more of the urgent symptoms in the chart that appears on page 31.

I'm afraid of what the doctor might find or do.

Usually, diagnosis and treatment are not as alarming as a teen imagines they will be. Tell your child about times when you felt a similar worry but felt so much better when a doctor explained the cause of a symptom that turned out not to be serious. In any event, knowing the truth is better than worrying in ignorance—and the sooner a problem is diagnosed, the easier and more effective the treatment is likely to be.

I can't pay.

Many families who are not insured through employers or Medicaid may qualify for other health insurance. For example, New York State offers free or low-cost government-funded insurance through the Child Health Plus (for newborns through age 18) and Family Health Plus (ages 19 to 64) programs. Ask your doctor, local clinic, or school nurse. Many clinics and other health providers, such as Planned Parenthood, offer services on a sliding scale.

I am having trouble making an appointment.

Many physicians and adolescent clinics have become sensitive to the need for more after-school, evening, and weekend hours. If the teen cannot obtain an appointment, an adult's assistance might make the difference. This is also an opportunity to teach the teen to be an assertive patient: "I need to see the doctor right away; this might be an emergency."

I'm worried about confidentiality.

Adolescents have many rights of confidentiality (see "Privacy and Confidentiality," page 23). They can ask a doctor or clinic about confidentiality policies. Public health clinics that treat sexually transmitted diseases honor confidentiality while also offering assistance for alerting sexual partners to seek treatment.

I can't get my parent or guardian to go with me.

Adults don't always realize that the "independent" teen in their lives might be desperate for their support and company. If parents cannot adjust work schedules, perhaps a favorite aunt or uncle, grandparent, or older sibling can go.

A Medical Consumer Prepares

Writing down symptoms and questions in advance helps teens focus and makes it more likely that they will get the answers they need. Encourage your teen to be specific and not be embarrassed. Whatever the problem, the doctor has probably treated it before.

To help teens feel confident in beginning to take charge of their health, they should:

- *Before the visit:* Write down their concerns. Describe when symptoms began, whether they have occurred before, and any ideas about what might have caused them (for example, allergy, medication side effect, injury, drug use, sexual contact).
- *During the visit:* Write down the doctor's diagnosis and advice. Put any prescription form in a wallet.
- *After the visit:* Fill prescriptions. Jot reminders in a calendar or electronic organizer about when to take medications. Call the doctor with any questions or if treatment doesn't help. Schedule a follow-up visit if necessary.

URGENT SYMPTOMS

See a doctor as soon as possible if you experience one or more of these symptoms:

- Unusual or ongoing fatigue, excessive sleeping, or insomnia
- Unexplained weight gain or loss, or loss of appetite
- Chronic feeling of depression or desire to harm oneself
- Persistent pain in the bones
- Pallor or unexplained bruising
- High fever or persistent low-grade fever
- Unusually severe or persistent headaches
- A sore or other injury that does not heal
- Change in a wart or mole; appearance of new skin growth or lesion
- Unexplained thickening or lump in a breast, testicle, or elsewhere
- Coughing that does not go away
- Persistent indigestion, heartburn, reflux, or vomiting
- Change in bowel habits, such as persistent constipation or diarrhea
- Intense or persistent pain or discomfort in the lower abdomen, testicle, or elsewhere
- Pain during urination or sexual intercourse
- Any unusual vaginal, urethral, or anal bleeding or discharge

---

An Ongoing Relationship

Whether at the initial visit, the annual checkup, or in between visits for specific health concerns, the adolescent and the doctor are building a relationship. Like any relationship, it becomes more familiar and comfortable over time. Some adolescents connect almost immediately with their doctor, while others might take years to really feel at ease. The parents' job as health partner is to encourage their adolescent to seek care when needed, to support the privacy of the doctor/patient relationship, and to maintain their own communication with the doctor.

HEALTH-PARTNERING TIPS FOR PARENTS

- *Discuss health issues with your child.* Share concerns. Read and discuss articles, pamphlets, and books. Watch movies and television shows about health. When health is a frequent topic of conversation, it's easier for the teen to feel comfortable raising a topic.

- *Acknowledge your own feelings about your changing role.* Talk with your child's doctor about any hesitation to allow your child to take charge of his or her own health. Ask how you can remain involved.
- *Articulate your concerns.* Don't hesitate to call your child's doctor after a checkup or about your concerns about issues such as school performance, sexual behavior, or worrisome changes in your child's diet. However, always tell your child before you call. You might say something like this: *I don't think you are eating enough nutritious food. I'll let you know what the doctor says.*
- *Request family meetings when necessary.* It is best to talk with the doctor with the child present.
- *Accompany your child to appointments.* Even if you don't meet with the doctor each time, your physical presence helps you and your child feel connected. It can be reassuring just to shake the doctor's hand and get a quick word about how your child is doing.

THREE: **The Basics:**
Nutrition, Exercise,
and Sleep

To go FAR in life, teens need the three health basics:

1. Fuel.
2. Activity.
3. Rest.

Yet many adolescents shortchange themselves. They skimp on nutritious food and they overload on junk . . . hang out for hours on end in front of a TV or computer . . . stay up late and never catch up on sleep.

Then they wonder why they are too heavy or too thin, lack energy, are irritable or depressed, and can't improve their grades.

Furthermore, the basics are as intertwined as the loops of a whole wheat pretzel. All three are necessary to be in truly good shape. Otherwise:

- An adolescent who eats poorly and does not exercise feels sluggish, even if he or she gets enough sleep.
- An overweight teen feels too awkward to exercise.
- A sleep-deprived kid reaches for too many sweets (or caffeine) for quick energy boosts that end up causing energy crashes (or caffeine addiction).
- A teen who exercises but doesn't get enough iron lacks the energy to achieve fitness goals.
- A young female athlete intent on lifelong fitness runs the risk of bone injury (fractures) now and in the future because she doesn't take in enough calcium.
- A motivated teen who stays up late to study never scores as high on exams as an equally smart friend who is in bed by ten.

Many adolescents know that they "should" change their eating, exercise, or sleep practices, but they need guidance, encouragement, and support. In this chapter are tips on how a few simple changes can make a real difference in a teen's short- and long-term health. Don't assume your child understands how

33

much the three basics of nutrition, exercise, and sleep affect how people look, feel, and learn. Adolescents often follow their friends' examples, but their friends are clueless, too.

When your child doesn't feel well, physically or emotionally, get into the habit of asking about the three basics. *What have you been eating? Are you exercising? How are you sleeping?* Fatigue, headaches, backaches, "spacing out" in class, having too many colds—all these and more may be linked to deficiencies in the basics. Very often, better nutrition, regular exercise, and more sleep help various ailments and negative moods resolve on their own.

Model good health practices for your children's sake and your own. Practicing what you preach lets you preach less. Your actions really do speak louder than words.

HEALTH BASIC #1: NUTRITION

The family dinner, where everyone sits together and discusses the day's events, can keep everyone connected. Yet today it can be difficult to achieve. Family members often have incompatible schedules and too little time. At mealtimes, therefore, many adolescents are left to fend for themselves. If they are uninformed about the importance of nutrition, and especially when a parent isn't around to plan, cook, or assist in preparing healthy food, teens tend to eat whatever is easy and fast, but not necessarily nutritious.

Yet good nutrition is especially important during adolescence. This is a stage of life characterized by rapid growth. It is a time to gain weight, increase height, and develop brand-new contours.

Growth Spurts in Weight and Height

Most people think of the "growth spurt" as an accelerated rate of increase in height, even though the weight spurt is even more dramatic.

The average (50th percentile) girl typically should gain about 50 pounds from age 10 to 15 or 16. This weight gain over five years of 10 pounds per year coincides with a height increase of slightly more than 2 inches per year. Weight increases by about 75 percent and height by about 25 percent. Therefore the increased curves that girls develop reflect the fact that their weight spurt exceeds their height spurt.

Boys gain even more weight. They start gaining weight at an accelerated rate later than girls do, at about age 13, but quickly make up for lost time. Every year, until about age 18, boys gain on average 10 to 15 pounds and 2 to 4 inches. The average boy's weight increases over 100 percent during this time (more than doubles) while height increases 25 to 30 percent.

The height spurt in girls usually occurs in early adolescence before a girl gets her first period, sometime between the ages of 10 and 14, and in boys between the ages of around 13 to 16, or older. The height spurt of most rapid growth continues for about a year. Girls continue to grow, at a slower pace, for a few years after the height spurt and their first menstrual period. Boys, however, often continue to grow considerable inches and for a longer stretch of time even after their phase of most rapid growth.

A Healthy Weight Gain

So adolescents face the important nutritional task of taking in enough calories from a wide enough variety of nutritious foods to support their growth. Yet this task is not so easy. "Weight gain" should be a neutral term, but in our thinness-obsessed society, even girls of normal, reasonable proportions often try to eat less than they might need so they can emulate the superslender shapes of popular actresses, singers, and models.

Boys are no less vulnerable. Eager for the "cut abs" or "bulging biceps" look, some boys strive to keep body fat low to better show off the effects of their weight lifting, which itself might become excessive and injure their developing bones and joints.

The challenge for parents is to help "normalize" eating, to help their children understand the importance of good nutrition and appropriate expected weight gain, to be on the alert for signs of eating disorders, underweight and overweight (see chapter 10), and to make healthy eating as easy and pleasurable as possible.

The Nutrients Your Adolescent Needs

Nutritionists always recommend a "well-rounded diet," but the term is not always well understood. The U.S. Department of Agriculture devised the Food Guide Pyramid (see page 37) to illustrate the recommended range and quality of foods.

- *Grains and Starches (6–11 servings per day)* are found at the pyramid's long base, attesting to their role as the foundation of a balanced diet. Breads, cereal, rice, and pasta are foods that many adolescents love filling up on. *They should get from six to eleven servings each day.* That doesn't mean six platefuls of spaghetti. *Each serving represents about a half cup or one slice of bread.* By far the best choice is whole grains, such as whole wheat bread, brown rice, and oatmeal. They have more nutrients and fiber than refined foods such as white bread and white rice. "Refining" usually involves stripping away the vitamin- and fiber-rich germ and bran layers of the grain. Foods made of refined grains might taste good, but they actually cheat you out of the full range of nutrients offered by whole grains.

- *Fruits (2–4 servings per day) and vegetables (3–5 servings per day)* share the pyramid's next level. Prime sources of vitamins and fiber, fruits and vegetables produce healthy teens. Steamed or stir-fried vegetables, green salads, and bowls of apples and plums come to mind. At minimum, teens should eat five servings of produce per day. A serving is one piece of fruit, three-quarters of a cup of juice, or one-half to one cup of cut-up fruits or vegetables.

- *Dairy products (2–3 servings per day) and other protein sources (2–3 servings of meat, poultry, fish, eggs, legumes, or nuts)* appear on the pyramid's next level. For many Americans, this part of the pyramid is counterintuitive. Our society tends to place a premium on protein, especially sources derived from animals. But instead of featuring chicken or a steak as the centerpiece of a meal, it is actually healthier to limit the size of a meat portion in order to accommodate larger amounts of the other categories in the pyramid. The total daily intake of protein should be no more than 15 percent of calories or about 75 to 100 grams per day. A serving is one cup of milk or yogurt; two ounces of cheese; three ounces of lean meat, poultry, or fish; a half cup of cooked beans; one egg; or two tablespoons of peanut butter.

- *Fats, oils, and sweets* crown the pyramid, relegated to the smallest part of the healthy diet. These are the only foods that do not have a designated number of servings per day. "Use sparingly," the pyramid advises. Many people crave sweets and fatty foods so much that they practically turn the pyramid upside down. Many teens eat greasy fast-food burgers and heaps of French fries, slather gobs of mayo on their sandwiches, and empty a bag of Oreos in less time than it takes to pour a glass of milk. But fat should comprise only 25 to 30 percent of calories in their diet (approximately 50 to 80 grams per day). Although it is healthy to limit fat in one's diet, a "fat-free" diet is definitely ill-advised. Fats are a nutrient and an important source of energy just like proteins and carbohydrates. The healthiest sources of fat are classified as "unsaturated," which includes plant-derived seeds, nuts, and oils.

It can be a very big adjustment for some teens to model their meals on the Food Guide Pyramid, reducing fats, minimizing sweets, downplaying proteins,

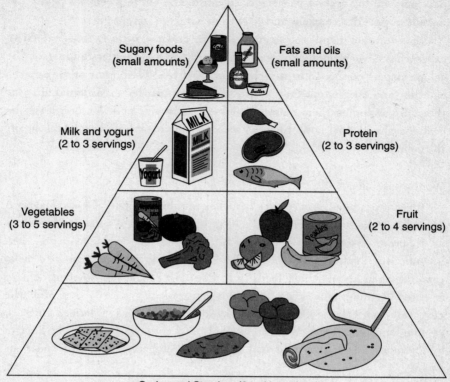

Sugary foods (small amounts)

Fats and oils (small amounts)

Milk and yogurt (2 to 3 servings)

Protein (2 to 3 servings)

Vegetables (3 to 5 servings)

Fruit (2 to 4 servings)

Grains and Starches (6 to 11 servings)

Source: Centers for Disease Control and Prevention

focusing more on vegetables and fruits, reaching for more whole grains. But learning to eat the pyramid way is a valuable lesson for lifelong health.

Calories per Day

Girls ages 11 to 18 need about 2,000 calories per day, and boys need about 2,500 to 3,000. Very active adolescents might need 600 to 1,000 additional calories, and sedentary teens somewhat fewer.

Not all growth happens slowly and steadily. As mentioned above, nearly every adolescent experiences "growth spurts," and calorie intake will naturally be higher at those times.

Help your child understand that if she wants energy, she has to take in enough calories to provide it. If teens don't consume enough calories, they will "run out of gas," experience fatigue, and even lose weight at a time in life when they are expected to gain. Weight gain is also crucial for supporting pubertal development and growth in height. So consuming too few calories might also impede normal development and growth in height.

On the other hand, too many calories—and too little exercise—lead to excess fat. Overweight adolescents might have little understanding of the caloric impact of the foods they eat. Keeping a food diary, then adding up the calories (and fat content) at the end of the day, can be a real awakening for them. By swapping their snack of cookies and whole milk for half a whole-grain bagel and skim milk, they can still feel comfortably full while taking off the pounds.

Worthwhile Calories

It is not practical or necessary to make every bite "count." Occasional servings of fries with roast chicken, a heap of chips with a tuna sandwich, or an ice-cream cone on a hot day are all fine and fun. Problems arise when low-nutrient foods are the norm and adolescents do not know how to make good decisions about which foods to choose. The concept of nutrient density is central to conscious eating. Nutrient-dense foods are those that offer the most value per calorie. They are high in such essentials as vitamins, minerals, protein, and fiber, but low in the fats, oils, and sweets that should be kept to a minimum. *The Health Nutrient Bible* offers this explanation of "nutrient density":

> It's sort of like comparison shopping for foods, but instead of thinking about price, you base your decision on what a food has to offer in the way of nutrition—both the negative and positive aspects. Say you're looking for a good source of calcium. Dairy products come immediately to mind—milk, ice cream, yogurt. Yet whole milk and rich premium ice creams offer that calcium at a high-fat cost. Skim milk, on the other hand, delivers the calcium without added fat and is therefore the better choice.[1]

"Empty calories" refers to foods like sweets, sodas, and chips that offer energy but little or no "added-value" nutrients. These foods might be fun to eat, but they don't really "earn" their place on the table.

Fiber

Adolescents need about 30 grams of fiber per day. Fiber aids digestion and elimination. Along with water, fiber helps keep constipation at bay. It also might help prevent colon cancer later in life. Good sources include pears, apples, grapes, and other raw fruits; dried apricots, prunes, and raisins; broccoli, frozen corn and peas, baked potato with skin, and other vegetables; bran cereal and whole-grain breads; and peanuts. One of the top sources is kidney beans, with 7 grams of fiber per cup.

Some adolescents think that eating bran cereal for breakfast takes care of their fiber needs for the whole day. But in fact they should select at least one high-fiber food at each meal and snack to ensure adequate fiber intake.

Iron

Especially among girls, fatigue might be due to inadequate iron. Their iron deficiency is probably due to eating too little of the right foods. Indeed, obese adolescents might eat a lot but still be prone to iron deficiency.

Iron is necessary in the manufacture of red blood cells, which carry oxygen throughout the body. Teens should consume 15 to 20 milligrams of iron per day. If a diet is too low in iron, anemia (low number of red blood cells) might result. Having an insufficient number of oxygen-laden red blood cells might cause fatigue. Girls with heavy or prolonged menstrual periods lose an excessive amount of iron and must be especially careful to include enough iron in their diets.

Good sources of iron are meat, poultry, seafood, legumes, seeds, raisins, spinach, and enriched breads and grains. Some breakfast cereals, such as Total, are fortified with the entire day's iron requirement and are a wonderful way to start the day.

Calcium

Calcium is the currency of bones. Just as pennies deposited into a savings account today can grow into many dollars years later, calcium deposited into the body during adolescence pays off in healthy adult bones.

Adolescents are literally sculpting their futures. Their calcium intake and weight-bearing exercise will dictate the shape and condition of their bones for life.

Bones strengthen until about age 30, when the body slowly reverses course and increasingly tends to lose more bone than it makes. That's why one researcher called the teen years a "window of opportunity for bone growth." [2] Of course, bones are not calcium's only beneficiaries. Calcium also supports teeth, muscles, blood clotting, and the nervous system. It is recommended that adolescents age 9 to 18 get 1,300 milligrams of calcium every day, which is higher than the 1,000 milligrams recommended for nonpregnant, nonlactating, nonmenopausal adults. [3] Good sources of calcium are all dairy products; leafy green vegetables such as spinach, kale, and broccoli; firm or soft tofu; and calcium-enriched orange juice.

Vitamins and Minerals: Via Nature or Supplement?

Getting enough vitamins and minerals is dependent on both the quantity and quality of the diet. Most health professionals would agree that the best way to get enough vitamin A, B vitamins (including folic acid, essential for preventing birth defects), and vitamin C—and minerals like calcium, iron, magnesium, and zinc—is through diet (with vitamin D accessed through enriched milk and sunlight). Eating a variety of the types of food and adhering to the numbers of servings recommended in the Food Guide Pyramid can cover an adolescent's vitamin and mineral requirements.

But many adolescent girls do not eat enough servings of the right foods to give them the vitamins and minerals they need. Careful to keep their weight down, they might deprive themselves of the nutrients they need for healthy bones, blood, and more. Therefore, taking a multivitamin-and-mineral supplement can be, as one dietitian put it, like a "little insurance policy," assuring that they get at least the minimum they need.

The problem tends not to be the same for many adolescent boys, who are famous for their unfettered appetites. However, boys who are also trying to keep weight low and do not consume enough calories might also benefit from a vitamin-and-mineral supplement.

And as described on page 42, some vegetarian adolescents might need to supplement their diets to replace key nutrients their diets do not provide, such as vitamin B_{12}, which is present only in animal-derived foods (which include dairy products and eggs).

Ask your child's doctor to evaluate his or her diet and advise on whether a supplement is, in fact, necessary. You might also want to consult a registered dietitian.

Nutrition Labels

In 1990 Congress passed legislation requiring food packages to bear nutrition labels. A cartoon published around that time showed a woman frantically racing from store to store, seeking food packages that were produced before the law went into effect and therefore lacked the new labels. She explained that nutrition labels would make it much harder to keep pretending that her favorite foods were low-calorie and low-fat.

Indeed, the labels remove illusions, putting the facts, so to speak, in your face. At a glance you can see, per the specified serving size, the amount of calories and the quantity of important nutrients, including total fat (and saturated fat), cholesterol, protein, carbohydrates, fiber, and selected vitamins and minerals, and the percentage of daily values provided. The label also shows the recommended quantities of the various nutrients based on total calories consumed.

By reading labels—and encouraging your child to do so—you can achieve a greater awareness of the nutrients your family is taking in (or not getting enough of).

Water

Water literally keeps life flowing. It comprises about 60 percent of our blood. Water is necessary for the proper movement of oxygen and nutrients through the bloodstream, and allows for sufficient flushing of waste through the liver and kidneys, and adequate sweating to modulate body temperature. Water lubricates joints, moistens tissue, aids digestion and elimination, and much more.

Every day adolescents should drink a minimum of eight glasses of water. Certain other fluids can count toward that amount, such as juices and broth. It is important to drink much more than eight glasses of water or other fluids that contain sugar and electrolytes (including sodium, chloride, and potassium) if adolescents are active in sports or other exertion or if the weather is hot, to provide extra energy and replace losses of water and salts in sweat.

Teens might also enjoy getting some of their eight glasses a day from peppermint, chamomile, and other herbal, caffeine-free teas. Freeze bottles of water for long car trips or days in the park.

Preventing Dehydration

Teach your kids "preventive" water drinking: *Drink before you get thirsty.* By the time people feel thirsty, chances are they are already somewhat dehydrated.

Acquaint your active children with the "urine test."

"Urine color is a good measure of hydration," says the website Kidshealth. org, sponsored by the Nemours Foundation, a nonprofit organization that specializes in children's health.[4] "If urine is clear or the color of pale lemonade, the hydration level is good. If a child's urine is dark, like the color of apple juice, however, he may be on the way to dehydration or heatstroke."[5]

Be aware of other signs of dehydration, too. If your child complains of a headache, dizziness, and lack of energy or appetite, give a drink containing sugar or salt, such as soup or juice, along with a nonsweet snack.

Young athletes must be especially aware of the risks of dehydration. They should avoid taking salt tablets (thought by some to improve performance) because they can cause dehydration and possibly harm the stomach lining. Active young people should get into the habit of drinking water (or sports drinks) before, during, and after exercise. It might be helpful to plan for beverage moments, such as between innings, and to make it a practice always to pack a bottle of water along with exercise gear.

Caution your child to avoid or minimize use of coffee and caffeinated teas and soft drinks. Caffeine can make people jittery or anxious, interfere with sleep, promote the loss of calcium and potassium, and contribute to dehydration.[6] Alcohol and sodas also contribute to dehydration.[7]

Don't let your family get caught in the soda habit. Sodas are expensive, have little or no nutritional value, and contain sugar (watch out for cavities), caffeine, and additives, including artificial sweeteners, colors, and flavors, that young people don't need and are better off without.

Vegetarian Teens

Much of the world favors vegetarian diets. They can be even healthier than conventional diets, offering just as much variety, nutrition, and dining pleasure. Many vegetarians can easily follow the food guide pyramid, removing meat from center stage and replacing it with beans and soy proteins, whole grains, fruits, and vegetables in starring roles.

A vegetarian diet has some special benefits. Eating few or no animal products can reduce blood cholesterol levels, lower blood pressure, and even aid in maintaining a healthy weight. A well-balanced vegetarian diet may reduce the likelihood of heart disease and certain types of cancer, such as breast and colon cancer.

There are many reasons adolescents cite for being vegetarians. Some have compassion for animals, taking a cue from such illustrious vegetarians as George Bernard Shaw, who said, "Animals are my friends . . . and I don't eat my friends."

Another renowned writer, Isaac Bashevis Singer, agreed. "I did not become a vegetarian for my health," said Singer. "I did it for the health of the chickens."

Many adolescents are concerned not only about killing animals but also about the harsh conditions in which some livestock are confined, raised, and slaughtered. They might also decline to eat meat out of concern for the environment, recognizing that raising grain for direct human consumption requires far less land and water than does raising grain for livestock. Vegetarianism shortens the food chain and aids in conservation.

Many parents may sympathize with their children's views but worry about whether youngsters will get all the nutrients they need from a vegetarian diet. Indeed, there are many ways to go vegetarian. The most common are:

- *Modified vegetarians* eat no red meat and little or no poultry, but do eat fish. By maintaining the kind of balanced diet shown in the Food Guide Pyramid, modified vegetarians can easily get all the nutrients they need.

- *Ovo-lacto vegetarians* eat no meat, poultry, or fish, but they do eat eggs ("ovo") and dairy ("lacto") foods. Some teens eat either eggs or dairy but not both. They can meet protein needs by eating at least two servings per day from the dairy/egg group, and should keep track of their calcium intake to make sure they get enough.

- *Vegans* eat no eggs, dairy foods, fish, or other animal products. They pose more of a challenge, but by planning their menus carefully, they may still get the nutrients they need. Ask your doctor if your vegan teen should be taking supplements of calcium, iron, and vitamins B_{12} and D.

- *Fruitarians* eat only fruits, seeds, and nuts. This very limited diet cannot provide all the nutrients adolescents need. Unfortunately, this is just one of a variety of quirky diets that teens might hear about and decide to try—all the more reason to acquaint your child with the reasoning behind the food guide pyramid.

The Knack of Vegetarian Meal Planning

Variety is both the spice and substance of life. Only through a varied diet composed primarily of nutrient-rich foods can adolescents get the fuel they need for energy, growth, and development.

Being a healthy vegetarian involves not only saying no to off-limit foods but also saying yes to the right vegetarian ones. Here are some ways to help your child get the knack of it:

- *Watch out for fat.* Vegetarians who try to compensate for eating no meat, poultry, or fish by getting protein through cheese and nuts might end up with a higher fat intake than is healthy. To keep fat content at no more than 30 percent of calories per day, buy low- or no-fat dairy products. Use nuts as a garnish rather than a main meal. Use cooking sprays instead of heavy coatings of oil in baking. Reduce butter and oil in sauces, dressings, and other recipes. In baked goods, replace much of the fat with applesauce, pureed prunes or bananas, or plain low- or no-fat yogurt.

- *Keep track of calcium.* Adolescents who shun dairy products must find other ways to get the calcium they need for their growing bones. Calcium-fortified orange juice, soy milk, and breakfast cereals are helpful. Natural nonanimal sources of calcium include leafy greens such as kale and broccoli; and also okra, tofu, and kidney beans.

- *Pursue protein.* People who often eat meat in large quantities get more protein than they need, but vegetarians often don't get enough. Beans, lentils, seeds, and nuts are good protein sources, but they are not "complete proteins" in the way that meat is. However, when they are combined with grains, the overall protein quality is boosted significantly. So while beans alone are good, rice and beans is even better. Go for a peanut butter sandwich on whole wheat instead of peanuts. And keep in mind that egg white is the "perfect" protein because it contains all essential amino acids.

- *Keep an eye on iron.* Meat offers a simple way to get iron. Vegetarians need to work a little harder to make sure they get the iron they need. It's a two-step process. First, they need to eat one of the many vegetarian sources of iron. These include leafy greens, dried beans and lentils, and whole grains or enriched cereals. Second, they should eat these foods with a source of vitamin C in order to help the body absorb the iron. Some examples: raw spinach salad with fresh orange sections and slivers of onion; brown rice with stir-fried broccoli; lima beans with chopped fresh tomato. Dried fruits are a terrific source of iron; tuck a small bag of dried apricots, prunes, or pineapple into your pocket for a quick snack.

- *Value vitamins and minerals.* Vitamin B_{12} is obtained only in animal-derived foods, so vegetarians have to make sure they take a supplement, eat foods that have been enriched with vitamin B_{12}, or eat sufficient servings of eggs and dairy products. The body makes vitamin D with the help of sunlight or fortified milk. If your child gets little or none of either, a supplement of vitamin D might be called for. Zinc can be obtained from such foods as garbanzo and other dried beans and peas, oatmeal, brown rice, and wheat germ (mix some with soy yogurt, sliced bananas, and a sprinkle of cinnamon).

- *Explore the possibilities.* Soy is a multipersonality food with endless possibilities. Tofu, for example, is a low-fat, low-calorie, high-protein food (and a good source of calcium) that cooperates with virtually any idea a cook can come up with. Check out the many vegetarian cookbooks at your library or bookstore. For example, *Tofu Quick and Easy*, by Louise Hagler, shows how tofu can be mashed into dips, chunked for casseroles and salads, tossed into soups, stir-fried with veggies, stuffed into jumbo pasta shells, hidden in cookies, and frozen to attain a chewy,

TIPS FOR BREAKFAST HATERS

- *Build in time for breakfast.* Get up earlier and make breakfast a special time. Talk with your family, savor the paper, read the comics, watch the sunrise.
- *Toast and cheese, a swig of juice.* Breakfast can be simple and quick. A minute or two is all you need to break the fast of night and give your day a good start.
- *Try breakfast shakes.* Throw skim milk or soy milk or yogurt, fresh or frozen fruit, and a little ice in the blender. Enhance the nutritive value by adding a spoonful of wheat germ or soy protein powder.
- *Combine breakfast cereals for variety.* Or jazz them up by adding fresh fruit, raisins, pumpkin seeds, or sunflower seeds.
- *Check out breakfast cookbooks.* Try *The Good Breakfast Book,* by Nikki and David Goldbeck. From granola to fish hash to Spanish eggs to griddle cakes with apricot topping, the Goldbecks serve up a smorgasbord of breakfast possibilities. They also offer timesaving shortcuts, such as advice on how to reheat leftover hot cereal. (Cover cooked cereal with a thin layer of water to prevent it from crusting, and refrigerate. To reheat, pour off water, stir in a bit of milk, and heat in the top of a double boiler or in a saucepan over low heat.)[13]
- *Eat leftover supper.* A casserole or a piece of chicken, tasty for dinner, is arguably even better cold the next day.
- *Save time.* Make a stack of peanut butter and jelly sandwiches on Sunday night, pack them in plastic bags, and snag one to eat on the way to school every morning.
- *Stock "grab-able" breakfast items.* Keep the following foods on hand: fresh fruit, hard-boiled eggs, whole-grain breads and muffins, containers of yogurt, cereal bars, plastic bags of cheese cubes or dried fruit and nuts.

meaty consistency that can be jazzed up with seasonings and served as "mock chicken" and other nonmeats.[8]

- *Taking the ham out of hamburger.* Supermarket freezers are stocked with all kinds of soy-based veggie burgers, from spicy black bean patties to mushroom burgers. Many are delicious and quick to heat in a skil-

BARRIERS AND BRAINSTORMS

Let your kids know that you are sympathetic to the fact that changing poor health habits can be hard. Collaborate with them in brainstorming some creative new strategies. Here are some examples of the barriers some teens have had and a number of approaches that can help.

Barrier: When everyone else is ordering burgers and fries, I feel conspicuous with a salad. Even though it's healthier, I don't like to feel different.
Brainstorm:
- Order a burger with salad instead of fries, or just a burger and have salad at home.
- Share a burger and salad with a friend.
- Order a salad and see how people react. They might be impressed.

Barrier: I don't have time for breakfast. I'm just not hungry.
Brainstorm:
- Get stuff organized the night before.
- Build up to the breakfast habit. Week 1: Eat just one piece of fruit. Week 2: Toast a frozen waffle, too. Week 3: Add milk!
- Cook something that smells really good, like a baked apple spiced with cinnamon.
- See "Tips for Breakfast Haters."

Barrier: It's not "cool" to eat the school cafeteria food, so I skip lunch or buy a candy bar in the vending machine.
Brainstorm:
- Join the school nutrition committee as a student representative and have a say in improving school meals (and vending machine fare).
- Take lunch to school. Keep your sandwich cool with a juice box you take out of the freezer in the morning.
- Ask a friend to eat the school lunch with you. If you say it's cool, it is.

let or microwave. But they can be expensive. Experiment with burger recipes from vegetarian cookbooks until you find some you like. In *The Tightwad Gazette II,* Amy Dacyczyn recounts her culinary quest in an article wryly titled "We Ate Lentils . . . and Lived." The winner of her home "test kitchen" attempts turned out to be a thrifty burger made with equal parts of cooked lentils and bulgur wheat; combined with bread crumbs, chopped onion and green pepper, milk, eggs or soy flour mixed with water; and flavored with herbs and garlic.[9]

• *Teen Support.* Teens can get good ideas on healthy vegetarian eating by reading books targeted to their age, such as *A Teen's Guide to Going Vegetarian,* by Judy Krizmanic. A subscription to *Vegetarian Times* magazine can give your child a monthly infusion of new ideas to share with the whole family.

Breakfast, a Brilliant Idea

The older kids get, the less likely they are to eat breakfast, citing lack of time or hunger. Yet research shows that students who eat breakfast get higher test scores and have fewer school absences and latenesses.[10,11] So compelling are the data that some school systems are taking "pro-breakfast" measures such as publicizing the breakfast-learning connection, marketing school breakfast programs more avidly, alerting parents to the need, and even serving breakfasts in classrooms during the first period of the day.[12]

By being aware of the nutrients adolescents need and making a few simple adjustments in the running of the household, parents encourage healthier food choices.

If your adolescent eats school breakfast, great. But at-home breakfasts can be even more enjoyable. Convert your breakfast hater into a breakfast lover by trying some of the tips in this chapter (see "Tips for Breakfast Haters").

Health-Partnering for Nutrition

• *Have dinner together as a family at least three times a week.* Leave the TV off. Use the time to catch up, cook together, and enjoy healthy meals.
• *Cooks like to eat.* Ask your kids what they like and enlist their help in planning, shopping, and preparing food. If your kids protest, remind them that learning to cook is a key skill for independent living. It prepares them for college life or eventually living on their own. Plus, if you make it a rule that the cook doesn't have to do the dishes, your kids might vie to take turns as chef.
• *Cookbooks for beginners.* Even if you own cookbooks, buy your teen his or her own cookbook as a holiday or birthday gift. Then be on hand to answer any questions or offer help as the chef experiments with recipes. Best are cookbooks with photos and step-by-step explanations. Many teens enjoy impressing their family and friends with their new gastronomic prowess. Julia, a 15-year-old in Washington, D.C., made lamb burgers with cucum-

ber sauce for Father's Day. The dish was such a hit that she began to cook regularly for her family.

- *Ambitious and delicious.* For teens who have been cooking a while, help them advance by buying them more specialized cookbooks that introduce them to new foods, new cultures, or new techniques. Julia's lamb burger recipe came from *The Encyclopedia of Cooking Skills and Techniques.* Another teen received the book *Cooking Under Wraps: The Art of Wrapping Hors d'Oeuvres, Main Courses, and Desserts.* He enjoyed learning nifty techniques for making burritos, beef *en croûte*, and strawberry empanadas.

- *First meal, first priority.* Since breakfast is so important, make it easy for your teens to eat it, either at home or on the go. Some families can't have dinner together but have family breakfasts so everyone can catch up on what's going on. Still no time for breakfast? One mom told her teens she would wake them earlier and earlier until time was not a problem. Suddenly breakfast was no problem.

- *Clearly available.* Store snacks in clear glass or plastic containers so foods are easy to see when kids are in a hurry. Opaque, unlabeled storage containers are probably a major cause of food wastage in many households. Incognito foods tend to vanish into the depths of the refrigerator, rediscovered only when it is too late to enjoy them.

- *Buy or make healthy snacks.* Some kids who won't pick up a piece of fruit will eat fruit salad. Pair raw or steamed vegetables with a small container of yogurt dip. Cut a block of low-fat cheese into cubes and slide a package of whole wheat pitas next to it.

- *Make extra dinner* so your kids can access the leftovers, heating them or eating them cold.

- *Experiment with foods from other cultures.* Sometimes a delicious, unfamiliar sauce gives fish, vegetables, and grains new appeal.

- *Consider calcium.* Use skim or low-fat milk in soups. Make oatmeal and other hot cereals with milk instead of water. Add a spoonful of dried milk to muffins and casseroles for extra calcium. Serve calcium-rich greens like broccoli and kale. Have various flavors of yogurt on hand. Ask your doctor about a calcium supplement if these calcium-rich foods fail to tempt your teen.

- *Serve salads with fun, flavorsome add-ons.* Use grated cheddar or Parmesan cheese; pumpkin, sunflower, or sesame seeds; cottage cheese; croutons; cold noodles; grated carrots or radishes; sprouts (buy a sprouting jar and have kids raise their own); chunks of chicken, meat, fish, or marinated tofu.

- *Advertise.* Post signs on the fridge: "Went to farmer's market—the peaches are so sweet!" Or put them on containers: "I asked the waiter to wrap this for me so you could try it."
- *Water, water everywhere.* Make water your family's number-one drink; it's essential, calorie-free, and inexpensive. Keep at least one pitcher of water in your refrigerator, as well as bottles of water that your kids can tuck into bookbags. When you buy bottles of water, refill them at home. Going to pick up your kids at soccer practice? Take some water bottles with you. Keep half-filled water bottles in the freezer; before leaving the house, add some water to the bottles and take them with you. They will melt gradually and provide cold water for several hours. Get into the habit of serving water at meals.
- *Drink UP.* When considering which beverages to buy and serve, think "Drink up"—that is, which beverages "up" your family's health versus which bring it down? After water, fruit and vegetable juices are a good number-two choice. Calcium-fortified orange juice is a must-have in many families. Round out your drink menu with skim or low-fat milk. If your kids will drink only flavored milk, such as chocolate milk, introduce them to new flavors through fruit shakes made with milk. One example: combine milk, banana, and a spoonful of chocolate syrup in a blender. Or introduce teens to the sweet (and iron-rich) appeal of a spoonful of blackstrap molasses stirred into milk.
- *Reduce or eliminate sodas.* Keep sodas, sweetened "fruit drinks," and sugary iced tea to a minimum. If you don't buy them, teens will drink the healthier beverages that you do have on hand. Combining juices and seltzer or club soda can be a satisfying alternative.
- *Liquid calorie alerts.* Drinking juice or milk as a primary thirst quencher can add up to many calories per day. An 8-ounce cup of milk or juice contains about 100 calories—or 800 calories per day for the person having that much each day. This is not a problem for the thinner teen, but for an overweight or obese teen, eliminating these particular thirst quenchers alone might result in weight loss. For that teen, calorie-free water is a much better choice, or 2 to 3 ounces of juice mixed with 6 ounces of club soda.
- *Steer active teens away from gimmick foods.* Athletic and other active adolescents need the same basic nutrients as others, but more calories and more water. It sounds simple, but young athletes are easily seduced by ads for bars, powders, and other supplements that promise better performance—often for a hefty price. They are better off with a variety of nourishing foods as their daily diet. Regular meals and healthy snacks are important for sustaining energy throughout the day. Complex carbohydrates such as

whole-grain pasta, cereal, and bread provide essential fuel—which is why
some athletes talk about "carbo-loading" before a major race or event.

- *Protect your active child from excessive concern with calories.* If your child
is active in a sport like gymnastics, or a performance art like ballet, which
prizes thinness, be especially aware of your child's attitude toward food.
Make sure your child eats a well-balanced diet and does not succumb to the
obsession with calories that afflicts practitioners of the "thin arts."

HEALTH BASIC #2: EXERCISE

Like nutrition and sleep, exercise is essential to good health. But unlike eating
and sleeping, staying fit can be postponed indefinitely. Day after day of good
intentions—or inattention—can add up to indolent years of lax muscles, excess
fat, reduced stamina, and a heart less hardy than it should be. Lack of exercise
also means missing out on the considerable psychological benefits. For stressed-
out adolescents, workouts can be an invaluable buffer zone that helps stave off
worsening funks.

Adolescents run the gamut in their attitudes toward exercise. Young athletes, dancers, martial arts students, and others regularly experience the charge
and challenge of goal-oriented, structured exercise. Teens who walk, bike, or
skate to school have an advantage over those in vehicles. But countless inactive
teens make more of an impression on couch cushions than on scoreboards,
stages, or sneaker soles. Alarmingly, the older adolescents get, the more likely
they are to stop exercising. The U.S. Centers for Disease Control and Prevention (CDC) reports, "Physical activity among both boys and girls tends to
decline steadily during adolescence. For example, 69 percent of young people
12 to 13 years of age but only 38 percent of those 18 to 21 years of age exercised
vigorously on at least three of the previous seven days, and 72 percent of 9th
grade students but only 55 percent of 12th grade students engaged in this level
of physical activity."[14]

An Epidemic of Obesity

Young people who do not get enough exercise are more likely to be overweight. In fact, according to the CDC, "overweight is at an all-time high
among children and adolescents."[15] Since many people's health habits are established during adolescence, teens' lack of exercise might lead to a sedentary
lifestyle and related health problems later in life. Operation Fit Kids, a nonprofit organization supported by the American Council on Exercise, reports
that "three-quarters of obese teens will remain obese in adulthood" and that
"80 percent of the kids tested in grades five, seven, and nine were unable to

meet the minimum standard to be considered physically fit during the 1999 California Physical Fitness Test."[16]

Exercise Can Heighten the Joy of Living

Exercise at its best is not a chore. It is a celebration of the body—all it can do, how good it can feel. Any auto aficionado knows the thrill of keeping a car well tuned so it hums along the highway. Fitness buffs go so far as to consider life hardly lived if they don't treat themselves regularly to a jog or swim or drum-accompanied dance class.

Horse trainers would not dream of keeping horses cooped up in their stalls, but are diligent about letting them roam and run. So should people of all ages crave and provide the same release for themselves. It may seem far-fetched to compare teens to horses—yet consider the small spaces in which many adolescents are confined for hours every day: the couch by the TV, the chair at the computer, the seat of a car, the desk in a school that neglects physical education in order to bring up math and reading test scores. Teens in unsafe neighborhoods stay inside rather than chance the unpredictable dynamics of neighborhood life, while those in safer neighborhoods often don't take advantage of the resources of their own backyards.

Georgia, a high school junior in New York City, complained to her doctor about headaches and fatigue, and said she had no time for exercise. The doctor pointed out that she lived just across Central Park from her school and could walk home every day instead of taking the bus. Georgia took the advice. These interludes in the fresh air eased her stress, made her headaches vanish, and gave her more energy.

At the Computer, Hours of Sitting Still

Computers are invaluable, wonderful tools, but as their use increases, so do the sedentary hours they occupy. In many schools, computers are essential for homework. Teachers post assignments, readings, and grades on-line, and expect students to do Internet research and hand in word-processed text that has been specially formatted, drafted, revised, and spell-checked. Term papers and special projects are like mini-marketing productions, resplendent with Power Point's telltale font changes and animated graphics. These are not necessarily negative developments. Who could argue with tools that foster good writing and creative presentations? And it's not just homework that tethers teens to computers. A kid can't keep up a social life these days without E-mail and instant messaging, not to mention on-line searches for movie schedules and music clips, on-line shopping, chat rooms, and more. All this activity makes for very little movement. While computer images dance, scroll, and zip around the screen, the teen in the chair just sits.

At School: More Sitting

Okay, but don't kids get their exercise in school? Some do, of course, both in classes and through team sports and after-school activities. But there has been a marked decline in the frequency of physical education classes, and parents cannot necessarily rely on them to counterbalance their children's many sedentary hours.

"Physical Activity and Health: A Report of the Surgeon General" noted that most middle and high school students are not getting the physical activity they need in school.[17] A CDC survey found that less than half of the nation's high school students were enrolled in a physical education class or played on a sports team.[18]

In many school districts a certain number of physical education classes might be required for graduation, but the grades are not counted toward the grade point average, nor are test scores included on student transcripts. Thus physical education essentially has second-class status. A class that doesn't "count" toward grade point average doesn't count as being particularly important. Indeed, many students, parents, and even educators regard physical education as being almost vestigial—a mandated "extra" that has to be shoehorned into schedules crammed with weightier topics like mathematics, language arts, and science.

Giving physical education short shrift is a shortsighted approach. Rather than distracting students from academic subjects, exercise "actively" complements them. Eric Jensen, a researcher on the role of movement in learning, believes that movement stimulates the brain and enhances learning through various mechanisms that include improving circulation and oxygenation of the brain, giving the brain rest periods to process information, and stimulating the release of neurotransmitters (such as noradrenaline and dopamine) that energize and motivate the learning process.[19]

Exercise is also a valuable aid to good mental health. It serves as a mood stabilizer and antidepressant. Some doctors "prescribe" exercise, finding that it enables many of their patients to avoid taking antidepressant medication. One study, in fact, found exercise even better than an antidepressant at keeping symptoms of depression from returning.[20] Aerobic activity such as running releases feel-good chemicals called endorphins that suffuse a person with a sense of well-being. Yoga centers the mind and contributes to a feeling of serenity and mastery.

In addition to all these immediate benefits, physical education classes can and should play a pivotal role in enabling students to identify and develop skills in fitness activities that they can enjoy for years to come.

Advocating for Improved Physical Education

Many school administrators are not aware of these findings on the value of physical education. While some say that they downplay physical education because of budget reasons or the need to enhance academic subjects, another reason may be that they never experienced good physical education classes themselves. They—like many adults—might recall experiences similar to those that are described in *Long Distance: A Year of Living Strenuously*, Bill McKibben's memoir of training as a competitive cross-country skier in his thirties. It was only as an adult that he understood how well suited he was to a sport that required enormous stamina and endurance. What a contrast to his "boyhood spent as a wimp . . . When I ran, I ran slowly; but no gym teacher ever explained that might mean I was built for distance, not sprinting. Instead, gym became a recurring bad dream . . . Soon I figured out a dozen ways to stand on the sidelines or make the most token effort. If I didn't try, I couldn't humiliate myself." [21]

The good news is that the field of physical education has progressed. Today's well-trained physical education teachers pay attention to such topics as the importance of cross-training. More diversified programs include not only team sports but also nontraditional classes such as yoga, aerobics, and tap dance. More emphasis is placed on equal opportunities for boys and girls. Noncompetitive teaching strategies eliminate "last one chosen" embarrassment for students who are less physically gifted.

School districts that avail themselves of these advances provide their students with a precious gift: the understanding that the body needs to move, that moving feels good and empowering, and that fitness benefits mind, body, and soul.

But school districts that are stuck in an "everybody plays volleyball for twenty minutes a week" mentality are in great need of informed parent advocacy. Just as parents should not tolerate mediocre math classes, they should not accept second-rate physical education classes for their children. Indeed, increased academic pressures virtually demand to be balanced by increased opportunities for exercise.

Within the context of exercise are countless discoveries to be made about oneself and others. For example, youngsters on sports teams develop a fine-tuned camaraderie, rejoicing in a teammate's great performance because it benefits them all. The players see their own efforts as contributing to a larger goal. They learn to be decision makers: At the bottom of the ninth, which pitcher is most likely to produce a win?

With good coaching, athletes learn to be close observers, supportive colleagues, gracious winners, and mature losers—lessons that are needed throughout life. A dancer who learns to leap higher by stretching in the air might incorporate the joy of intensified effort in other aspects of life. Exercise can hone self-discipline and increase responsibility; no adolescent wants to be the cause of having to forfeit a game due to late arrival. Adolescents who struggle in other areas of their lives can find in the physical arena opportunities to feel good about themselves and to relate constructively with others.

Three Forms of Fitness

Adolescents, like adults, should participate in a variety of exercise activities that enable them to achieve in the three major fitness areas: cardiovascular fitness, strength training, and flexibility.

Cardiovascular Fitness

Cardiovascular fitness is achieved through aerobic exercise that increases the flow of oxygen to the heart and other muscles, strengthens the heart, increases stamina, and burns fat. At a minimum, adolescents should exercise aerobically twenty to thirty minutes, two or three times a week,[22] ideally on alternate days to permit rest and recovery. Exercises include biking, running, ice and roller skating, aerobic dance, cross-country skiing, swimming, basketball, soccer, lacrosse, rowing, and hockey (field, ice, and roller). And don't forget brisk walking as a great aerobic activity. Walk instead of ride. Climb stairs instead of taking an elevator. Simple steps like these can add up to heart health.

Strength Training

Strength training, also known as weight training or resistance training, helps prevent injuries, support the joints, improve metabolism, and sculpt the body. Exerting the body against resistance strengthens bones and helps protect against osteoporosis.

Strength training includes toning and isometric exercises as well as lifting with free weights and machines. Bodybuilding takes strength training to a different level, as athletes use weight training techniques to shape and define their muscles for competition. The American Academy of Pediatrics policy statement on strength training recommends that adolescents participate in strength training only if (a) they are supervised by well-trained adults who will "plan programs appropriate to the athlete's stage of maturation, which should be assessed objectively by medical personnel," and (b) they have achieved Tanner stage 5 maturity (see chapters 2, 5, and 6), which usually is reached by ages 14 to 16.[23] If your child wants to get started earlier, encourage strengthening activities that do not use weights, such as push-ups, pull-ups, and abdominal exercises such as crunches.

Proper strength training includes learning correct form, always making time for warm-up and cool-down stretching, alternating and gradually increasing intensity of exercises for different muscle groups, and alternating days for weight training and rest.

Flexibility

Flexibility exercises keep the body supple, improve balance and focus, and reduce injuries. Activities that enhance flexibility include yoga, ballet, gymnastics, and martial arts.

It is important to warm up before and after stretching to reduce the chance of strain and cramping, and to take it slow. Some goal-oriented adolescents might be so eager to do a backbend or touch their toes that they'll rush it—and pull muscles. Achieving flexibility must be a gentle though persistent pursuit.

Naturally, there is crossover among these types of exercise. Certain types of yoga have cardiovascular benefits and build muscle. Biking can build strength as well as aerobic fitness. Dance can increase flexibility as well as provide an aerobic workout.

As with any good thing, exercise can be overdone. Lean adolescents who seem to exercise excessively might be trying to lose weight; keep an eye out for any signs of an eating disorder (see chapter 10). Competitive athletes who seem to train obsessively might be under the stress of having to prove themselves to teammates, coaches, or others. Overtraining might cause injuries (see chapter 12), or it might be a sign of disproportionate, possibly self-imposed pressure (see chapter 11 for a discussions of teens' stress levels).

Health-Partnering for Exercise

- *Prescription: exercise.* Ask your child's doctor to evaluate his or her capacity to exercise, identify any limitations, talk with your child about the importance of exercise, and collaborate with your child on making an exercise plan. On subsequent visits, make sure the doctor follows up on this conversation.
- *F is for fitness.* Grade your child's school on its physical education program. How many times a week does your child have physical education? Does the school system offer a variety of activities? Does your child seem engaged? Does the school offer team sports and other fitness activities? Does the school have well-maintained facilities and equipment? Work

through the school's parent association to ask these questions and advocate for improvements.

- *Model motion.* Make fitness a priority for yourself. Your child will notice and be more likely to do the same. Let your child see you doing those crunches and push-ups, following workout videos, taking your bike for a spin, and setting off on walk-and-talk dates with your mate or friends.

- *Take a hike.* Invite your children to walk, with or without you, to do errands, or just get some fresh air.

- *Family discount?* Join a health club—and try for a family membership. Alexandra, age 14, joins her mom for kickboxing classes every Sunday and Wednesday evening, a great activity for togetherness and fun. The classes give Alexandra and her mom a lot to talk about, too. Alexandra says they laugh about "the people who stand there and sweat watching *you* do the exercise."

- *Home gym.* Buy new or gently used exercise equipment and videos for the whole family to use. Stationary bikes, treadmills, and steppers promote cardiovascular fitness. Free weights (very light ones if children are under 15) are inexpensive. Or use homemade weights such as soup cans or plastic milk bottles filled with different levels of sand. Exercise balls are fun ways to tone muscles and improve flexibility and balance. Some balls come with pumps for easy deflation (since they can take up a lot of space). If you have a driveway, put up a basketball hoop.

- *Car gym.* Keep balls and Frisbees in the trunk for impromptu stops at parks for games of catch. Outfit your car with a bike rack. Toss skateboards or skates in the car and set off on searches for smooth new surfaces to enjoy.

- *Carpool to the pool.* Join with other parents to plan fitness activities for your children and theirs. One mom rounded up her son and his pals for ice skating in August. They had the indoor rink almost all to themselves. It was the very coolest way to cope with a hot summer day.

- *Buffed floors, buff bods.* Household chores are fitness opportunities in disguise: vacuuming, mopping, turning mattresses, mowing, gardening, car washing, even hauling laundry to and from the Laundromat. It's all in the attitude. If you have the money to hire a cleaning person, think twice. Why should the cleaning person have the benefit of all that exercise when your children need it, too? Can't resist the professional's touch? Reduce the frequency and have the family clean during the cleaning person's time off. Choose a weekend morning or a more modest goal of one room a day.

- *Limit TV and computer time.* Don't let these machines lure your child into sedentary living.

- *Become involved in your child's activities.* Volunteer to coach or assist with your child's team. Showing up at games is an equally important way to express your support and interest (even if you don't always understand the subtleties of the sport).
- *Downplay winning.* Sure, it's fun to win. But give your child the consistent message that what's most important to you is that your child participate, learn, and have fun.
- *Fold fitness into community activities.* Work within your community to encourage the development of fitness programs for adolescents. Petition your parks department to clean up the local playground and basketball courts. Ask your religious institution to plan fitness-oriented activities and trips. The California Adolescent Nutrition and Fitness (CANfit) Program issues competitive grants for fitness and nutrition programs for adolescents in diverse low-income communities, such as hip-hop dance for African American girls, parent/child fitness programs in Saturday Korean language schools, and soccer leagues for Latino youth.[24]
- *Plan fitness weekends and vacations.* Hiking, biking, skiing, camping, and swimming (with or without dolphins) can be part of many vacations. Equipment can often be rented if you don't want to take it along.
- *Encourage, don't push.* Support your adolescent's interests but be open to changes. If your child is on the swim team in eighth grade but abandons the backstroke for biking the following year, go with it. Don't come on too heavy about staying with a sport a child doesn't want to do. The more adolescents enjoy and choose fitness activities for themselves, the more likely they are to stay active.

HEALTH BASIC #3: SLEEP

Adolescents seem to sleep either too little or too much. A teen might even do both: sleep-starve on weeknights, sleep-binge on the weekends. Teen sleep can be such a seesaw thing, it almost would be funny if it didn't have such serious health implications. Researchers are so concerned that the National Sleep Foundation and other organizations have convened conferences and issued sober reports on the sleep deficiencies and the "problem sleepiness" that are rampant among this age group. Sleeping too much might indicate physical or mental health problems that should be evaluated by your doctor. But most likely, excessive sleep is a weekend or after-school phenomenon that results from insufficient sleep on weeknights and an erratic sleep schedule.

The many adolescents who skimp on sleep see it as a luxury, a frill, or a nuisance. In their overcommitted lives, they almost resent the need for sleep. Shut-eye shuts out life. It cuts short cramming for the history exam, hangs up the phone, and shrinks the hours available for after-school jobs. The need for sleep almost seems like a design flaw. Does it make sense to have to surrender 8 hours a day—a third of your life!—to *sleep*?

Only 15 percent of adolescents get an average 8.5 or more hours of sleep on school nights. More than 25 percent of adolescents sleep only 6.5 hours or less.[25] Some brag about how much they pack into their days on only 5 hours of sleep.

Most figure they'll catch up on the weekend. By then they're so sleep-deprived that an alarm clock and a bucket of cold water combined could not rouse them at the hour they would normally get up for school. The average adolescent sleeps more than 2 hours longer on weekends.[26] Some, in fact, seem to sleep much of the weekend away. The problem is, sleeping in on the weekends (combined with staying up late) throws off a teen's sleep pattern, making it even harder to get up and go to sleep earlier on schooldays.

Most adolescents do not realize what "healthy sleeping" is, why it is so important, or how the lack of sleep affects their lives.

Adolescents' Sleep Needs

Sleep experts recommend that adolescents get 8.5 to 9.25 hours of sleep every night. Since that is much more sleep than most adolescents get, it's worth taking a look at the reasons that the brain earns its right to that much rest, and the consequences if the brain's demands are not met.

Why do people sleep, anyway? In the report "Adolescent Sleep Needs and Patterns,"[27] the National Sleep Foundation (NSF) sums it up nicely: "Sleep is food for the brain." Sleep is *not* a time when the brain shuts down and goes on strike. The brain uses this "down time" to adjust its chemical levels and process memories and experiences. If the brain is deprived of the amount of sleep it needs, it will not, so to speak, take this lying down. The brain is "relentless in its quest to satisfy its needs," says the NSF.

When Sleep Needs Are Not Met

Adolescents who have not had sufficient sleep are likely to feel drowsy or slowed down, lack energy, not think clearly, and have to fight off the urge to sleep. Sleep enables people to function; lack of sleep is disabling. Like driving with the emergency brake on, getting by with too little sleep can be done, but it slows you down, doesn't feel right, and is bad for your body.

Citing a National Institutes of Health Study, the NSF says that "excessive sleepiness is also associated with reduced short-term memory and learning ability, negative mood, inconsistent performance, poor productivity, and loss of some forms of behavioral control."

So if your adolescent is forgetful, cranky, depressed, volatile, or not performing to his or her ability in school, insufficient sleep might be the culprit, or at least a contributing factor.

As teachers—especially of early classes—can tell you, many sleepy teens might show up in class, but their sleep-craving brains prevent them from being truly present. In the middle of class their eyelids droop and their heads fall back. Sleep researchers call this "involuntary napping" or "microsleeps," and say that sleepy people often have "gaps in processing information and in behaving reliably." [28]

Sleep-deprived adolescents are sometimes misdiagnosed with attention deficit hyperactivity disorder (ADHD) because the symptoms of sleep deprivation mimic those of ADHD: difficulty staying focused, sitting still, and completing tasks, and a greater likelihood of aggressive or impulsive behavior.

Fatigue increases the effects of alcohol, so adolescents who drink are more likely to get intoxicated and out of control if they don't get enough sleep.

Sleepy teens who drive are asking for disaster. According to the National Highway Traffic Safety Administration, drivers age 25 and under account for more than half of all crashes linked to fatigue. [29]

According to an NSF poll:

Drowsy driving causes approximately 100,000 car crashes annually. Statistics show that fall-asleep crashes are most common among younger people, with peak occurrence at age 20.

- Half of the nation's adults (51%) report driving while drowsy during the past year.
- 60% of 18- to 29-year-olds have driven while drowsy, with 24% reporting that they dozed off at the wheel at some point during the past year.
- Among younger adults, 22% drive faster when they're tired, compared to 12% of the general adult population. [30]

It is essential that teen drivers understand that driving when tired may be as dangerous as driving when drunk. In a twist on a famous slogan, the NSF advises teens, "Remember: friends don't let friends drive drowsy." [31]

Healthy Sleep Patterns

Healthy sleep is not just a matter of racking up the hours but also of establishing a pattern that the body can rely on. There are many gears in the "biological clock," and the sleep schedule is one of them. Regular sleep patterns assure both quantity and quality of sleep, and fortify the mind and body for better functioning throughout the day.

Adolescents' sleep patterns are not the same as those of younger children or adults. Researchers have found that adolescents have a natural tendency to fall asleep and wake up later in the day. Eleven o'clock at night is the hour when most high school students most readily fall asleep. That would mean that their natural waking time would be between 7:30 and 8:15 A.M. Yet that would make most of them late for school.

When High Schools Wake Up

The disparity between adolescents' natural time clocks and high schools' schedules has inspired some school districts to assess and revise their hours to be more accommodating of adolescents' biological realities.

Changing school hours is not a simple thing. Schools must take into account a myriad of factors, including coordinating transportation and food service with lower-level schools in the district, taking into account commuter traffic for school staff, assessing the impact of later home arrival times for students who stay after school for athletic and other activities, considering safety issues pertaining to daylight and darkness, and more.

Also, later start times have both negative and positive implications for family life. Getting home later might impair a teen's ability to supervise younger siblings or do household chores. However, as a plus, it decreases the amount of unsupervised time that adolescents have until parents get home from work. After-school hours are high-risk times for teens; they might be more likely to get into trouble, have sex, and use alcohol and drugs. Reducing the "witching hours" might add up to improved adolescent health in ways that transcend increased sleep.[32]

Insomnia

There are various reasons why some adolescents suffer from insomnia, the inability to fall or stay asleep.

BEDTIME IS TOO EARLY. Some parents are so eager for their children—especially early adolescents—to get enough sleep that they give them unrealistic bedtimes, such as 8:30 or 9:00 P.M. The adolescent gets into bed and can't fall asleep; the parents might not even know that he or she is up, tossing and turning or reading with a flashlight under the covers. If an adolescent requests a later bedtime for this reason, add an hour as an experiment, to see if the teen falls asleep more easily and is still able to feel alert, energetic, and cheerful the next day.

EVENING ROUTINE IS UNCONDUCIVE TO SLEEP. Evening activities should have a flow that takes into account an adolescent's need to "wind down" before going to sleep. It often helps to "re-order" the evening so that an adolescent doesn't get too stimulated right before bedtime.

For example, Andrew's typical evening involved doing homework, practicing his violin, chatting on-line with friends, then going to sleep—or trying to. He found that he lay in bed, unable to sleep, all jazzed up from his chats with friends. His doctor suggested that he change the order of activities to do homework first, then talk on-line for an hour, then practice the violin. The music was more relaxing, and his insomnia disappeared.

Other activities that help an adolescent unwind before bedtime include gentle yoga, taking a warm (not hot) bath, listening to soft music, writing in a diary, or reading an enjoyable book or magazine that is not related to schoolwork.

WORRIED ABOUT WORRYING. An adolescent who develops temporary insomnia might become so anxious about not being able to go to sleep that the anxiety prolongs the insomnia. Changing evening activities or—in some instances, and preferably with the doctor's permission—trying a drowsiness-inducing antihistamine such as Benadryl for a few evenings can break the cycle and restore sleep.

ANXIETY AND DEPRESSION. An inability to get to sleep or persistent awakening during the night or very early in the morning might be "red flags" signaling depression or anxiety that should be evaluated by parents and then brought to the doctor's attention. (See chapter 11.)

Sleep Disorders Associated with Excessive Sleep

While too little sleep is a problem for many teens, too much sleep is a problem for others. These adolescents dive into sleep as if into a whirlpool, quickly immersed in oblivion. Sleep might be their refuge from stress, their respite from boredom, or their response to depression. When their parents fight, they sleep to escape the tension. When overwhelmed, they go under the covers.

School might wear them out. Some adolescents with learning disabilities have to work harder and are prone to fatigue. Teens who are out of shape but somehow get onto a sports team collapse from overexertion when they get home.

Or an adolescent might sleep a lot in order to shake off a cold or while recovering from an illness such as mononucleosis. Iron deficiency anemia is another possible culprit that a doctor must rule out.

A sleep disorder might also be a cause of excessive sleeping.

- *Delayed Sleep Phase Syndrome* can make it impossible for adolescents to wake up in the morning because they also find it impossible to go to sleep before 2:00 A.M. or 3:00 A.M. The problem is that their internal "sleep clock" has been thrown off by puberty, and they haven't been able to reset it to more normal hours. A sleep specialist can help them recalibrate their sleep schedules by devising a new bedtime pattern over a few weeks, or by instructing them on how to use bright lights to waken at specific times in the morning.

- *Narcolepsy* is a tenacious sleepiness that progresses to sudden, deep sleeps. Generally an inherited condition, narcolepsy is often misread as a lack of interest in activities, as depression, or as attention deficit disorder (ADD). It can be treated with medication—but only if diagnosed properly.

- *Obstructive Sleep Apnea* is the temporary cessation of breathing during sleep. Symptoms include snoring and bed-wetting. The splintered sleep prevents people with apnea from really feeling rested, even if they "got" eight hours of sleep. Apnea is often caused by allergies or by obstruction of the airway by enlarged tonsils and adenoids. Treating the allergies or removing the tonsils and/or adenoids relieves the apnea. However, apnea is not always promptly diagnosed, and in some instances has even been misdiagnosed as ADHD.

Neither assume that your child has a sleeping disorder nor dismiss the possibility. If your child seems to sleep too much, to be unrefreshed by sleep, or to have erratic or problematic sleep, describe the problem to your child's doctor, preferably in the company of your child so you can address the issue together.

Health-Partnering for Sleep

- *Find ways to explain the importance of sleep in language your teen can relate to.* For example:
    » *Byte-Size Info.* Is your teen's computer programmed to "defrag" and "disk-clean" overnight? Explain that the brain needs downtime to clear up gaps and reset itself so it's ready for the next day's challenges.
    » *Weight Lifters' Manifesto.* Teens who are into weight lifting know that muscles respond best and are less vulnerable to injury if lifting is alternated with rest. So it goes with the brain. After "mental lifting," the brain needs respite before returning for another round.
    » *Sleep on It.* Budding writers know that something magic happens when they put a story in a drawer for a day or so before

revising it. When they look at it with fresh eyes, they can see rough spots that escaped them the first time around. Sleep is the magic drawer that refreshes the mind, sharpens the eye, and inspires new ideas.

- *Evaluate the situation.* Talk with your child about the signs of sleep deprivation identified by the NSF. It might be a problem if your child:

  » Has a hard time waking up in the morning. A person who has had enough sleep will awaken fairly easily and naturally. A sleep-starved teen might not even hear an alarm clock that's right next to the bed.

  » Gets cranky (or crankier) as the day wears on. Remember how your child's behavior as a toddler tended to deteriorate around dinnertime? The pattern repeats in a sleepy adolescent.

  » Nods off at quiet times, such as when a film is shown in school or on the bus or train ride home.

  » Sleeps for long stretches on weekends.

- *Invite an experiment.* Suggest that your teen keep a "sleep diary" to explore the correlation between how many hours he sleeps and how he feels. For a week or so, don't change anything. Follow with two weeks of going to bed one to two hours earlier, maintaining this sleep schedule over the weekend. Does he feel more energetic, less irritated, better able to concentrate? What's going on at school and with homework? (See the National Sleep Foundation's sleep diary at http://www.sleepfoundation.org/publications/diary.html.)

- *Driving dreams.* Alert your teen to the link between drowsiness and car accidents. Before lending the car, ask your teen how much sleep they got last night. Consider making sufficient sleep a condition for car privileges.

- *Power naps.* Because many adolescents are so tired, they nap after school. But what many working parents don't know is that their adolescent is conking out for two, three, even four hours, making it almost impossible to fall asleep by 10 or 11. Talk with your child about taking a twenty-to-thirty-minute "power nap" instead. This amount of sleep is restorative, will refresh a teen for homework or other activities, and will not interfere with a reasonable bedtime.

- *Wake-up calls.* Have your child call you when she gets home, and offer to call her back in twenty or thirty minutes to wake her from her "power nap." It's a nice way to know when your child is home from school, have a chance to touch base, and support your child's sleep health.

- *Sunday night syndrome.* Many kids—and adults—have a hard time falling asleep on Sunday nights. For one thing, they might have slept in until noon.

And they might be nervous or anxious about a test or social situation to confront at school the next day. Talk about Sunday night syndrome with your adolescent and brainstorm ways to ease tensions and prepare for the week ahead. Setting out clothes, taking a Sunday night walk, imposing phone curfews, organizing the backpack, taking a bath, or just chatting about what's coming up over the coming week might be helpful.

- *Appliance alert!* Certain appliances are notorious for tempting adolescents to prolong their days and resist sleep. Consider a "gadget bedtime," by which the following must be turned off: TV, radio, CD player, phone, computer, and lights. Of these, the computer might be the appliance teens beg you hardest to spare. There's always one more website, one more song, and ten more instant messages to respond to. But even though computers never sleep, people must. Set a time after which the answering machine will pick up any calls, the lights will be dimmed, and the house quieted so that everyone can wind down their day in time for a refreshing night's sleep.

- *Plump your own pillow.* To aid your adolescent in signing off and going to bed, set an example. Get sufficient sleep, take power naps if you need to, and pull off to the side of the road for a nap if you're tired while driving.

- *Synchronized sleeping.* Talk with your child about maintaining consistent sleep patterns, even on weekends. Sleep and wake times should not deviate by more than an hour or so, and changing the schedule for two or more nights in a row should be avoided. Offer support in returning to the schedule after vacations and other time shifts. To make this work, your child must make sleep a priority. It won't be easy, given competing demands or temptations. But the sleep diary should provide a compelling incentive by giving evidence of how much better your child will feel every day with sufficient sleep.

- *Edit time.* With your teen, take a close look at how he or she spends time. Are there activities that could be cut? Job hours that could be reduced or rescheduled? Homework that could be better organized to free up time? Could regular reviews reduce or eliminate the need to cram before a test? Are there preslumber relaxation opportunities that could be added? Ask your child how you can help.

- *Explore reasons for insomnia or excessive sleep.* Consult the doctor if your child is sleepless or oversleeping for extended stretches of time.

FOUR: Common Health Problems of Girls and Boys

Pimples are often thought of as the most common teen health issue. But in fact, adolescents experience a much wider array of health problems. Some of their illnesses or symptoms afflict people of any age—such as the flu, constipation, or headaches. Others are more specific to adolescence, such as scoliosis or delayed puberty (see chapters 4 and 5). And a host of health problems results from choices adolescents make, such as sexually transmitted diseases (see chapter 8) and infections from tattoos and piercing.

ILLNESS IN CONTEXT

A common illness or symptom is often less an isolated incident than an outcome of other things that are going on in an adolescent's life:

- *Check out the "three basics."* Adolescents are most likely to get sick when their resistance is down. A healthy diet and sufficient exercise and sleep (discussed in chapter 3) go a long way toward keeping illness away. Giving short shrift to any of the three can temporarily compromise the immune system, giving germs a chance to work their mischief.
- *Assess stress.* Like sleep deprivation or a junk-food diet, stress can push the immune system beyond its limit. Adolescents may get stressed out from pushing themselves too hard, coping with family or peer problems, or using alcohol or other drugs. An illness signals the need to take time out.
- *Consider the level of susceptibility.* Adolescents with allergies, asthma, or other chronic conditions need to be extra-attentive to their health and environment. For example, highly allergic people may be more susceptible to the complications of colds and flu (such as sinusitis, ear infection, or bronchitis) because their respiratory tracts tend to be more swollen and inflamed in reaction to allergens (such as dust or pollen), which in turn interferes with drainage and clearing of infection.
- *Connect the dots.* Always consider the adolescent's lifestyle and behavior. If an adolescent complains of abdominal pains, it might be constipation, an ulcer, gastroenteritis, or appendicitis. But if that adolescent is female and

sexually active, a range of other possibilities must be considered, too, such as pelvic inflammatory disease or ectopic (tubal) pregnancy (see chapter 8).

THE ONE BEST WAY TO PREVENT ILLNESS

A healthy diet, regular exercise, sufficient sleep, and a moderate stress level are essential to keeping the immune system strong. But even they do not qualify as the health practice identified by the U.S. Centers for Disease Control and Prevention (CDC) as *the single most important way to prevent disease*. That honor goes to the simple act of handwashing.[1]

Colds and other airborne diseases, conjunctivitis and other bacterial or viral diseases, hepatitis A, meningitis, and infectious diarrhea—all these and more can be transmitted on the hands. Many people are not aware of how often they touch their eyes, nose, or mouth. These are entryways through which germs on their hands can enter and infect their body.

How and When to Wash Hands

The CDC recommends washing hands:

- Before eating.
- Before, during, and after preparing food.
- After using the bathroom.
- After touching animals or animal waste.
- When hands are dirty.
- When you or someone near you is sick.

To wash hands effectively, wet hands thoroughly, wash with soap for ten to fifteen seconds, making sure to reach every part of the hands and nails, rinse well, and dry.

Washing Hands in School

Many school bathrooms do not provide adequate soap or paper towels, or they run out by the end of the day. Some adolescents avoid school bathrooms altogether. To maintain proper hand hygiene, adolescents can buy packets of wipes, or carry a liquid hand sanitizer such as Purell, or pack wet soapy paper towels from home in "zippered" plastic bags so they can cleanse their hands and wipe their face during the day.

Washing Hands at Home

Keep a bottle of liquid soap in every bathroom and by the kitchen sink. Wash towels frequently or use paper towels. Give your adolescent a nailbrush and demonstrate how to use it. Keep soap, a jug of water, and paper towels in the car, too. If your adolescent needs reminders, post signs in the bathroom, by the kitchen sink, and near the cat's litter box or the dog's leash.

BODY ODOR AND OTHER HYGIENE MATTERS

"My son used to smell so sweet," mused the mom of a young adolescent boy. "Now he smells *rank!* I don't know what happened!"

What happened was that hormones activated by puberty sent his sweat glands into overdrive. Armpits, crotch, and feet are suddenly funky presences to be reckoned with. And although it is very obvious to you (and others within a one-mile radius) that something must be done about these scents, don't take it for granted that your adolescent has noticed them. When smells are one's own, they're not so bad.

So it falls to the parent to broach the delicate subject of stink: "I think it's time you started using a deodorant, dear. Here, I bought this one for you. See what you think." Start with an unscented deodorant. Your adolescent might want to try different kinds: scented or unscented, roll-ons or sprays or sticks— and perhaps one that is not only a deodorant (stops odor) but also an antiperspirant (stops sweating). A more powerful antiperspirant, if needed, can be obtained with a doctor's prescription.

But deodorant alone will not do the job. Bathing regularly and wearing clean underwear and clothes are crucial components of this clean-up campaign. Young adolescents seem to fall into two camps when it comes to hygiene. They are either oblivious or obsessed. It is not unusual for adolescents to strew their clothes all over their room, put on whatever jeans and T-shirt they see first (even if worn daily over the last four days), and head out the door. It is time for your adolescent to do his or her own laundry, and shower or sponge-bathe every day.

Hygiene or Style?

It can be hard for parents to accept the unkempt and shaggy appearance of their teen who seems not to care. But there is a difference between hygiene and style. Body odor, filthy clothing, untrimmed nails and dirt-filled undernails, unbrushed hair, and a neglected beard are about hygiene and good health. On the other hand, torn and baggy jeans, long and stringy hair, although aesthetically not pleasing to the adult, may be very cool among teen peers, and the style preferred by your child. Parents need to choose their battles about style, can insist (or try to) on a reasonable degree of good hygiene, and should also be alert to whether the poor hygiene could possibly be a symptom of depression or your teen's feeling overwhelmed (see chapter 11).

SKIN AND HAIR

Skin, hair, and nails can be mirrors, reflecting stress and lifestyle, diet, and hormonal changes related to puberty. Some adolescents are blessed with barely a blemish, while others curse their skin daily, watching it erupt with acne or flake from dryness.

ACNE

More than 80 percent of adolescents suffer from acne. This skin disorder is caused by a combination of factors, all put into play by the hormones of puberty. Androgen hormones, including testosterone, are present in both males and females. These hormones stimulate the oil (sebaceous) glands in the hair follicles of the face, chest, shoulders, and back to produce sebum, a fatty substance. Dead skin cells on the surface of the skin combine with the sebum and they plug the pores (follicles). Enter a third culprit: *Propionibacterium acnes (P. acnes)*, skin bacteria that feed on the triglycerides in the sebum and normally cause no problems. But when pores are clogged, the bacteria contribute to inflammation and the dreaded zit.

Acne is so common, it's practically a rite of passage. By the early twenties, acne usually subsides. But the prospect of eventual relief might not be that comforting to an adolescent who wants to put his or her best face forward. During a stage of life when young people are self-conscious anyway, acne makes "facing" people even harder.

How to Talk with an Adolescent About Acne

Blemishes can ruin a party or make a teen want to stay home from school. In an American Medical Association survey on acne and teenagers' self-esteem, one third of teens said that they believed "pimples were the first thing people noticed about them."

More than three quarters of teens said they are very aware of the appearance of their skin, and about one fifth cited acne as contributing to depression.[2] It is not unusual for teens to worry that everyone is noticing, maybe even talking about their acne. Using their hair as a veil or a mask, they assume a head-down, eyes-averted posture, as if avoiding eye contact makes them less visible, less vulnerable to other people's critical gaze.

No matter that their peers have skin problems, too. Indeed, teens might need to be reminded that they are not alone. Even so, they still feel unlucky, singled out, cursed. Pimples are like outside evidence of problems inside, announcing, "There's something wrong with me." For adolescents who just want to blend in with the crowd, acne is the enemy.

How cruel that the very same hormonal changes that stir sexual feelings also create skin problems that make it hard to flirt convincingly. How's he going to notice your sparkly eye shadow if he keeps glancing at the whiteheads on your chin? How's she going to take you seriously as a man when your zits announce that you're still a kid?

Internet bulletin boards attest to teens' anguish:

I'm growing acne that looks like it has faces on it . . . sometimes I hear voices inside my head telling me stuff like, "Hi, I'm your pimple," and "It's me, that big red thing on your face," and sometimes even stuff like "I'M ALIVE!" It's scaring me!!! Please help! They're growing bigger and bigger each day.

Okay . . . I had this big red zit on my face and it was bothering me and I just wanted to pop it! So I came on the message board and tried every-thing!!!! I did the saltwater, the toothpaste, the tea bag, the washcloth, and nothing worked!

Guys—this sounds really gross, but I read in a magazine that if you have a pimple and you need to get rid of it fast, put a little tiny dab of Prepara-tion H on it, but it has to be the cream kind. I know it sounds sick but I had to do it for a school dance . . . and all the redness was gone the next morning and you could hardly see it! Sorry, it's gross but it helps!

Why do people seem to think that the reason we get acne is because we don't wash our faces! Come on!

How Does *Your* Teen Deal with Having Acne?

Teens cope with acne in various ways. Consumer-culture teens buy every new skin-care product. Diligent teens follow a strict regimen of morning, after-noon, and evening cleansing. Internet-savvy teens research and check into chat rooms. Some suffer in silence; others complain constantly.

Find out how your adolescent feels. This may seem obvious, but many par-ents assume that their children will feel as they did at that age. Herb had been a shy kid who found acne unbearable. So when his son Joey developed acne, he insisted that he go to a dermatologist. But Joey was so busy with school, base-ball, and a close circle of friends, he did not want to be bothered.

"I don't have time to go to a doctor," Joey told his dad. "Anyway, who cares that I have pimples? Everybody has some. They'll go away eventually." Indeed, they did—and Herb got a good lesson in not projecting his own concerns onto his son.

By the same token, if you were blasé about blemishes when you were a teen, do not put down your child for being upset by a single, ill-timed pimple. Acne is a big deal for many adolescents. Their already shaky image is at stake. Acne is literally a surface concern, but its impact is anything but superficial.

Do not minimize your child's concern, but don't feel that you need to match his or her level of intensity, either. Sympathize, but also say that you consider your child as attractive, appealing, and lovable as ever. Beauty may be skin deep, but assure your child that love is not.

Abigail's mother, Joyce, was aghast at the pimples that spotted her child's lovely face, and kept careful track of their response to treatment. Every morning, Joyce cupped Abigail's chin in her hand and said, "Let's see how we're doing today, honey." At first Abigail did not mind, but as the weeks dragged on, she resented the fact that her mother now rarely talked about anything else. Joyce was reading up on treatments, urging her daughter to drink lots of water ("I read about this, honey, maybe it will help you"), and sending away for cleansing lotions and concealers featured in late-night infomercials.

Finally, Abigail exploded: "Enough, Mom! Leave me alone!"

"But I'm just trying to help," said Joyce.

"All you end up doing is making me feel like an ugly freak," Abigail sobbed. "I feel like no matter what else I do, it won't matter until my skin is cleared up."

How Can You Help? Ask Your Child

Young people desire and tolerate different levels of parent involvement.

Karen told her mother that she wanted her company in the drugstore, "But don't say anything, just be there."

Lisa wanted her mom to help her evaluate cleansers and cover-up creams.

Henry asked his dad to find him a dermatologist and drive him to appointments.

Don't own the problem. No matter how the sight of your child's blemishes pains you, ultimately skin care is your child's responsibility. Avoid admonishing your teen to cut bangs, to ditch the French fries, to lay off the makeup. Nagging never motivates.

Be sensitive to your child's level of embarrassment, if any. Adolescents— and families—differ in their comfort level with discussing acne. For Kurt's dad, it was fine to say, "I put some cleansing pads in the bathroom, thought you might like to try them for your skin." Another parent might find it better to quietly leave cleansing pads in the bathroom and let the teen discover them.

Initiate conversation if your child does not. Let your child know it is okay to talk about acne: "I notice that you and your friends have been breaking out a bit. That's very normal for kids your age. It happens because your hormones are changing. If it bothers you, we can make an appointment for you to see a doctor. Or maybe you don't think about it."

Or, "I had some skin problems when I was your age, and my mother always told me not to worry, acne would go away. I worried about it anyway, but she was right. By the time I left for college, the pimples were gone."

Your child might be relieved that you brought it up. But if you sense resistance, back off.

Offer to schedule a doctor's appointment. Mention any special concerns to the doctor privately. For example, you might ask the doctor to initiate a conversation about acne if your shy child will not do so.

Ask the doctor how treatment will affect your child. At the very beginning of September, Sandra's mother took her to the dermatologist. Bad idea. The dermatologist extracted sebum from plugged follicles and Sandra's skin was embarrassingly red the very next day, which also happened to be the first day of high school. The doctor never mentioned the possible side effects, nor did he consult Sandra or her mother about the timing. This experience became a lesson in how to be a medical consumer: Ask questions.

Be patient and encourage your child to be patient. It takes time for treatments to work, for doctors to adjust them if necessary, and for hormones to settle down. Keep in touch and work collaboratively with the doctor. Don't give up or switch doctors if the first treatment doesn't work. Meanwhile, life goes on. Help your adolescent identify special interests that will help keep acne in the background.

What to Do About Acne

Acne may be noninflammatory or inflammatory. Noninflammatory acne lesions are clogged pores called comedones. There are two types of comedones.

A *blackhead,* or *open comedone,* is a pore that is clogged with sebum and dead cells at the skin's surface. Its dark color is not due to dirt but to pigment in the sebum.

A *whitehead,* or *closed comedone,* is a pore that is plugged below the skin's surface. It appears as a fine bump and is the same color as the skin (not white).

If a comedone ruptures under the surface of the skin, and in the presence of *P. acnes* bacteria, an inflammatory lesion results. A red "pimple" is called a *papule,* a white pus-filled lesion is a *pustule,* and larger, deeper, and even painful lesions (prone to result in scarring) are called *cysts* and *nodules.*

Acne may occur on the face, shoulders, back, chest, or upper arms. An acne-like outbreak can also occur on the buttocks.

At times of stress acne might flare up, perhaps as a result of hormone fluctuations. Similar fluctuations occurring during the menstrual cycle often affect the degree of acne severity, typically worsening during the week or two before a period. Various medications, including certain anticonvulsants, steroids, and some types of birth control pills, might exacerbate or cause acne eruptions.

Contrary to popular belief, acne is *not* caused by hot fudge sundaes, pizza, or other foods, or relieved by masturbation or other sexual activity. Pollution or high humidity can make acne worse. Teens who work in gas stations, parking garages, and fast-food restaurants might also be exposed to grease and oil that can contribute to acne. A tendency to acne may be inherited.

Basic acne management and prevention include the following:

- *Keep skin clean.* Wash in the morning and evening, as well as after heavy exercise and sweating, with a mild soap. Using the fingertips (not a brush), wash the whole face, from under the jaw all the way to the hairline. Also wash any other areas of the body, including the chest and back, where acne appears. Be gentle. Rubbing too hard can irritate the skin and make acne worse.
- *Shampoo regularly.* Keep hair off the face to limit contact with oils in the hair. Keep hair pomades and other preparations away from the skin.
- *Avoid heavy, oil-based makeup,* as well as skin creams, suntan or sunscreen products, and hair pomades that can choke pores.
- *Avoid tanning and sunburn,* both from natural sunlight and tanning salons.
- *Keep hands off.* Picking at blackheads, papules, or pustules can further inflame them and delay the healing process. Scabs generally form over picked-at pimples that make them stand out even more.
- *Do not wear tight bras or other clothing,* hats, or backpacks. They can irritate acne.

How Can Acne Be Treated?

Dermatologists generally follow the basic principles of acne treatment. First, try topical agents (products used on the surface of the skin). If they do not adequately help, then try systemic agents (medications taken by mouth). Because adolescence—the time when people are most susceptible to acne—lasts so long, it is important to minimize exposure to systemic medications that might have harmful side effects.

Topical Agents

The key ingredient in familiar, over-the-counter products such as Clearasil and OXY 5 and 10 is benzoyl peroxide. It helps unplug sebaceous follicles, decrease sebum production, and kill bacteria. Gels and solutions are more potent (but also more drying) than creams and lotions. Benzoyl peroxide preparations (both over-the-counter and by prescription) are available in concentrations of 2.5 to 10 percent and are usually used once a day. Start with the lowest concentration cream or lotion. If that doesn't help, graduate to higher concentrations or try a gel.

Apply the medication daily by placing a pea-size amount in the palm of one hand and from this quantity place a series of dots of medication over the entire affected region (e.g., the whole face or upper back, not on individual pimples). Then spread the dots into a thin layer, avoiding the eyes and the corners of the mouth.

Benzoyl peroxide might irritate the skin and trigger an allergic reaction in a small percentage of people. It is important to follow directions and do a patch test (apply the medication to a small hidden area first to check for any reaction). Use only mild soaps, such as Dove or Neutrogena, or a nondrying cleanser such as Cetaphil. Harsher soaps or astringents can excessively dry the skin and cause peeling.

If benzoyl peroxide alone doesn't help enough, ask your doctor about other topical medications that may be combined with benzoyl peroxide or replace it (but will require a prescription). The selection of prescription topical medication depends on the type of acne you have. For example, retinoids (Retin-A, Differin, Avita, Tazorac) are especially effective for noninflammatory comedones, whereas topical antibiotics (erythromycin, clindamycin, and others) work best against papules and pustules. Several preparations combine benzoyl peroxide with an antibiotic in a single gel (Benzamycin and Benzaclin). The doctor will give you instructions for proper usage, such as whether to use the medications once or twice a day, alone or in combination.

Acne treatments do not work instantly, so a patient attitude is part of the regimen. Your child should see some improvement in four to six weeks. At first it might even appear that the acne is getting worse as the skin adjusts to the new treatment. The key to successful treatment of acne is finding a doctor to work with over time whom the adolescent likes and trusts. Acne generally lasts for at least a few years, during which time treatments must be continued and continuously reevaluated.

Systemic Treatments

Oral antibiotics fight *P. acnes* bacteria and relieve inflammation. In the past they were more frequently prescribed, but advances in topical therapy have reduced the need for them. The antibiotic prescribed most often for acne is tetracycline, starting with a dose of 500 to 1000 milligrams daily, then gradually decreasing to 250 milligrams daily or every two days. It should be taken on an empty stomach because food interferes with its absorption. Children under age eight should not use tetracycline because it can cause discoloration of their teeth. People of any age who are taking tetracycline (or similar preparations of minocycline or doxycycline) must be very careful to avoid intense exposure to sunlight, which will more seriously burn their skin while on this antibiotic. Other effective antibiotics against acne include erythromycin, azithromycin (Zithromax), and cephalosporins (such as Ceftin or Duricef).

Antibiotics might lead to vaginal moniliasis (yeast vaginitis) or gastrointestinal side effects. They might also interfere with the effectiveness of birth control pills, so a woman on an antibiotic who is sexually active and taking the Pill should always use a backup method of contraception, which generally would be a latex condom, which her partner should be using anyway.

The Pill, in fact, is often prescribed as a treatment for severe acne in females, because the hormones in most Pills effectively diminish the effect of androgens (such as testosterone), which stimulate sebum production and induce acne. If an adolescent girl is sexually active and also has acne, the Pill would be an especially good choice of contraception for her (see also chapter 7).

Accutane (isotretinoin) is a highly effective and somewhat controversial oral treatment for severe cystic-nodular acne that has not responded to other forms of treatment. It is thought to reduce the size of sebaceous glands, diminish the growth of *P. acnes* bacteria, and lessen the shedding and stickiness of hair follicle skin cells. Its chief advantage is that often it can almost miraculously erase the acne after about five months of daily treatment, and thereby prevent permanent scarring. But it also might have serious side effects, including marked drying of the lips, the lining of the nose (causing nosebleeds), and the surface of the eyes; increased susceptibility to sunburn; musculoskeletal and chest pains; gastrointestinal problems; temporary increases of blood cholesterol; and other side effects. PREGNANT GIRLS AND WOMEN MUST NEVER USE ACCUTANE, WHICH CAN CAUSE SEVERE BIRTH DEFECTS. Some dermatologists insist that ANY female taking Accutane also be on the Pill during the months of treatment.

A highly publicized suicide in May 2000 (the victim was the teenage son of a U.S. congressman, and he was taking Accutane at the time) brought to the fore a previously noted concern that Accutane might cause depression. The U.S. Food and Drug Administration is currently investigating whether Accutane increases the risk of depression and suicide or whether depression and suicide potential co-exist at a higher rate among teens with severe acne. Until this question is resolved, all teens on Accutane should be made aware of this concern and also be closely monitored by their parents and their doctor for any signs of depression, with appropriate action taken in a timely fashion if it is needed.

Despite the various problems and worries with Accutane, most adolescents who have taken it consider it a "miracle" drug that rescued them from the many stresses and hassles of their acne. Accutane may be considered as an option for the small group of teens for whom all else has failed, the acne is severe, and it will be prescribed by a dermatologist experienced in its use.

DRY SKIN

Advice on coping with dry skin might seem counterintuitive. The very remedies adolescents try—hot showers, lingering baths—are the very things that make dry skin worse. Hot water, especially for prolonged periods of time, steals the skin's natural oils. As water evaporates, it takes moisture away.

To help combat dryness, adolescents should:

- Take short, warm (not hot) showers, and avoid baths altogether.
- Use nondrying soaps like Dove or cleansers like Cetaphil.
- After bathing, pat skin dry and use a hypoallergenic face and body moisturizer, such as Eucerin or Lubriderm or Curel.
- Drink at least eight glasses of water a day. Although exposing skin to water can be drying, drinking water benefits skin by keeping it well hydrated.

Tough Guys in Winter

Winter makes dry skin worse, as harsh winds, cold weather, and indoor heating reduce environmental humidity. Frequent bathing and inadequate moisturizing exacerbate the loss of the skin's natural oil barrier and contribute to the abnormal dryness known as "winter itch."

Further complicating the problem is adolescents' resistance to dressing sensibly against the cold. It is not unusual to see adolescents spurning gloves, hats, scarves, and even umbrellas. They complain that hats flatten their hair, producing the dreaded "hat hair." Or they believe that "real men" don't need to bundle up against the cold. Somehow, by going hatless and wearing their jackets open, they think they appear more macho. But they can end up with red, dry skin, not to mention a reduced resistance to illness. To combat winter dryness, in addition to the suggestions above, adolescents should:

- Bathe less frequently (but to prevent body odors, daily sponge-bathe armpits, crotches, and feet; and use deodorant).
- Limit showers to a minute or two, and use as little soap as possible.
- Protect skin against the cold and wind. Convince your adolescent to tuck a pair of gloves and a hat into his jacket pockets or bookbag. If the weather becomes especially ferocious, at least he'll be prepared, even if he only wears these items when his friends are not around. (Oh, and what about that "hat hair" problem? Maybe your adolescent will agree to try loose head scarves, earmuffs, or oversize turtlenecks that can be pulled up to cover the lower third of the face.)

DERMATITIS

Dermatitis is an all-purpose word for skin inflammation. There are several types and causes of dermatitis that can cause erythema (redness), pruritis (itching), edema (swelling), xerosis (abnormal dryness), scaling, flakiness, and other symptoms.

Contact Dermatitis

Contact dermatitis is a temporary inflammation caused by contact with a substance to which an individual is sensitive or allergic. Among the products that adolescents might react to are scented soaps, lotions, cosmetics or other grooming products, laundry detergents, jewelry containing nickel, or fabrics (such as wool or polyester). The location of inflammation on the body is the best clue to what is causing it . . . for example: wrist (metal jewelry), waistline (fabric), face (cosmetic). In general, opting for unscented soaps, hypoallergenic cosmetics, nonnickel jewelry, and natural fiber clothing is likely to solve the problem.

Contact dermatitis is often caused by an allergic reaction to common plants such as poison ivy, poison sumac, or poison oak, which rub against the skin while a person is on a hike or sitting on the ground.

Adolescents with contact dermatitis should:

- Become "medical detectives," trying to identify and then avoid "sensitive" products, and testing other products to find those tolerated. Ask a physician to recommend products least likely to cause a reaction.
- Wear gloves when working with potentially irritating substances—for example, when doing housework or painting. If wearing gloves is not practical, substitute protective "barrier" ointments.
- Learn to identify and avoid the distinctive three-leafed poison ivy or other plants that have caused dermatitis, and in the future wear long pants, socks, and closed shoes when hiking.

Eczema (Atopic Dermatitis)

Atopic dermatitis, better known as eczema, is a chronic skin condition that often runs in families and afflicts individuals with asthma, hay fever, or other allergies. The patchy skin rash appears red, raised, dry, sometimes blistery, and shows scratch marks (because it itches). It often results in the skin becoming thickened and darkened in color. Eczema most often appears in skin creases at the elbows, behind the knees, around the neck, behind ears, and on the hands, but it can appear anywhere on the body.

Eczema might flare up for various reasons, including:

- An increase in dryness of skin, especially in winter (see page 75).
- An "allergic reaction," but unlike contact dermatitis, the reaction is not due to contact and the allergic trigger might be difficult or impossible to identify.
- Stress, anxiety, or depression—although it is fair to say that this might be a chicken-and-egg situation: Which came first, the eczema, causing stress, or the stress, causing eczema? Most sufferers would say the stress came first.

Some adolescents with dry skin have a condition similar to eczema called *keratosis pilaris*. Inflammation of tiny hair follicles creates areas of tiny red dots, usually on the upper outer surface of the arms and the front of the thighs. This totally benign condition can be upsetting to any adolescent who would naturally crave smoother skin.

Coping with Eczema and Keratosis Pilaris

Adolescents with eczema or keratosis pilaris should follow the same suggestions offered above for dry skin, including short (not too hot) showers, judicious use of nondrying cleansers and moisturizers, and use of protective gear against the cold and wind. In addition, they should:

- Consult with their regular physician or a dermatologist for advice, medication, and other treatments. Especially for eczema, a corticosteroid cream or ointment is likely to be prescribed.
- Try, on their own, to identify factors that contribute to eczema flare-ups, such as hot water, harsh soaps, sweating, and emotional stress.
- Stay alert to possible skin infections that might result from scratching or other causes of breaks in the skin's integrity, and notify their doctor promptly.
- Seek treatments for the itching if it is not well controlled, to prevent infection, skin discoloration and thickening, sleep deprivation, and general malaise.

• If the problem is severe, consider how recreational and occupational choices might affect the eczema. In some cases, adolescents are counseled to steer clear of career choices that require frequent handwashing, such as beautician, nurse, doctor, or restaurant worker.

Seborrheic Dermatitis

Seborrheic dermatitis often begins in adolescence, its most common form being scalp dandruff. Scaly, red, itchy skin inflammation flares in areas rich in sebaceous glands, such as the scalp, face, chest, eyebrows, and eyelashes. A yeastlike organism might play a role in this disorder.

Medicated, over-the-counter lotions and shampoos containing selenium sulfide, antifungal, or other substances are highly effective. But if the dermatitis worsens, becoming red, scaly, or crusty, consult a dermatologist (or ophthalmologist if on eyelids).

SUNTANS ARE "SKINJURY"

Adolescents who love to get a tan are taking a chance with their health. Excessive sun exposure may cause sunburn, sun poisoning, or skin cancer.

Tanning lamps and booths are no safer and should be avoided at all cost. Some claim that they only emit UVA ("good") ultraviolet rays, and not UVB ("burning") rays. But in fact both UVA and UVB rays can cause damage. Furthermore, any malfunction of timing devices can increase the risk of prolonged exposure. Failure to use goggles can cause eye damage. (Rays can penetrate through closed eyelids.)

The reason? Tanning—like sunburn—is literally a form of skin injury. When ultraviolet rays penetrate the skin, they stimulate the production of melanin, a pigment produced by skin cells to prevent further injury. Dark-skinned people are less likely to burn, since they have a larger natural supply of melanin, though they, too, can burn. People with fair skin are at greatest risk. Those who work and play outdoors and do not take precautions, like many farmers and sailors, can have permanent skin damage. Such is the meaning of "weathered skin." Their exposure to the weather—to sun and drying winds—makes skin age and wrinkle faster, and increases their likelihood of skin cancer.[3]

To protect against skin damage and skin cancer, adolescents should:

• *Never use sun lamps or go to tanning salons!*
• *Never use a sun reflector!*
• *Avoid all commercial and home tanning devices*—but adolescents who insist on using one should at least carefully read all instructions and pre-

cautions. A buddy system is also a good idea, so that a friend can double-check that timers are in good shape and exposure is limited.

- *Use lotions and lip balms with sun protection factor (SPF) of 15 or higher.* This applies to people of all skin tones.
- *Reapply sunscreen every two hours and after swimming or sweating.* Pay special attention to parts of the body that tend to burn fast, including the nose, ears, shoulders, and lips.
- *Avoid exposure when the sun is at its strongest,* between 10:00 A.M. and 4:00 P.M. Sun can burn not only at the beach, but also on cloudy days or when glinting off snow.
- *Reduce the amount of skin exposed to the sun* by wearing long-sleeved shirts and long pants or skirts, wide-brimmed hats, and sunglasses.

PIERCING AND TATTOOS

A people may be both painted and tattooed, and the motive for this may be simultaneously sexual, social, and magical.

—Robert Brain, *The Decorated Body*

The current popularity of piercing and tattooing amounts less to innovation than to a rediscovery of ancient arts. Around the world and since prehistoric times, people have pierced, tattooed, painted, scarred, reshaped, or otherwise marked their bodies. The reasons vary among individuals and cultures. People mark their bodies in order to beautify, to proclaim a point of view, to display membership or role in a group or society, and to express individuality.

Some adolescents want to pierce or tattoo both to rebel and to conform:

Susie's dad let her get a navel ring.

Greg got a tattoo and his parents don't mind.

Lisa has five holes for earrings—and so does her mom.

The beauty of piercings and tattoos is definitely in the eye of the beholder. Parents might find themselves slamming up against two opposing views:

View #1—Let adolescents decide for themselves:
"Teens' bodies are their own and they should be allowed to express themselves." (A variation: "I don't like the idea, but I pick my battles, and this isn't one of them.")

View #2—Adolescents are not ready to make an informed decision:
"Adolescents aren't mature enough to decide on something that will mark

their bodies forever. And how will an employer feel about that stud in my kid's tongue?" (A variation: "I'm worried that this means that my child is getting into a gang, using drugs, or hanging out with a risk-taking group of kids.")

Parents who wrestle with what to do might want to delay giving an immediate yes-or-no answer, and address the issue with their adolescents in a non-judgmental way:

- *What's behind this decision?* What makes you want a tattoo/piercing? What are peers' experiences? How will it affect your life? Do you think you would be willing to wait? What if you change your mind?
- *Are you getting a tattoo to prove your love for a boyfriend or girlfriend?* Is he/she pressuring you to do that? If so, what does that say about your relationship? What will happen if you break up? (It's one thing to wear your heart on your sleeve, but quite another to become weary of the heart you wear on your arm.) How about finding another way to express your love?
- *Is the procedure legal here?* Some states or cities outlaw tattoos or require customers to be above a certain age.[5]
- *Have you explored what the procedure involves?* Many tattoo and piercing studios do not use anesthesia.
- *Have you checked out the tattoo/piercing studio?* Even with a reputable provider, complications can occur. It is essential to make sure that the practitioner is licensed and that the studio uses new needles, pigments, gloves, ink cups, and other materials for each customer.[6] All other equipment should be sterilized in an autoclave, and blood safety rules must be followed.
- *Are you aware of the health risks?* Both tattoos and piercings can lead to infections, allergic reactions to inks or jewelry, scarring, tetanus, or injury. Tongue piercing can cause infections, swelling, breathing problems, speech impediments, chipped teeth, or choking from swallowed jewelry. The American Dental Association notes that a pierced tongue might swell so much that it can block the airway, and that oral piercings can cause nerve damage and uncontrollable bleeding.[7]
- *Are you prepared to take precautions against infection?* Because tattoos and piercings are wounds, they must be cared for diligently during the healing process to prevent infection. Will an easily distracted adolescent remember to keep a tattoo or piercing clean?
- *Have you considered that the results might not be what you hoped for?* Eyebrow, nose, and other facial piercings will always be part of your appear-

ance, even if you stop wearing jewelry. Tattoos can fade or might not be as appealing as you thought they would be.

• *Are you aware of how difficult, painful, and expensive it can be to get rid of a tattoo?* Laser or other removal of tattoos can be expensive, time-consuming, and painful. Afterward, the skin might still not look as it did before you got the tattoo.

HAIR LOSS

Hair loss from the scalp is a fairly common occurrence, and although quite frightening at first to the teen, it rarely results in an ongoing serious problem. Often while washing hair in the shower or brushing it, a teen notices that more than the usual few hairs are coming out. This results in a generalized thinning of the scalp hair (usually mild, called *telogen effluvium*) or sometimes the loss of hair in only one or two discreet areas *(alopecia areata)*. This kind of thing most often occurs about one to three months following an emotional or physical stress, which causes growing hairs to go into a resting phase and then fall out prematurely. Alopecia areata and telogen effluvium generally require no treatment once the diagnosis has been made, but on occasion may be treated with topical or injected steroids. Without treatment the condition continues for approximately three to six months, rarely more than a year.

Hair loss may also be associated with eating disorders such as anorexia nervosa, use of certain medications (such as chemotherapy for cancer), allergic reactions to hair products, hormonal changes following childbirth or rarely with birth control pills, scalp infections, iron deficiency, thyroid disorders, or autoimmune diseases such as lupus.

Alopecia totalis is a much more severe condition in which hair is lost from the scalp, eyebrows and lashes, pubic and other areas, and should prompt consultation with a physician (usually a dermatologist). Treatments are helpful, but the condition often recurs.

Adolescents who tightly pull back or braid their hair may find themselves losing hair from breakage. Some teenagers acquire the nervous habit of actually plucking or breaking off hairs from the scalp, a condition called *trichotillomania*. Trichotillomania may result in small patches of hair loss, often hidden by the hair above, or in severe instances, very short broken hairs covering most of or the entire scalp.

EYES

VISION TESTING

Visual acuity often changes during adolescence. Teens are old enough to recognize and report when suddenly they are having trouble reading the blackboard, or when objects in the distance appear blurry, or when reading requires squinting and results in headaches. At such times a thorough eye examination by an ophthalmologist (a medical doctor/eye surgeon with expertise in disorders of the eye) or optometrist (a nonphysician specialist in eye disorders) is in order. Teens with no difficulty seeing may be screened by their regular doctor using a simple eye chart either annually or every two years. Vision screening may also be done at school or when applying for a driver's permit or license.

EYE AILMENTS

Adolescents should see their regular physician or request a referral to an ophthalmologist or optometrist if they have any of the following symptoms:

- *Inflammation of the eye.* Redness (or "pinkness") of the eye, accompanied by pain, crusty discharge, and/or swelling of the eyelids, usually indicates conjunctivitis, a mild infection (viral or bacterial) or allergic reaction of the invisible membrane that covers the eyeball and insides of the eyelids. Warm soaks and sometimes antibiotic or antiallergic eyedrops are prescribed. If redness, pain, or light sensitivity continue beyond a few days, then examination by an ophthalmologist is needed to investigate the possibility of more serious disorders of the eye involving the cornea (white area) or iris (colored area).
- *Inflammation of the eyelid.* Blepharitis is a bacterial infection of the eyelid margin and is characterized by redness, crusting, and sometimes eyelash loss. Treatment includes lid cleansing with baby shampoo on a Q-tip and application of antibiotic ointment. A stye is an infected eyelid gland that swells with pus. Applying warm compresses alone may relieve pain and release pus. Treatment with an antibiotic ointment or even drainage by an ophthalmologist may infrequently be needed.
- *Trauma to the eye.* Trauma may take various forms and is often an emergency. Injury to the various parts of the eye may result from chemical or fire/smoke burns, blunt or perforating injuries, or foreign bodies. Trauma to the globe of the eye may cause a subconjunctival hemorrhage, which looks horrific (the entire white part of the eye turns bright red) but, in fact, heals on its own without any intervention. On the other hand, far more serious injuries requiring emergency surgery may not produce as dra-

matic an effect. Consultation with an ophthalmologist should always take place following eye trauma.

EYE CARE

Adolescents can do some basic things to protect the health of their eyes:

- *Keep contact lenses clean.* Follow cleaning instructions, never clean lenses by putting them in the mouth, and don't sleep in contact lenses unless they are the extended-wear type. Never attempt to tint contact lenses with food coloring or anything else. It can lead to infections or other serious problems.
- *Wear protective goggles* for baseball, hockey, and other sports; wood or metalworking; welding; use of pesticide sprays.
- *Take eye injuries seriously.* Seek medical attention promptly.

EARS

All humans need quiet time, as well as restful sleep, for the body to recuperate, to repair itself. Without such time, we risk physical and mental breakdowns. That is true for children as well. They need a quiet time and place to study, to read, to reflect, to think, and to slow down.

However, we and our children cannot depend on tranquility at home. There are so many noises invading our living space—noise from helicopters and jets, from nearby bars and discos, from construction, from traffic, from jet skis, from leaf blowers. How might this loss of tranquility affect us and our children?

—Arlene L. Bronzaft, Ph.D., *Hearing Rehabilitation Quarterly*[8]

We live in a noisy world, and adolescents often make it even noisier. Loud music in their rooms and ubiquitous headphones underscore the importance of music in their lives.

But if the music is loud enough it might diminish their ability to hear. Adolescents who habitually surround themselves with sound might become increasingly desensitized to the effect of constant noise on their hearing. Playing music loudly might itself be a sign of hearing loss.[9] Many adolescents sustain temporary or permanent hearing loss from attending loud concerts.

Constant noise can also affect adolescents' peace of mind, whether they are creating the sound themselves or there is always a TV or radio on in the home. This "background noise" not only obliterates quiet, it also can impede family communication and learning.

Hearing loss may also result from accumulated fluid in the middle ear (following a middle ear infection, or from a cold or allergy) or from blood that pools in the middle ear after a fight or sports trauma or in connection with scuba diving. Hearing loss may also result from wax clogging the ear canal, but a doctor should treat this. No Q-tips in the ear allowed!

To protect their hearing, adolescents should:

- Listen to music at lower volumes, whether music is ambient or through headphones.
- Give their ears a rest after exposure to loud noise, such as a concert.
- Wear earplugs or protective earphones if they perform with a band or attend loud performances or travel on screeching subways.
- Get their hearing checked annually by an otolaryngologist (ear, nose, and throat specialist) if they frequently listen to very loud music, or any time they are having problems hearing conversations or understanding teachers in school—or parents at home.

ORAL HEALTH

Oral health cannot be considered separate from the rest of children's health and well-being, just as the mouth cannot be separated from the rest of the body . . . Oral diseases are common, and many of them—such as caries—can be prevented with early cost-effective interventions. Despite the availability of such measures, and improvement in children's oral health in recent decades, many children still lack needed dental care—more in fact, than lack medical care.

—David Satcher, M.D., U.S. Surgeon General, *The Face of a Child*, Surgeon General's Workshop and Conference on Children and Oral Health [10]

Which illnesses make adolescents stay home from school? Many people might be surprised to learn that dental problems account for about 52 million lost school hours per year, according to the U.S. surgeon general.[11]

When most people think of dental needs and adolescents, they think about braces—and indeed orthodonture is very important. But oral health care is important for a number of reasons.

DENTAL CARIES

According to the U.S. Surgeon General's Report, the most common chronic childhood disease, affecting more than 80 percent of children by late adolescence, is dental caries (cavities). Two excellent and cost-effective ways to prevent cavities are water fluoridation and the application of dental sealant. Yet only 15 percent of 14-year-olds have had sealant applied to permanent molars.[12]

BAD BREATH (HALITOSIS)

The horror of halitosis is that it can turn a person into a pariah—and nobody tells you why!

Is that guy really scurrying away because he has to file grocery coupons for his mom—or does my breath smell?

When she turned her head so I'd kiss her cheek instead of her mouth, did she really develop a sudden cough—or did my breath turn her off?

Malodorous breath may be caused by bacteria in the mouth, gum disease, residual scents of strongly flavored foods like garlic, gastric reflux, sinusitis, or smoking. Mints and chewing gum are good in a pinch, but they don't heal the problem or last long. To banish bad breath, it is essential to practice good oral care (see below) and address any underlying medical or dental problems.

GUM DISEASE

Gum disease is not just a grown-up problem. In fact, according to the American Academy of Periodontology, gingivitis (gum inflammation), which is the first stage of gum disease, is frequently found in adolescents. If teens do not practice good oral care, they can develop periodontal disease, the main cause of tooth loss in adulthood.[13]

The academy notes that the hormonal changes of puberty increase adolescents' risk of gum disease. Progesterone and possibly estrogen send more blood to the gums, making them more sensitive to trapped food particles, plaque, and other irritations.[14]

BRACES

In the film *My Stepmother Is an Alien,* Kim Basinger, playing a beautiful creature from outer space, gazes admiringly upon an adolescent boy wearing braces.

"Mouth jewelry!" she exclaims.

She might have been an alien, but she was on the right track. Although it is not so pleasant to walk around with a mouthful of metal, braces do assure a lifetime of straight teeth, and greater self-confidence in having an attractive smile. Adolescents who balk at wearing braces should be made aware that their teeth announce their state of beauty and health. They will never feel sorry later that they wore braces as adolescents.

But braces are not only worn for aesthetic reasons. They also produce a healthier bite. Malocclusion—a "bad bite" resulting from having crowded, extra, or missing teeth, or jaws that do not line up properly (overbite and underbite)—makes braces a necessity for health reasons.[15] Left uncorrected, malocclusion can lead to gum disease, tooth decay, or tooth loss.

Advances in orthodontic materials and techniques have given wearers of braces more options than they used to have. Some adolescents opt for brightly colored rubber bands on their braces to match their school colors or those of a favorite sports team. Other teens are grateful for the option of wearing clear, ceramic, mini-, or "invisible" braces that attach to the inside of the teeth.

Braces Pay Off, But You Might Have to Pay

Some types of dental insurance may cover only the least-expensive metal braces (but probably do not restrict the colors of rubber bands worn with them). If your insurance does not cover braces, it is still important to explore how you can manage to pay for them, given their importance to your child's self-image and health. Orthodontists might have payment plans or sliding scales available. Some employers permit payment for braces out of pretax dollars through a "flexible spending plan" benefit, according to the American Association of Orthodontists.[16] There might also be a lower-cost clinic, such as one connected with a dental school, to which you can take your adolescent for braces.

Special Care Protects Braces

Braces take an average of two years to work their magic.[17] During that time, oral care is more important than ever. Not only do wearers of braces need to follow the basics of oral care (see page 87), but they must be aware that if they skimp on brushing they can end up with permanent stains on their teeth from the braces, wires, and other components of the braces. In addition to their regular orthodontist visits, they need to visit the dentist for a thorough cleaning at least every six months, or more often if recommended.

Safeguarding braces also involves staying away from certain hard, crunchy, or sticky foods such as hard candy, mints, and nuts; chewing gum, and sticky foods like Tootsie Rolls, caramels, fruit leather, and taffy; popcorn; and hard pretzels. Instead of biting into an apple, pear, or carrot, cut it into small pieces.

Adolescents who participate in team sports such as baseball and basketball should wear a mouthguard to protect braces and prevent injury. Ask your orthodontist to recommend one.

When Braces Come Off

Once the braces are off, that does not mean the care ends. The orthodontist might prescribe wearing a retainer, either full- or part-time, to make sure teeth "retain" their new alignment. By this time, most adolescents are so happy to be rid of their braces they do not want to be bothered with a retainer. They need to understand that it will assure that their years of wearing braces were not in vain.

To increase the likelihood of your adolescent's compliance with the retainer, consider asking the orthodontist not to remove braces before your child goes off to summer camp. Out of your sight, your child is likely to put that retainer out of mind. At least if the orthodontist waits until school resumes, you have the ability to check and remind your child to wear it.

THE BASICS OF ORAL CARE

To keep their breath sweet, their mouth healthy, and their smile beautiful, adolescents should follow this advice:

- *Learn to love brushing*. Most in-a-hurry adolescents brush their teeth for half a minute and don't bother to floss. To sweeten their breath, they need to invest the time. Brush at least twice a day, using a fluoride toothpaste. Brush for a minimum of three minutes, using a soft toothbrush with a small head that can reach every surface of every tooth.
- *Gently brush the gums and tongue, too*. They can harbor lots of bacteria. (This goes double for teens with tongue piercing.)
- *Floss at least once a day*, to get at the bacteria a toothbrush cannot reach. If you do not know how, ask your dentist for instruction.
- *Avoid relying on mouthwash*. It may temporarily disguise bad breath, but does not substitute for good dental care. Mouthwash with alcohol can even dry the mouth, which can encourage certain bacteria to grow.
- *Rinse the mouth after eating if you can't brush*. Or carry a travel toothbrush and interdental stimulators (toothpicklike sticks for removing food trapped between the teeth).
- *Don't smoke*. Smoking and spit tobacco make the mouth a smelly place. Along with all their other ill effects, they also stain the teeth, contribute to periodontal (gum) disease, and increase the risk of cavities, candidiasis (oral yeast growth), and oral cavity and pharyngeal cancers.[18]
- *Visit a dentist for a checkup and cleaning at least twice a year*, or as recommended.
- *Rule out other causes of bad breath*. Still have a problem with breath despite conscientious oral care? Gum disease, sinusitis, or gastric reflux might be the culprit.
- *Don't try to diagnose your own bad breath*. Breathing on your hand is not a reliable way to smell your breath. Breath exhaled while talking carries odors from the throat, which can't be detected by oneself. (Also, people have a built-in tolerance for their own odors; they are less charitable

with other people's.) Ask a trusted parent or friend if you suspect a breath problem.

• *Avoid sugary treats and sodas.* Or at least rinse your mouth or chew sugar-less gum afterward.

Helping Your Adolescent Stay Motivated

Adolescents might say that brushing is boring and flossing is "gross." But these activities are nothing less than an investment in their future. So much oral disease is preventable. Help your adolescent understand that spending a few minutes a day now can prevent countless hours in a dentist's or periodontist's chair later.

If your adolescent insists that flossing is "gross," point out that it doesn't matter—nobody sees behind the closed bathroom door.

Multitasking might help make tooth care more tolerable. No time to floss? One woman reported this time-management strategy to the business section of her local newspaper: Floss in the shower after putting on hair conditioner. The flossing gives the conditioner just the right amount of time to do its job, and teeth and gums get an excellent workout.

Toothbrushing is boring and takes too long? Use a timer so you don't have to keep an eye on your watch, then use these few minutes to do squats and heel raises, read a magazine article, or think through the day's plans.

As with other good health practices, modeling good oral health care yourself will mean more than any admonitions you utter. Stock up on floss, buy everybody in the family a new toothbrush every few months, allow your adolescent to choose a favorite toothpaste and rubber band colors for braces, and admire the resulting healthy smiles.

RESPIRATORY PROBLEMS

COLDS

They call it the "common cold," as if it were a single, simple thing. But in fact, about 200 viruses can cause infections of the upper respiratory tract (nose, throat, ears)—which is why it has been impossible to find a "cure" for the common cold.

Symptoms of a cold are most likely to occur when an adolescent is run down and stressed out. Common cold viruses are coughed or sneezed into the air all year round, but they infect and cause a bad cold in only those people whose resistance is down. A cold is payback for too many late nights running around or catching up with a stressful buildup of schoolwork. Colds are also spread by the hands—a good reason to wash hands frequently—and are more likely to strike and persist in a person who smokes.

Most people know all too well how it feels to have a cold: runny or stuffy nose, sneezing, teary eyes, clogged ears, sore throat, cough, low-grade fever, achiness, fatigue. All you want to do is crawl under the covers and sleep. And that's just what the doctor orders, along with drinking plenty of fluids (water, chicken or vegetable broth, any kind of juice) and perhaps taking a few over-the-counter remedies just to feel a little better. A remedy should be chosen to target a specific symptom. The icky-achy feeling and sore throat at the beginning of a cold are relieved by acetaminophen (Tylenol) or ibuprofen; lozenges, cough drops, and a hot steamy shower also ease the pain and dryness of a sore throat. A simple decongestant such as pseudoephedrine (Sudafed) and a nose drop or spray, used no longer than three days, help the nasal and ear congestion, and an expectorant such as guaifenesin might ease a cough. Combination medications with three or four or more ingredients might be more than needed and often contain an antihistamine, useful for an allergy but only exacerbating the fatigue and sleepiness of someone with a common cold. A dab of petroleum jelly on the nostrils helps keep the nose from getting too red and sore.

One great strategy to avert a cold just coming on (those earliest signs of scratchy throat and mild fatigue) is to get a few extra hours of sleep that night . . . and wake up with those bugs having been fought off by your own immune system. Most colds, once established, last about a week and move through stages where first sore throat, then nasal/ear symptoms, and finally a cough predominate. If symptoms and fatigue persist beyond two weeks, this cold might have graduated to something more serious (as described below).

SINUSITIS AND OTITIS MEDIA

Behind and above the nose and cheekbones are air-filled openings in the skull known as sinuses. When the membrane lining these spaces becomes inflamed and swollen (along with the lining inside the nostrils during a cold), mucus that normally drains through the nose and throat accumulates in the sinuses. The pressure from this mucus (and sometimes also pus) produces a feeling of soreness and pain inside and behind the nose, under the cheekbones, and/or above and around the eyes (this area might also swell a bit). At this point, the common cold has progressed into a sinus infection, called sinusitis. A similar phenomenon might occur in the middle ear, also an air space that drains through the eustachian tube into the back of the throat behind the nose. If fluid and pus build up inside the middle ear, a feeling of clogging, decreased hearing, or intense pain may indicate a middle ear infection, called *otitis media*. Sinusitis and otitis media are common complications of the common cold, are most often caused by various bacteria invading in addition to the cold virus, require diagnosis by a doctor, and are treated with antibiotics.

BRONCHITIS

Bronchitis is an inflammation of the bronchial tree, the complex system of branching tubes inside the lungs that carry inhaled air into and exhaled air out of the lungs as we breathe. The inflammation causes swelling of the inside of these bronchi, thus narrowing the bronchial tubes and making it a little harder and more painful to breathe. The mucus (white or yellow or green) stimulates a "wet" cough, which may bring it up from the lungs. These symptoms of bronchitis may be accompanied by headache, a low-grade fever, and wheezing. In the otherwise healthy teenager, such symptoms may simply need a little time and rest to abate with the help of an expectorant (such as guaifenesin) and cough suppressant at night.

Guaifenesin is the ingredient in Robitussin and many other over-the-counter cough preparations. It is an expectorant—that is, it loosens coughs but does not suppress them. Robitussin DM contains guaifenesin combined with dextromethorphan, which is a mild cough suppressant. The two ingredients work well together to loosen the mucus but suppress the tickle.

If bronchitis is more severe or persistent an antibiotic may be prescribed to cover the possibility of a bacterial infection. Sometimes, an inhaler (albuterol) is suggested to ease the cough, tight breathing, or wheeze.

Many smokers have chronic bronchitis. The smoke itself irritates and can permanently damage the bronchial tubes and other parts of the respiratory tract. Teenage smokers who get a cold are much more likely to end up with bronchitis, which is difficult to shake, than a teen nonsmoker who fights off a cold in a few days. Secondhand smoke can cause similar problems.

PNEUMONIA

Pneumonia is an infection of the lung tissue itself, not limited to the inside of the bronchial tree. It can be a severe illness resulting in death (rarely), or be quite mild and never even diagnosed as such. If it occurs in both lungs it may be referred to as "double pneumonia." If it is a mild case, meaning that one can walk around and pursue normal activities, it is called "walking pneumonia."

Most cases of pneumonia are caused by viruses, but some are caused by various bacteria, and rarely by a fungus or parasite. The most common bacteria infecting an adolescent is called mycoplasma. Pneumonia may or may not follow a cold. Teens with pneumonia generally feel sicker than someone with bronchitis, and often have fever, chills, chest pain, difficulty breathing, cough, and profound lassitude. Whereas a chest X ray appears normal with bronchitis, pneumonia produces shadows on the X ray that confirm its presence.

Treatment with an antibiotic is generally prescribed. Most teens recover in a week or so and feel fine soon thereafter.

FLU

"The flu" is caused by the influenza virus, types A and B. In addition to this real flu, other viruses cause "flulike" illnesses of moderate to high fever, chills, severe muscle aches, headache, nasal congestion, cough, and profound malaise. Occasionally the flu is complicated by pneumonia. The flu season in the United States lasts from late fall to early spring and peaks during the winter. Healthy adolescents generally recover after one to two weeks, but this is an eternity for most teens eager not to miss out on school and other pursuits. If diagnosed within two days of the appearance of symptoms, medication is available that somewhat shortens the length of the illness. But most adolescents simply rely on acetaminophen (Tylenol) or ibuprofen, lots of rest, and fluids to get through this ordeal. Aspirin and other salicylates should be avoided at all costs with the flu to prevent the risk of developing Reye's syndrome, an often-fatal liver disorder.

Adolescents with asthma and other lung disorders, diabetes, immune deficiencies, and other chronic illnesses are advised to receive a "flu shot" immunization each fall. Healthy adolescents, especially college or boarding school students living in dormitories, might opt to get the vaccine as well. The flu shot only protects against the influenza virus, so unfortunately it does not guarantee a totally healthy winter.

MENINGITIS

Fortunately, meningitis is *not* a common health problem of adolescents, but parents frequently worry about this serious illness. Parents should be aware of the symptoms and the three types (viral, bacterial, fungal) of meningitis.

Meningitis is an infection of the meninges, a membrane that covers the brain and spinal cord. Meningitis can be caught from an infected person, especially through coughs and sneezes. Meningitis can also occur, but very rarely, when a person's existing infection, especially upper respiratory, ear, or sinus, spreads to the nearby meninges.

The symptoms include fever, malaise, nausea, vomiting, headache, and a characteristic stiff neck. The stiff neck results from an extreme resistance to movement due to severe pain.

A virus or bacterium accounts for 80 percent of meningitis infections. *Viral meningitis* has no specific treatment, but in most cases runs its course without causing any lasting damage.

The type of *bacterial meningitis* most likely to affect adolescents is caused by the bacterium *Neisseria meningitides*. *Meningococcal meningitis* can progress very rapidly—within a day or two, or even in a matter of hours—from wellness to death or, in about 30 percent of cases, to permanent brain damage.

Meningococcal meningitis often begins with a petechial rash, small red spots due to breakage of small blood vessels in the skin, and is accompanied by the other symptoms listed on page 91. Fortunately, when antibiotics are prescribed early in its course, most patients recover.

Meningococcal meningitis spreads most easily among young people living in close contact with each other, such as in college dormitories and in the armed services, and somewhat less so at day schools. People who have been in close contact with an infected person should immediately receive prophylactic (preventative) antibiotics and the Menomune vaccine. This vaccine is also now recommended for students going off to college and has been used for years in the military. Boarding high school students might also benefit from receiving this vaccine.

Fungal meningitis, the rarest form of meningitis, is caused by cryptococcus and primarily affects people with severely compromised immune systems, such as those with AIDS. Antifungal antibiotics are used to treat this form of the disease.

INFECTIOUS MONONUCLEOSIS

Infectious mononucleosis, or "mono," is nicknamed the "kissing disease" because it can be transmitted through saliva. But mono can be passed without a single pucker. Infection with the Epstein-Barr virus (EBV) causes most cases of mono, and adolescents and young adults are the usual sufferers. The reason for this is that many children unknowingly become infected with EBV without becoming very sick, and then acquire lifelong immunity. Those adolescents never previously infected, and therefore not immune, are the ones most susceptible to coming down with mono.

Infectious mononucleosis is a very distinctive illness consisting of severe tonsillitis/pharyngitis, marked swollen glands (especially along the front and back of the neck), fever, and a characteristic blood test showing "atypical lymphocytes." Teens with mono start out with a few days of a generally mild "flu-like" illness, which progresses into the classic symptoms above. The severe swelling (and pain) of the tonsils and back of the throat makes eating and drinking difficult. If the swelling also interferes with breathing, then steroids are used for several days to shrink the tissue and ease breathing. Usually treatment is supportive, as with the flu, consisting of pain medication (such as ibuprofen), lots of rest, and an effort to maintain adequate fluid intake to avoid dehydration.

Most adolescents can gradually return to school and other activities after a week or two. Roughly half of teens with mono get an enlarged spleen for several weeks or longer, and are advised to avoid activities (such as skiing, contact sports, or sports played with a bat or stick) that potentially could traumatize and cause rupture of this organ. Although heralded as a disease that causes profound and prolonged fatigue, in fact, only a minority of adolescents do not feel completely well after a few weeks. Teens who are simply very fatigued do not have mono and should be evaluated for other causes of their debilitation. (See discussion of fatigue later in this chapter.)

GUT FEELINGS

People take their food processing for granted until the stomach or bowels call attention to themselves. When the stomach hurts or the bowel balks, suddenly nothing else matters. An active life can screech to a halt until the guts are put right again.

Every person has his or her own normal pattern for bowel movements. Some people defecate once or more daily, while for others a bowel movement every couple of days is the norm. However, a normal bowel movement should not be painful, excessively dry, or liquidy.

CONSTIPATION

Constipation occurs when stool is hard, dry, and difficult to pass. Gas, bloating, and an urge to strain are typical. Constipation may occur from inadequate liquid and fiber in the diet, inadequate exercise, stress, travel, or rarely a disease. If bowel movements are postponed (for example, out of a desire to avoid a school bathroom), constipation may result.

While some teens use laxatives to cure constipation, this is rarely a good idea. It is far better to prevent constipation by improving diet (see page 95), exercising, and if necessary using a natural fiber source, such as Metamucil.

DIARRHEA

Diarrhea is the overly frequent, urgent passage of liquidy stool, sometimes accompanied by chills and sudden in onset. Diarrhea may occur from food poisoning, viruses or bacteria, parasites picked up from contaminated water or food, reaction to antibiotics or other medication, and often stress. Diarrhea usually goes away by itself within one to three days; if it persists, contact a doctor.

Diarrhea can be treated with over-the-counter Imodium or Pepto-Bismol. Usually no treatment is necessary, but it is important to maintain good fluid intake. Juices, soda, and clear soups are especially good. A minimum of eight to ten cups per day should be drunk over a twenty-four-hour period to provide adequate hydration. Drinking only water, if you are not eating any food, will result in profound weakness since water contains no calories and is therefore not a source of energy. Foods that can be safely consumed without exacerbating diarrhea are often referred to as the BRAT diet (bananas, rice, apples, toast, and similar items). Milk and milk products can make diarrhea worse and should be avoided for at least several days after it stops.

PERSISTENT SYMPTOMS AND IRRITABLE BOWEL SYNDROME (IBS)

If symptoms persist, such as abdominal pain, heartburn, bloating, gas, diarrhea, or constipation, they may indicate such problems as gastro-esophageal reflux (GERD), ulcer gastritis, parasitic infection, inflammatory bowel disease, or rarely cancer.

But far and away more likely, the situation is irritable bowel syndrome (IBS), also known as irritable colon or recurrent abdominal pain (RAP). IBS is a common problem among teens, causing great distress in an otherwise healthy person. IBS tends to hang around for years, waxing and waning, while the child grows and thrives normally . . . in contrast to more serious intestinal disease that may impede weight gain, pubertal development, and growth in height.

Ease of digestion and elimination are taken for granted by most people, like breathing and the beating of the heart. However, for people with IBS, each day presents a new adventure and uncertainty about how they will feel. Painless digestion and elimination depend in part on the integrity of peristalsis, the rhythmic, muscular motion through which bowels push food along. Constipation and a buildup of gas (bloated feeling) in the intestinal tract occur when movement is too slow, diarrhea and cramping when movement is too hasty.

The diagnosis of IBS is based on certain characteristics of the pain and other symptoms, an essentially normal physical examination, and a laboratory evaluation that is also normal. Typically teens with IBS are growing normally and not losing weight. They describe the pain as occurring throughout the abdomen or at various locations. Their pain typically does not awaken them from sleep and is often exacerbated by stressful situations.

Other than active bowel sounds the exam is normal, although sometimes there is mild diffuse abdominal tenderness. A lab evaluation usually can be kept to a minimum, such as routine blood count and chemistries, and a stool exam for parasites. If abdominal sonograms, X rays, or endoscopic procedures are done, they are normal.

The best treatments are those listed below for promoting healthy digestion. Sometimes antispasmodic medications (such as donnatol) are helpful. If the teen has trouble increasing fiber and tends to be constipated, then drugstore preparations such as Metamucil, in powder or wafer form, may help. Laxatives are not recommended. Sometimes psychotherapy to deal with stress is very helpful.

Promoting Healthy Digestion

To prevent problems with digestion and elimination, adolescents should:

- *Eat diets that are low in fat, high in fiber* (see chapter 3). Fiber keeps stool bulky and attracts water that keeps stool soft and easy to pass.
- *Drink at least eight glasses of water (or other fluids) a day* to prevent constipation and keep stool soft.
- *Exercise regularly* to stimulate the digestive process and ease elimination (exercise also reduces stress).
- *Find ways to reduce stress and anxiety,* which may contribute to indigestion or erratic bowel patterns.
- *Make it a personal policy to "obey the call of nature."* When the urge to defecate occurs, go to the bathroom as soon as possible. This can keep the bowel functioning well, especially the muscles in the anal area that serve as a trip mechanism. When weighed down with feces, they trigger the urge to defecate. If repeatedly ignored, the muscles "forget" to relax appropriately, contributing to constipation.
- *Eat breakfast every day, and allow time after breakfast to go to the bathroom.* This is especially important for adolescents who do not like to go to the bathroom in school.
- *Eat lunch and dinner and one or two snacks per day, and eat consistently from day to day.* This will stimulate the bowel in a regularized way, which promotes a stable environment in the intestinal tract.
- *Reduce intake of foods and beverages that cause diarrhea, constipation, or indigestion.* Everyone is different; adolescents need to know their own digestive tracts. Which foods agree with them, and which do not? Do they tolerate dairy products well? How about nuts, chocolate, cookies, and caffeine? Do fatty foods make them sorry afterward? And could all that gas be coming from too much soda?

ENURESIS AND ENCOPRESIS
BED-WETTING (ENURESIS)

Bed-wetting is the unlikely topic of conversation between a boy's possessive mother and his prospective girlfriend in the decidedly adolescent film *The Water Boy*, starring Adam Sandler. The mother seizes upon her son's bed-wetting as a surefire way to break up his romance. Pointing to a yellow circle on her son's bed, she slyly asks the girl if she knows about his "problem." But the ploy fails to scare the girl off. A little bed-wetting cannot dampen her love.

Bed-wetting is not uncommon during adolescence, and is somewhat more common among boys. The problem seems to run in families (small comfort to one boy whose father confided that he wet the bed throughout adolescence, during his stint in the army, and up until shortly before his wedding night).

Adolescents who wet their beds often believe it's an indication that inside they are still immature little boys. They feel ashamed and have a poor self-image. They are afraid to sleep over at a friend's house or to travel with a school group. Parents don't help when they scold their child for "ruining" the sheets again, or insult them for being "too lazy to get out of bed."

Bed-wetting is not an emotional or learning problem.[19] It may result from a sleep disorder (failure to awaken from a sound sleep in response to an urge to urinate), inadequate bladder capacity, or insufficient production of ADH, a hormone that limits the quantity of urine produced by the kidneys.[20]

To help your adolescent:

- Ask your doctor about bladder-control exercises, hypnotherapy, moisture alarm systems, medications, and other treatments.
- Encourage your child to drink less fluid for several hours before bedtime (especially cola and other caffeinated beverages).
- Set an alarm clock for one to two hours after bedtime to awaken him to get up and void.
- Avoid punishing your child for bed-wetting. Support his efforts to comply with treatments, and be encouraging.
- Show your child how to strip the bed and wash the sheets on his own. (He can start washing his clothes, too.)
- Reassure your child that most adolescents outgrow the problem by age 15.
- Consider the possibility of a psychological explanation that may benefit from therapy.

ENCOPRESIS

Encopresis is the involuntary leakage of liquidy stool from the anus. It occurs primarily in children and adolescents who are chronically constipated and have been in the long-term habit of postponing bowel movements due to the difficulty and discomfort of passing hard, impacted stool. Over time, the anal muscles that sense the presence of stool and signal the urge to defecate become less sensitive and grow lax. Liquid bowel contents slide past the stool that is lodged in the rectum and leak out of the weakened anal opening and onto the child's underwear. Children feel embarrassed and ashamed, and may not realize the connection between encopresis and their chronic constipation.

Adolescents with encopresis should:

• Consult a physician to rule out diabetes, hypothyroidism, Hirschsprung's disease, and inflammatory bowel disease; and to advise on whether impacted stool should be removed and a stool softener or medication prescribed.[21]
• Increase exercise.
• Improve dietary and bathroom habits (see "Constipation," page 93).

SCOLIOSIS

In some adolescents, a growth spurt during puberty brings a new problem: scoliosis. The vertical path of the spine veers off-course, curving sideways in one or more places, creating a C shape or an S shape. In some cases the spine also rotates. Although the problem can also occur among younger children, most cases surface after age 10 and throughout puberty. Seventy percent of adolescents who develop scoliosis are girls. (Judy Blume memorably describes a girl with scoliosis in *Deenie*, a novel for teens.[22])

The severity of scoliosis is measured and expressed in "degrees" on a plain X-ray film of the spine. Most teens with scoliosis don't even know they have it, either because it is so mild and imperceptible or because their slightly asymmetric shoulder heights are thought to be due to slouching or from heavy backpacks. If caught early, while the spine is still growing, progression of the scoliosis can be prevented with appropriate treatments, described on the following page. If scoliosis is left untreated, an adolescent may develop pain and deformities later in life.

Diagnosing Scoliosis

Checking for scoliosis is an important part of the physical exam for both girls and boys. First the doctor stands behind the upright adolescent looking for any asymmetries between the levels of the shoulders, shoulder blades, hip-bones, or buttock folds. Next the adolescent is asked to bend forward with legs straight and to touch the toes. The doctor looks for any curves in the spine or asymmetry in the height of the right and left sides of the back. Scoliosis most often appears in the thoracic (upper) part of the back and less commonly in the lumbar (lower) region. If a significant curve is detected, an X ray and/or an orthopedic consultation is obtained to further evaluate the extent of the problem and whether treatment is necessary.

Treatment

In mild cases, the doctor recommends repeated screenings every six months or so to see if the scoliosis has progressed (gotten worse). Progression of the curve is most likely in an adolescent who is still growing. A small number of adolescents will need treatment with a lightweight and flexible brace that holds the spine as straight as possible as growth continues. Rarely is surgery necessary to correct a severe curve. The key is early detection in the pre- and early adolescent, regular visits to check for progression, and early bracing when needed.

BACK PAIN

It is not unusual for teens to complain of discomfort, pain, or tightness somewhere in the upper, mid, or lower back. Although scoliosis is relatively common among adolescents, it is rarely, except when severe, the cause of back pain. Most often back pain is due to muscle spasm (tightening) in the paraspinus muscles that travel vertically along either side of the spine. Sometimes the muscles that run down the neck and toward the shoulders are the source of muscular pain.

Many teens complain of back pain that comes and goes, worsening at times of stress or exertion. Sometimes muscular back pain starts suddenly as the result of an acute injury during a sport or other activity (such as moving heavy furniture or boxes) or even during an illness with strenuous coughing. Carrying a heavy backpack, especially on one shoulder, can cause or worsen back pain, and adolescents should be urged to "prune" backpack loads every night. They should also be advised to carry their backpacks on both shoulders, even if they don't think it looks as cool.

Some girls with large breasts experience shoulder and back pain. A supportive bra is so important that it might be worth the extra money to get a high-quality bra and have it professionally fitted. Exercises to strengthen abdominal and back muscles will also help. Breast reduction surgery is often considered by older adolescents with very large breasts (see chapter 5).

Acute (sudden) back pain is likely to be due to back muscle strain (tearing of a muscle) followed by muscle spasm. In this case, applying ice to the sore muscle (for fifteen minutes out of an hour, whenever possible) for the first forty-eight hours and taking an over-the-counter painkiller such as ibuprofen will generally result in improvement within a few days. Most teens with muscular back pain will benefit from learning exercises (from a coach, trainer, or physical therapist) that gently stretch out tight muscles and strengthen back and abdominal muscles to reduce the chances of recurrence.

Much less frequently, back pain in an adolescent is due to a "slipped disc." Discs are "cushions" of cartilage located between the vertebrae. If a disc slips or herniates, it might put pressure against a spinal nerve and cause shooting pains down a leg or arm (if the disc is at the level of a neck vertebra). *Spondylolysis* is a stress fracture of a vertebra and may be the cause of back pain, especially in teen dancers, gymnasts, skaters, and volleyball players who place a great deal of stress on their lower back.

Back pain that is severe, limits function, or persists beyond two weeks (and is not improving) should always be checked out by a doctor. Rarer causes of back pain in adolescents include rheumatoid diseases, bone or disc infections, tumors, or endocrine disorders.

HEADACHES, DIZZINESS, FATIGUE

Headaches, dizziness, and fatigue are among the most common complaints of teens. Because they may portend something very seriously wrong with one's health, parents often become concerned or alarmed. Home from school every day with a headache, jumping out of bed each morning feeling dizzy, or frequent napping and droopy, tired eyes . . . What can this be? Concerned parents, of course, will call the doctor for advice. The teen, more often than not, seems less worried and is reluctant to visit the doctor. He knows he's had these feelings before, they always get better, and they make sense considering the load of work, erratic eating, stress among his friends, and little sleep he's had the past few weeks or months. Sometimes, however, the tables are turned, and the parents are unconcerned while an anxious teen quite eagerly seeks medical care.

Luckily, the worry among parents or teens that headaches may be due to a brain tumor, brain infection, or other very serious problem is very rarely the case. However, if the pattern or feel of the teen's headaches changes, or an adolescent who never had headaches suddenly starts getting severe and unrelenting ones, consult a doctor immediately.

TENSION HEADACHES

The most common type of headache is called a *tension headache*. This means it feels as if the muscles surrounding the head and neck are in a state of increased tension or contraction, like a band or belt tightening around the entire head, or only in the region of the forehead or the upper neck. Many people experience this type of headache occasionally, and some teens get tension headaches a lot. Typically they can occur at any time of the day, from awakening with one in the morning to feeling one late at night, before bedtime. Very often among teens tension headaches come on in school, either in late morning or late afternoon. This may be due to a particularly stressful class or social situation at school, which may trigger the headache, or perhaps to not having eaten anything for several hours, another possible trigger.

Tension headaches are usually relieved with a simple painkiller such as acetaminophen (Tylenol) or ibuprofen, and generally do not interfere with daily activity. Eating regular meals and snacks might help to prevent them.

MIGRAINE HEADACHES

Some teens suffer from a generally more severe type of headache called *migraine*. Most teens with migraine headaches have a close relative who also gets them.

"Classical" migraine headaches are preceded by an "aura," such as a visual disturbance (flashing lights, blind spots, blurry vision), weakness or tingling of an extremity, or hallucinations. The headache that follows is typically on only one side of the head, usually around the eye, forehead, or temporal area, and is described as pounding or throbbing. The headache is accompanied by nausea and often vomiting, sensitivity to light or sound, and is exacerbated by movement. Therefore, the migraine sufferer does best to lie down in a quiet and dark room until the headache abates.

"Common" migraine headaches are the same, but not preceded by an aura.

Why do migraines occur at certain times and not others? The answer varies from person to person. It can be helpful to keep a journal, noting days and circumstances when headaches occur, in order to identify (and ultimately avoid) factors that seem to trigger a headache. Stress, a change in sleep schedule, medications, season, weather, or environment may lead to migraines. As with tension headaches, some girls find they get more migraine headaches during the week just prior to their period.

Some people find that certain foods or beverages trigger migraines. Among the most common triggers are alcohol (especially red wine and beer), aged cheeses that contain the chemical tyramine, food additives such as monosodium glutamate (MSG—found in some Chinese food, canned soups, and other processed foods) and sodium nitrite (found in hot dogs and lunch meats), chocolate, and coffee.

Medication may be prescribed to treat migraines. Some medicines should be taken just as a headache comes on. Other medications may be taken daily to try to prevent these debilitating attacks for people who experience them frequently.

DIZZINESS

Teens who complain they feel dizzy most often are experiencing light-headedness, a feeling of being off-balance, faint, or about to fall down. More rarely they may have vertigo, a feeling that they or their surroundings are spinning.

Almost everyone has experienced a brief moment of light-headedness when jumping too quickly out of bed in the morning or suddenly changing the body's position from lying flat to standing upright. This feeling is the result of a temporary decrease in blood flow to the brain until the circulation adjusts to a position change, which requires greater force of blood flow against gravity. Generally the dizzy feeling lasts a few seconds. A more severe feeling of faintness (sometimes accompanied by nausea) may come on at certain times of stress, sudden fear, if dehydrated or in a very hot or stuffy environment, after use of alcohol or drugs, or if standing in one place for a long time such as in church or on a crowded subway train. In these situations, called *vaso-vagal attacks*, the decrease of blood flow to the brain is more prolonged and may result in a full faint or brief loss of consciousness. Upon falling into a lying-down position, the blood flow to the brain improves, and the individual wakes up. If this feeling comes on it is sometimes possible to prevent fainting by sitting down and placing one's head between the legs or lying down with legs raised.

If dizziness or fainting occur during exercise, or without any clear explanation (such as being in a hot stuffy room or sudden fear or pain), or if the symptom is accompanied by a spinning sensation (vertigo), then a doctor should be consulted to rule out any heart, neurologic, inner ear, or other explanation. Dizziness can be a symptom of anxiety, sometimes related to hyperventilation. Such a possibility should also be discussed with a doctor.

FATIGUE

Whether due to their rapid growth, which saps some energy, or a lifestyle of burning the candle at both ends and getting little sleep—or the stresses imposed on them by parents, school, and peers, or a host of other possibilities—it seems that all teenagers complain of fatigue frequently or from time to time. The fatigue might feel like needing more sleep, or more rest, or more space-out time, or an inability to concentrate or complete a task. If the teenager is not sick (no fever, no sore throat, not achy), just tired, and the feeling seems to come and go (more so in late afternoon on schooldays, and not at all on Saturday night), then the fatigue is unlikely to be due to a medical cause. If the fatigue is persistent over several weeks or months, however, then it becomes important to understand why. It is likely that a persistently fatigued adolescent is chronically sleep deprived, depressed, or overly stressed out. These possibilities need to be defined and treated (see also chapters 3 and 11), and a doctor should be consulted, too, to make sure a serious medical problem is not overlooked.

CHRONIC FATIGUE SYNDROME

A condition called chronic fatigue syndrome (CFS) is occasionally diagnosed in an adolescent. Specific case definition criteria of CSF include the recent onset of persistent or recurring fatigue lasting at least six months in the absence of any specific medical condition that could be causing the fatigue (based on a thorough medical evaluation), and at least four of the following: sore throat, tender lymph nodes, muscle aches, joint pain, headaches, unrefreshing sleep, malaise following exertion, and impaired memory and concentration. There is no specific laboratory test that confirms CSF, and its cause is unknown. Most important for the adolescents who might have this condition is to be cared for by a doctor they trust who can help them through it with a range of strategies. Most teens feel better after one to two years.

HEALTH-PARTNERING TIPS FOR PARENTS

- *Keep liquid soap and a towel by every sink in your home.* Emphasize the importance of handwashing after using the bathroom and before preparing or eating food.
- *Advocate for well-stocked, clean bathrooms in your adolescent's school.*
- *When your teen seems to be run down, return to the basics.* Remind your teen that healthy eating, exercise, and sufficient sleep go a long way toward maintaining health and fighting illness. Reducing stress also helps the immune system stay capable of thwarting germs.
- *Help your teen keep a sense of perspective.* If, due to illness, your teen is upset about having to miss a basketball game or a math test, sympathize but also note that "this, too, shall pass." Assure your teen that a return to normal routines will happen faster and more firmly if not attempted prematurely. Alternatively, after a debilitating illness such as mono or the flu, help your teen consider a *gradual* return to most important activities first

as perhaps a better approach than resuming them all at once. This allows a teen to take an important test or attend a special event without being overwhelmed by a full schedule, and risking a relapse.

- *Take seriously symptoms that bother your teen.* Even if acne, constipation, cough, headaches, dizziness, or other problems do not seem particularly significant to you, if they concern your child, allow the child to consult a doctor. The doctor might have some useful suggestions, simply reassure your child that all is well, or engage him or her in a discussion of other related matters (such as sources of stress) that need to be addressed.

FIVE: Health Issues for Your Daughter

So long ago, your small daughter splashed in her bath, nestled in your arms at bedtime, and wore without complaint the turquoise-and-red-striped pajamas you bought on a whim. Then one day, with an air of imperious disdain, she spurned those pajamas as if they carried a contagious disease. In some girls, the first signs of adolescence seem to appear years before puberty, when they suddenly sprout a sense of style and say their parents have none.

The flowered overalls (you) versus black velour skirt (her) is a preview of wrangles to come. During department store debates with your opinionated girl, strangers sidle up and whisper warnings: "You're going to have your hands full when she's a teenager!" *Gee, thanks—just what I needed to hear.*

But indeed many parents dread the teen years around the corner. They have heard how nasty some adolescent girls can be, and might have seen their friends become frustrated, tearful, or just plain sad as their daughters seemed to turn on them or just turn away.

Some people claim that boys are easier to raise, less complicated, and less competitive, at least with their moms. Girls, on the other hand, bristle with *issues*. Suddenly, everything's an issue:

My best friend is mad at me.

My teacher hates me.

You hate my friends.

You never let me go anywhere.

You don't trust me.

You're overprotective.

You still think I'm a little girl.

You're always on my back.

Leave me alone.

Where's my sweater?

Isn't that wonderful! What a communicator! Right out there, eager to connect with you. She might bristle, but she's engaged. She needs you as much as ever, values your opinion, wants to be close.

Your daughter's testing, snapping, and rebelliousness do not negate her love and attachment. As her hormones swirl and her body changes and her moods switch at the speed of strobe lights, she is in a reactive, not a reflective, mode. She often doesn't even understand what she is reacting to.

Puberty not only introduces major physical developments, it also reshapes a girl's fundamental concept of who she is. Menstruation affirms that she is no longer a child; now she is capable of *having* a child. But she is not yet a woman, either. In the push-pull between wanting to sit on Mom's or Dad's lap or wanting to wear Mom's clothes or gain Dad's approval of a new outfit, she is constantly adjusting to changes in how she feels physically and emotionally, what she wants out of life, and what she thinks is expected of her. When talking with her about how her body is changing, it is important to emphasize that these changes are normal and wonderful. Whether or not she chooses to become a mother someday, puberty is all about the concept of potential. As her body changes, she will think not only about looking like a woman, but also about what kind of woman she wants to be, what kind of goals she will hope to achieve en route to adulthood.

THE PUBERTY EXPERIENCE FOR GIRLS

Puberty is a process that begins well before the onset of menstruation and continues for several years thereafter. Between the ages of 8 and 13, the hormones from the hypothalamic and pituitary glands, which are attached to the underside of the brain just behind the nose, set puberty in motion. The hypothalamus stimulates the pituitary gland, which starts manufacturing the hormone FSH, or follicle-stimulating hormone, and sends it to the ovaries. The follicles it stimulates there are tiny sacs that enclose the eggs (ova). The ova—hundreds of thousands of them—have been there since before birth. FSH essentially awakens them and nudges the follicular cells to begin production of another hormone, estrogen.

Estrogen is the key that unlocks the womanly development of many parts of the body. Estrogen causes nascent breasts to bud, hips to become more curvaceous, and eventually the menstrual cycle to begin.

TANNER STAGES FOR GIRLS, AND RELATED CHANGES

There is a wide range of ages at which onset of puberty is considered normal. To assess a girl's development, doctors measure height and weight (see chapter 2), and note the age of menarche (menstruation onset). They also use the Tanner stages to assess a girl's stage of sexual development. The Tanner stages rubric, which divides sexual maturation into a five-phase process, is named after Dr. James. M. Tanner, a physician at the University of London who defined these stages in the early 1960s.

The Tanner stages are useful because they confine assessment to two sets of visible clues: pubic hair growth and breast development. Of course, there are other changes that are occurring at the same time, and these together constitute a true portrait of pubertal change.

Tanner Stage 1 (prepuberty): Before puberty, a girl has no pubic hair and her chest is flat.

Other Features: A girl looks and sounds childlike, with straight body contours, often stick-thin or baby-fat chubby, and petite in height.

Tanner Stage 2 (early puberty): Sometime between 8 and 13 years of age, the areola (area around the nipples) widens and may appear puffy and the tissue behind the nipples thickens (feels firm), making the breasts appear to "bud." This onset of breast bud development is known as *thelarche*. The first isolated tendrils of pubic hair usually appear along the top of the labia major or slightly above on the lower abdomen. The hairs are straight or perhaps somewhat curly, but lack the coarser texture that will come.

Other Changes: She is growing more rapidly (more inches per year), and shoe size is more quickly outgrown. Estrogen from the ovary stimulates the first signs of vaginal secretions, which begin to stain the panties or feel a little wet between the legs. Underarm hair begins to grow.

Tanner Stage 3 (mid-puberty): Breast tissue enlarges and forms a mound that spreads well beyond the edges of the areolae. Pubic hair darkens and thickens, and begins to grow over a wider area both laterally and upward onto the lower abdomen.

Other Changes: Height continues to increase rapidly and the body begins to fill out into a more womanly silhouette, with hips broadening. Menarche, the onset of menstruation, is soon to happen.

Tanner Stage 4 (preadult stage): The breast tissue continues to grow and blend more smoothly with the surrounding chest wall. The areolae, however, seem to protrude slightly from the surrounding breast tissue. Pubic hair becomes bushier and coarser, and covers a larger area, but not onto the inner thighs.

Other Changes: Growth in height continues but at a slightly slower pace as menarche happens. (The first period comes approximately two and a half years after the onset of breast budding.) Ongoing weight gain results in softer curves and supports the maintenance of menstrual periods.

Tanner Stage 5 (adult development): The breasts achieve their adult contour and the areolae no longer protrude from the breast tissue. Breast size may still increase with weight gain after Tanner 5. Pubic hair now extends onto the inner thighs.

Other Changes: The girl has not quite finished growing, although the rate of growth is slowing down. Her body has reached its adult proportions, but weight gain (and increase in height) continues for a few more years before leveling off.

LEARNING ABOUT THE FEMALE BODY

The artist Georgia O'Keeffe's giant paintings of flowers seem to suggest that flowers are woman's botanical counterpart. Her biographer wrote:

> Her trembling, feathery, unfurling petals reminded people of genitalia
> . . . One woman who owned a big O'Keeffe flower painting was shocked
> to discover someone teaching a child the facts of life from it. When she
> hastily rehung it in her bedroom, a friend remarked, "Oh, I'm so glad you
> moved that vagina out of the living room."

—Laurie Lisle,
Portrait of an Artist: A Biography of Georgia O'Keeffe[1]

O'Keeffe herself denied that her flower paintings were intended to have that particular significance. But perhaps the fact that so many people see them as such indicates a common desire for artwork that acknowledges women's inherent beauty and power. Today, when pornographic magazines feature artless images, O'Keeffe's grand blossoms seem almost an antidote. What a pleasing way to talk to a daughter about reproductive organs: as petals surrounding a "powerful center of inner gravity."[2]

Why Your Daughter Needs to Learn How Her Body Works

Many adolescent girls are unaware of the intricacies of their reproductive anatomy, even though they might have touched themselves while bathing, out of curiosity, or while masturbating. Some girls even find their genitals repellent or shameful, and refuse to touch themselves. Lacking knowledge of her body directly affects a girl's health, self-esteem, and sexual well-being. But learning about her anatomy can help a girl appreciate her own changes and cycles, practice good hygiene, feel more confident of her sexuality, and recognize when she might have a health problem.

She Can See for Herself

One basic way to learn about one's body is simply to look at it. Health practitioners who conduct pelvic exams sometimes hand a girl a mirror so she can see what the inside of her vagina looks like when a speculum is used. For many girls, this is the first time they have ever used a mirror to look at their genitals. Yet a first pelvic exam usually does not occur until a girl is in her teens and is sexually active. It would be good if long before that time she would have felt comfortable enough to look at herself—to get to know her own body, a form of "hands-on learning."

Many girls think that touching themselves would be "gross." It is not unusual for girls to think that the female genitals are "unclean" (an idea that douche manufacturers profit from). So these girls refuse to touch themselves—but there are unfortunate ramifications. For example, a girl who cannot bear to touch herself will never know the freedom of using a tampon. She will refuse to use a hands-on contraceptive such as the diaphragm. She will not learn to recognize how monthly variations in the texture of her vaginal secretions indicate when she is most fertile. She will be less likely to detect bumps, rashes, or other indications of sexually transmitted diseases. She will not learn about her sexuality through masturbation. By denying herself that form of sexual exploration and release, she might be more likely to engage in sexual relationships before she is emotionally ready.

Of course, a parent or teacher instructs a girl about her anatomy through discussion, books, videos, or by showing or sketching diagrams. But you may also mention to your daughter, "If you look at yourself with a mirror sometime when you're by yourself, you will be able to identify these parts of your body." Don't expect her to say, "Oh, cool, great idea." She will be more likely to scoff, at the very least. But you will have conveyed the idea that her body is her own, that it is hers to know and appreciate. You might also want to ask (or suggest to her that she ask) her health care provider to review anatomy with her, perhaps encouraging her to look in a mirror during an exam of the external part of her genitals and surrounding structures.

External Genitalia

Many people mistakenly refer to a girl's external reproductive organs as her "vagina." More accurately, the vulva is the most external part of the female

External Female Genitalia

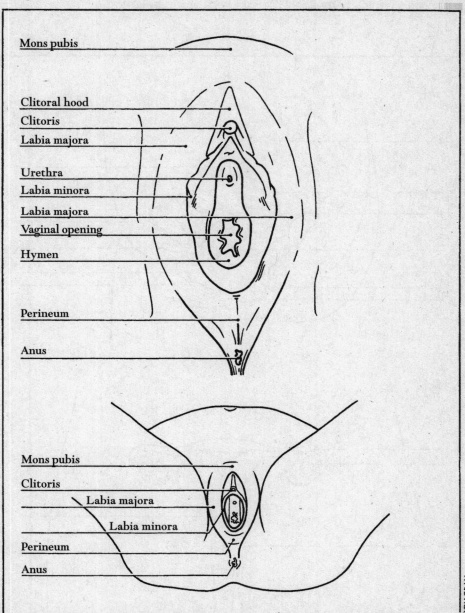

Mons pubis

Clitoral hood
Clitoris
Labia majora

Urethra
Labia minora
Labia majora
Vaginal opening
Hymen

Perineum

Anus

Mons pubis
Clitoris
Labia majora
Labia minora
Perineum
Anus

DIAGRAM

Female Internal Organs

A. Side View
B. Front View

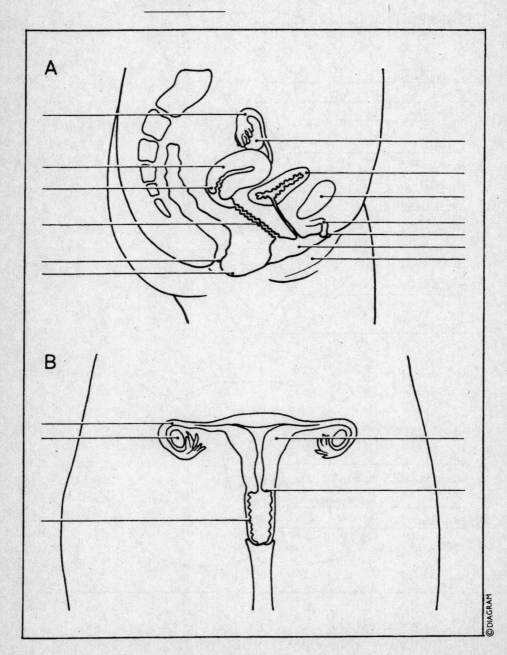

genitalia, encompassing all visible (external) parts of the female reproductive system. The vulva includes:

- The *mons pubis*, the rounded triangular portion of fatty tissue that covers the pubic bone, located at the base of the abdomen. During the course of puberty, pubic hair will grow on the mons pubis and the labia majora.
- The *labia majora*, the two fleshy outer lips of the vulva between the thighs.
- The *labia minora*, or the inner lips, hairless folds of skin located within the labia majora.
- The *clitoris*, a small, sexually sensitive, nerve-rich organ located at the top (if standing upright) part of the vulva, just above the labia minora and beneath a curve of skin called the *clitoral hood*. The clitoris, like the penis, has erectile tissue and swells when it is engorged with blood during sexual excitement.
- The *urethra*, the opening to the urinary bladder, through which urine passes. If standing upright, it is located just above the vagina and below the clitoris. It is the highest of the three openings between a girl's legs.
- The *vaginal opening*, the middle opening, is the vagina's sexual entrance and its exit for menstrual blood and vaginal discharge. During childbirth the vagina is the birth canal.
- The *hymen* is a flexible, thin piece of skin that lines the inside edges of the vaginal opening and partially narrows its circumference. There is nearly always enough open space for menstrual blood to exit through the hymen and for a tampon to be slipped into the vagina. An intact hymen is said to be proof of virginity. When having sexual intercourse for the first time, the hymen may be torn or stretched, causing bleeding and discomfort. However, this does not happen with all virgins. Some girls have a very minimal hymen or one that has been gradually stretched open, for example, by tampon insertion. Rarely, a hymen covers the entire vaginal opening or has only a pinpoint opening, permitting no passage of menstrual blood and making insertion of a tampon impossible. This condition, imperforate hymen, must be surgically corrected.
- The *anus*, the lowest of the three openings, is the exit of the rectum, through which feces pass.
- The *perineum* is the space (approximately 1 inch long) between the vaginal opening and the anus.

Internal Organs

- The *vagina* is the muscular, 3- to 5-inch tube that extends from the vaginal opening to the cervix. Most of the time the vaginal walls touch, but they are remarkably elastic. The vagina stretches to embrace a penis during intercourse, and to permit the passage of a baby during childbirth.
- The *cervix* is the lower neck of the uterus that protrudes into the vagina where the vagina ends (its "ceiling"). The *cervical os* is the opening in the cervix through which menstrual blood exits and sperm enter the uterus. During childbirth the os dilates, or stretches, to ten centimeters, letting the newborn pass into the birth canal.
- The *uterus* is a pear-shaped organ, about the size of a girl's fist or a large lemon. During pregnancy the uterus is called the womb, and its thick muscular walls stretch to accommodate the growing fetus and the placenta. After birth the uterus gradually contracts back to its original size.
- The *fallopian tubes* extend laterally from each side of the uterus, echoing the shape of arms extending from the torso. At the ends of the fallopian tubes are fingerlike projections called *fimbria*.
- An *ovary*, each about the size of a walnut, is located at the end of each fallopian tube just beyond the fimbria. The fimbria catch the eggs stored and released by the ovary, and the ovary is also the source of female hormones, estrogen and progesterone.

Anatomical Differences Between Adolescent Girls and Women

A young adolescent girl's internal organs are not the same as those of a late adolescent or a woman. Although puberty initiates changes in the organs, a girl's vaginal walls are thinner and less elastic than those of an older female's. If she is sexually active, she is more susceptible to injury (vaginal abrasions from sexual friction). She is also more likely to contract a sexually transmitted disease. STD organisms can pass more easily through her thinner mucous membranes. They also can gain easier entry to cervical cells. This is because during early adolescence, a girl has cervical ectopy—that is, her cervix has more fragile "columnar" cells exposed on the outside of the cervix, which makes her more susceptible to acquiring a sexually transmitted infection. As she matures, these columnar cells move inside the cervical os and tougher squamous cells cover the outside, more exposed, portion of the cervix.

Understanding that full internal sexual maturity does not occur until later in adolescence might offer your daughter another way of understanding that younger adolescents are literally not ready to engage in sexual intercourse.

THE MENSTRUAL CYCLE: PREPARATION, RELEASE, RENEWAL

The very first menstrual period (called menarche) doesn't really come out of the blue, and to some extent can be predicted. Menarche is a relatively late event in puberty, usually occurring between Tanner stages 4 and 5, when breast and pubic hair development are nearly complete. For most girls menarche occurs approximately two and a half years after the onset of breast budding (see Tanner stages, above), and in the United States this is at an average age of 12½ years. An early and rapid developer might get her period as early as age 9 or 10, and a later developer as late as age 16 or 17. The range of normal is extremely broad, and the age when menarche occurs often resembles that of other members of the family.

"Be prepared" is a two-word way to explain menstruation. Every month a woman's body prepares for pregnancy. If she does not become pregnant, menstruation is her body's way of creating a fresh start for the next month. Menstruation is an announcement from within: *My body is capable of someday creating and supporting new life.*

The world's many cultures and religions have explained and responded to menstruation in many different ways. For example, menstruation can be considered a time when a woman is "unclean" or "impure." Or a solemn, even sad, time because it signifies that, this month, no new life has been created. Or a time when a woman should be set apart. Within our own society, menstruation is often described in pejorative terms—as a "curse," or as a time when a girl loses her right mind in her monthly battle with PMS (premenstrual syndrome, see page 118). Happily, however, some girls refer to their menstrual period as their "friend."

Whatever your cultural or religious beliefs, the fact is that menstruation is going to be a part of your daughter's life for a long time. She might welcome this change more if you can help her appreciate the biological elegance of the menstrual cycle. Menstruation is literally life affirming. Through a woman's monthly cycle, she *prepares*, *releases*, and *renews* her capacity to begin and support life.

Preparation

Every month, the uterus prepares for the potential of pregnancy. The hormones estrogen and progesterone cause the uterine lining, the *endometrium*, to thicken with nutrient-rich cells that can support an implanted fertilized egg.

Meanwhile, an egg has ripened and is released from an ovary. This is called *ovulation*. Ovulation usually occurs approximately mid-cycle, if the cycle (from day one of a period to day one of the next period) is the classic length of twenty-eight days (four weeks). Ovulation usually occurs fourteen days (two weeks) before day one of the next period. Therefore, a girl with a long cycle (for example, every thirty-five days) will ovulate closer to her next period than the previous period. A girl with a short cycle (for example, twenty-one days) will ovulate about seven days after a period begins, and might still be bleeding from her period when she ovulates.

When the egg leaves the ovary, it is first "grabbed" by the fimbria and then moves along the inside of the fallopian tube. If sperm enter the uterus and then swim into the fallopian tube during the approximately forty-eight hours that the ovum happens to be there too, a sperm may fertilize the egg. If that happens, the fertilized egg will pass into the uterus and attach to the wall of the uterus. The cells of the thickened endometrium will nourish the egg until a placenta forms.

Sometimes an ovary releases more than one egg. If two or more eggs are fertilized, the result is twins, triplets, or more. Because all are created from separate fertilized eggs, they are *fraternal* twins, triplets, etc. *Identical* twins and triplets originated as a single fertilized egg that split into halves or thirds.

At the time of ovulation vaginal and cervical fluids thicken, attaining a slippery "raw egg white" consistency that makes it easier for sperm to wiggle-swim up into the uterus.

Release

If the egg is not fertilized, the endometrium that had built up in anticipation of a possible pregnancy dissolves. It becomes the menstrual flow. The microscopic unfertilized egg disappears, passing from the body hidden within the menstrual blood.

Renewal

The cycle begins again. The endometrium slowly thickens. An egg begins to ripen. The vaginal fluids are thin and watery until close to ovulation, when they will thicken again. As far as the uterus is concerned, this is a fresh start, another chance to anticipate the creation of new life.

There is something inherently hopeful about this process of preparation, and something inherently accepting about the process of release. When a woman does not want to be pregnant, the sight of menstrual blood is cause for celebration. When she is trying to get pregnant, the blood is proof that next month she and her partner must try again.

Some Things About Menstruation Your Daughter Should Know

- *Menstruation is not always monthly or "regular."* As with many pubertal changes, menstruation can take a while to get started and establish itself. Timing is likely to be irregular for the first months or even years. Although the average menstrual cycle—the time from the onset of the period to the beginning of the next one—is twenty-eight days, cycle lengths may vary widely from girl to girl or an individual girl's cycle may vary from month to month. A cycle of fewer than twenty to more than forty days may be entirely normal. Because a girl will not always know when she will get her period, it is a good idea always to carry a pad or tampon in her purse or bookbag.

- *It is important to keep track of one's menstrual cycle.* Encourage your daughter to get into the habit of circling the first day of her period on a calendar. Keeping track of periods lets her chart her menstrual patterns, predict when she'll get her next period, and figure out whether she has missed one. She will also be prepared to answer her health care provider's questions about when her LMP (the date of the first day of her last menstrual period) was or any irregularities she is concerned about.

- *Certain events and circumstances may affect menstruation.* The reproductive system, like other parts of the body, is sensitive to what is going on in one's life. Travel, stress, weight loss or gain, even changes of season, can delay a period.

- *Periods and pregnancy are not necessarily incompatible.* It is possible to get pregnant before ever having a period, because ovulation sometimes precedes menstruation. It is also possible to get pregnant *during* a period, especially if you have a short cycle and ovulation occurs while you are still menstruating.

- *An abdominal pain may be "mittelschmerz."* Most girls are usually unaware of the moment when an egg slips out of the ovary, embarking on its journey through the fallopian tube. But occasionally ovulation announces itself by causing a sharp pain on the side of the body whose ovary is releasing an egg. This pain is known as *mittelschmerz*, a German word that means "middle pain." The pain is caused by a small leakage of blood into the lower abdomen from the follicle that releases the egg. Some girls feel this every month and recognize it. Others may be puzzled by it and seek medical attention if it is severe.

- *Not everyone has menstrual cramps.* Cramps and discomfort do not necessarily go hand in hand with menstruation; a period is a very personal thing, and women experience it differently. (See discussion of premenstrual syndrome and dysmenorrhea on pages 118 and 119.)

• *The menstrual flow changes during the course of the period.* It may start off heavy the first day, then taper off starting with day two, or start off light and get heavier the second day. Some girls' periods typically last only a couple of days, others' for five or six days or longer.

Pad or Tampon?

Pads and tampons are made in a variety of absorbencies, thicknesses, and designs, scented or deodorized or not, with different absorbencies targeted to days of heavier or lighter flow.

Many girls use pads when they first begin their periods, then learn how to insert tampons if and when they are ready. But some girls want to use tampons from the very beginning so they do not feel limited in their activities or self-conscious about odor or having a pad show.

Other girls would like to use tampons but might have heard some incorrect information that must be cleared up. For example, they need to know that a tampon cannot get lost. The cervical os is not big enough to admit a tampon. Once a tampon is in the body, a girl can always reach in to retrieve it with her fingers, even if the string has worked its way inside the vagina.

Using a tampon also will not damage a girl's hymen or make her "lose her virginity." Only having sexual intercourse will do that. If there is room within the hymen for menstrual blood to come out, then there is room enough to insert a tampon. For most girls it works out best to have someone supportive and encouraging teach them how to insert the tampon. This may be a mother, friend, favorite aunt, or older sister (or even their doctor). It helps to start out with the narrowest tampons available, which are covered in a plastic (rather than cardboard) sheath, and to spread some lubricating jelly on the tip to help it slide in more easily. The tampon is inserted at a slight angle pointing downward toward the small of the back. Some girls insert it too straight in and it seems to get blocked easily by the vaginal wall before it is completely inside the vagina. Being patient and staying calm are important to initial success with a tampon. Then it becomes easy.

Whether to use a pad or a tampon should be a girl's personal choice. If she does want to use tampons, it is important for her to know how to use them safely.

Toxic Shock Syndrome and Safe Tampon Use

There is something especially chilling about a disease associated with an everyday object on which people confidently rely. Rely, in fact, was the name of one of these objects, a superabsorbent tampon made with a new amalgam of cellulose and polyester foam. The tampon fostered the growth of the deadly

Staphylococcus aureus bacterium. Like a number of other bacteria, *S. aureus* is normally present in the nose or vagina. Most people develop effective antibodies to counteract it. But when certain conditions lead the bacterium to proliferate, it can release toxins into the bloodstream, leading to Toxic Shock Syndrome (TSS). By the time Rely and similar tampons were identified as culprits (and withdrawn from the market), hundreds of women had become ill and about forty had died.[3] (TSS is not limited to menstruating women; also susceptible are diabetics and people suffering from HIV infection or chronic lung or heart disease.)

Today, tampons, which are regulated as medical devices by the Food and Drug Administration, are made of rayon or cotton or both. TSS is now very rare, but the epidemic had a lasting impact on tampons and their packaging. Package inserts alert women to seek medical attention immediately if they experience the symptoms of TSS.

Symptoms of Toxic Shock Syndrome

- Sudden high fever (102 degrees or higher), possibly with chills.
- Diarrhea.
- Vomiting.
- Low blood pressure, indicated by dizziness, light-headedness when standing up, or fainting.
- A sunburnlike rash.
- Headache.
- Fatigue.

How to Reduce the Risk of TSS

- *Do not wear tampons, or do alternate their use with pads.* For example, wear a tampon during the day but a pad at night. Or wear pads most of the time, using tampons only during activities like swimming, dance, gymnastics, or other sports, or when wearing clingy or white clothing.
- *Wear the lowest-absorbency tampon needed for the menstrual flow.* Wear "super" only on heavy-flow days, "regular" or "junior" when flow is light. Wearing a pad or panty liner along with a tampon provides "insurance" in case of leakage.
- *Change tampons every four to eight hours, or more frequently if needed.* However, changing tampons too often may cause irritation. A heavy flow is hard to ignore. But especially when the flow is light during the last days of a period, some girls and women tend to forget to change their tampon. Figure out a reminder system, such as sticking a note onto your alarm clock or looping a ribbon around your keys.

- *Avoid wearing two tampons at the same time.* Some women forget they are already wearing one or wear two for double protection. Not a good idea, since infection can result.
- *Use tampons only during your period.* Do not wear tampons to absorb normal vaginal fluids the rest of the month. Use a panty liner instead. If vaginal fluids are excessive or foul-smelling, or if bleeding occurs between periods, contact a health provider to make sure you do not have an infection or other problem.
- *To prevent reinfection, never use tampons if you have had TSS.*

MENSTRUAL CONCERNS AND DISORDERS

Some girls are proud or relieved to get their period. Others resent or resist the experience, especially if they have cramps or other menstrual discomfort or problems. But whether girls take menstruation in stride or wail about it, at least they know their periods are normal. They don't realize how lucky they are to be able to take their periods for granted. Girls who mature later than their friends may feel left behind and anxious about when or whether they will catch up.

For girls who never begin to menstruate, or stop menstruating, have painful periods, or bleed between periods, menstruation is a matter of deep concern. Menstruation is such an integral part of a girl's health that any of these irregularities should be checked out by a doctor. They may stem from a variety of underlying problems—ranging from lifestyle, to disease, to a girl's genetic makeup.

CRANKY AND CRAMPY: PREMENSTRUAL SYNDROME

Premenstrual syndrome (PMS) is a distinctive group of physical and emotional changes that may occur within a week or two before getting a period. Not all girls will get PMS, but those who do will recognize a similar set of symptoms every month.

Physical symptoms include fatigue, bloating, weight gain, breast soreness, headaches, skin breakouts, cramps, and cravings for certain foods (especially chocolate or salty foods like corn chips).

Emotional symptoms include mood changes, irritability, depression, tearfulness, anxiety, or a reduced ability to concentrate.

PMS can be very disorienting, giving a girl a feeling that she is simply not herself, not in control of her body and feelings. Although the cause of PMS is not known, there are a number of things a girl can do to reduce the severity of symptoms.

- *Keep a journal to discern your own patterns.* See if there is truly a repetitive relationship between your period and days when you feel uncomfortable or upset.
- *Reduce stress.* Get enough sleep every night, exercise (preferably aerobic), and do yoga, stretching, meditation, or some other calming activity every day.
- *Relax through guided imagery.* Sit or lie in a relaxed position with eyes shut and imagine a restful, repetitious scene: On a beach, observe the waves moving in and out . . . or watch a bird flying a smooth figure eight in the sky . . . or in the woods see a leaf drift from a tall tree onto the ground. Guided imagery can also be sequential images, not necessarily repetitious ones. These images can be self-imagined or listened to on tapes, which can be purchased.
- *Eat three small meals and three snacks every day, and limit salt, sugar, caffeine, and alcohol intake.* Large meals and salt can contribute to bloating. Sugar, caffeine, and alcohol can contribute to mood swings.
- *Try different ways to relieve cramps.* Cramps may begin even a day or two before menstrual flow, but typically are most prominent during the first one or two days of the cycle. (See dysmenorrhea section, below, for how to cope with menstrual cramps.)
- *Ask your doctor about medications for PMS.* Birth control pills may help. Ask your doctor about a relatively new pill, Yasmin, which has diuretic qualities and might diminish bloating associated with PMS and also help modulate mood. Another option is antidepressants such as Zoloft (sertraline) or Prozac (fluoxetine), taken daily or only during the week or two of PMS. Or a doctor may prescribe a mild diuretic.

CRAMPS AND DYSMENORRHEA (PAINFUL MENSTRUATION)

Menstrual cramps are contractions of the uterus brought on by the hormone prostaglandin to help expel menstrual blood. The uterus is about the size of a clenched fist. If you take your fist and squeeze it very tightly, the feeling resembles a menstrual cramp. For some women, simply visualizing the uterus clenching and releasing makes any menstrual discomfort more tolerable.

There is a continuum of ease, discomfort, and pain associated with menstruation. Generally speaking, menstruation should not hurt. However, transient and treatable menstrual cramps are common. Dysmenorrhea is the presence of severe pain during a period. It is distinguished from common cramping by its severity and duration.

Primary Dysmenorrhea

Primary dysmenorrhea is caused by somewhat excessive production of prostaglandin and other hormones. When these hormones are in proper balance, they stimulate the uterus to contract just enough to expel menstrual blood. The pain is tolerable and easily managed with gentle painkillers (see below). However, in some girls the uterus seems to go into overdrive, and more powerful tools are needed to relieve the pain.

The good news is that dysmenorrhea is a normal occurrence and marks the onset of more mature periods associated with ovulation. Only about a third of girls will ovulate and have pain during the first year, up to three quarters of girls by the fifth year of menstruation. Having normal ovulatory cycles means your daughter is growing up, has the potential for parenthood, and therefore has to be sure to take appropriate measures to prevent it if she is not ready.

Treatment of Menstrual Pain

Nonmedicinal Treatment

For many women with menstrual cramps, discomfort is not debilitating and is easily relieved—for example, by taking a warm bath, using a hot water bottle or heating pad, or kneading the abdomen gently with the hand. One woman swore by the phone book method: lying on the floor with her knees bent, she placed a phone book on her abdomen and said its weight helped suppress the cramps. Aerobic exercise, yoga, or the relaxation techniques described above may also prove sufficient.

Over-the-Counter Medications

If pain is not relieved by the methods discussed above, ask your doctor to recommend over-the-counter or prescription medication. First try acetaminophen (Tylenol). If this does not provide enough relief, try ibuprofen (Advil, Motrin, etc.) or naproxen (Aleve).

The key here, if cramps are severe and resistant to pain medications, is to start the medication even before the cramps begin. This is possible if you learn your pattern of premenstrual symptoms (such as breast tenderness and fullness) or have very regular periods (approximately the same number of days between periods, chartable on a calendar). When the symptoms or the calendar indicates that a period is imminent, start the medication. With Advil, for example, take two tablets three times a day, beginning one or two days before the expected period. With Aleve, take two tablets twice a day in advance. Once the period begins, and if cramps still occur (likely less intense than if no medication had been taken), take two Advil every four hours, or two Aleve every six to eight hours.

If it is not possible to tell when a period will begin, start taking these painkillers as soon as the bleeding begins.

Prescription Medication

Depending on the severity, primary dysmenorrhea can be treated with more powerful prescription medicines in the same family as ibuprofen, or more serious painkillers like Tylenol with Codeine.

Oral contraceptives also provide relief. They are an especially good choice for a sexually active girl who has bad cramps, but may also be considered for a teen who is not sexually active.

Secondary Dysmenorrhea

Secondary dysmenorrhea occurs in conjunction with an abnormality of the anatomy of the uterus or surrounding structures, or as the result of an illness (such as pelvic inflammatory disease), ectopic pregnancy, congenital anomaly causing obstruction to blood flow, cysts, or fibroids. It may also be a miscarriage in disguise.

Secondary dysmenorrhea may also be caused by endometriosis, a condition more often diagnosed in adults. Endometrial tissue is normally found only inside the uterus; endometriosis is the growth of this tissue beyond the uterus, such as on the outer surface of the uterus, or on the fallopian tube, ovary, or rectum. An early form of endometriosis may be diagnosed in a girl, but diagnosis requires a gynecologist or surgeon to look inside the lower abdomen with an instrument called a laparoscope. Although not major surgery, this procedure is not likely to be suggested for an adolescent unless the dysmenorrhea is very severe, debilitating, and not manageable with painkillers and/or birth control pills. Treatments of endometriosis include painkillers, birth control pills or other hormonal medications, or in some instances, surgery.

AMENORRHEA

Amenorrhea is the absence of menstruation. Either periods never started (primary amenorrhea) or they prematurely stopped coming (secondary amenorrhea).

Primary Amenorrhea

Since the first menstrual period is an event that occurs late in puberty, its arrival is not expected until approximately two to three years after the onset of breast bud development. Many girls may not remember exactly how old they were when breast buds first appeared, but may more easily remember what grade they were in or that buds first appeared at camp or on a family trip or around a special holiday or event.

A girl should be evaluated by a doctor if by age 13 she has not shown any signs of puberty (breast and pubic hair growth), or if by three years after the onset of breast development (or by age 16 if she was a late developer) she has not gotten her period. The doctor must first rule out pregnancy, since occasionally a girl ovulates before ever menstruating. In most instances she is not pregnant, and there are many other causes to explore.

Family history may provide a clue. If a mother did not menstruate until after her sixteenth birthday, the chances are good that her daughter won't either. Knowing early on that she might be "genetically programmed" to be a late bloomer might ease a girl's anxiety and help her cope with the delay.

Low weight, eating disorders, and obesity can cause amenorrhea. Young girls who are naturally very thin but normal and healthy may have a delay in onset of menstruation. Those with anorexia nervosa typically fail to menstruate. So might girls with bulimia nervosa or those who are extremely obese (see chapter 10).

Excessive exercise—especially among avid runners, cyclists, ballet dancers, and gymnasts—is often combined with inadequate intake of calories, causing such a low percentage of body fat that a girl fails to produce estrogen. The hypothalamus and pituitary glands are not stimulating the ovaries, and the role played by fat cells in estrogen production is also affected. As a girl progresses through puberty and adolescence, not only her weight but also the percentage of her weight that is fat must gradually increase in order to initiate or sustain periods. (See "The Female Athlete Triad" on page 125.)

Anatomical abnormalities should also be explored. If a girl has progressed normally through puberty, is healthy, and is not excessively exercising or stressed, then the possibility exists that her hymen is not open enough to allow the outflow of menstrual blood. An imperforate hymen is a layer of skin that completely covers the vaginal opening, obstructing the flow of blood, which builds up inside the vagina and often causes periodic pain. A simple operation opens the hymen and solves this problem.

Rarely, more serious congenital malformations of the vagina and uterus might be the reason for primary amenorrhea.

Chromosomal abnormalities, while rare, must also be ruled out. Turner's syndrome (one of the two X chromosomes is completely or partially missing) is considered in a girl who fails to grow normally in height and to develop breasts and who fails to menstruate. Girls with Turner's syndrome have undeveloped ovaries and do not produce estrogen and progesterone. Although there is no cure, estrogen and progesterone replacement therapy stimulates breast development and menstruation.[4]

A girl with testicular feminization is, in fact, chromosomally male (XY) but appears from the time of birth and throughout childhood to be an anatomically normal girl and is raised as such. At puberty she develops breasts but scant pubic hair, and never gets her period. It is usually not until she is evaluated for primary amenorrhea that this chromosomal factor is realized. Her gonads are within the abdomen but are not true ovaries and are best removed because of the risk of cancer.

A true vagina can be surgically constructed, and although lacking a uterus, most girls in this situation choose to continue their lives as female. The challenge of coping with this sudden realization can be overwhelming to a young woman's fundamental sense of identity. More than ever before, there are media articles, Internet discussions, and support groups for people with a wide variety of sexual anomalies and identity concerns.

A variety of *endocrine gland disorders*, originating in the hypothalamus, pituitary, thyroid, or adrenal gland, or in the ovaries, can result in a delay of onset of menstruation. Each may be associated with other symptoms (such as headache, visual disturbance, excessive weight loss or gain, fatigue) or might only cause amenorrhea. The precise nature of an endocrine gland disorder should be evaluated by an endocrinologist.

Chronic illnesses, known or undiagnosed, may cause amenorrhea as a prominent symptom, especially if the illness has been poorly controlled and the girl has been recently sick. Such chronic illnesses include inflammatory bowel disease, diabetes mellitus, cancer, cystic fibrosis, or lupus.

Some medications used to treat some of these illnesses, or certain antidepressants or tranquilizers used for psychiatric care, and certainly various street drugs, may impede the onset of menstruation.

Secondary Amenorrhea

She menstruated, perhaps only for a year and irregularly, perhaps monthly and for several years. Then the periods stopped. Where did they go? The chromosomal and anatomic abnormalities discussed above are usually specific to primary amenorrhea. However, many of the other causes of primary amenorrhea can also be the reason for cessation of periods that have already started. Eating disorders, other nutritional factors, excessive exercise, a chronic illness, an endocrine disorder, medications, and drug abuse are all possibilities.

Pregnancy is much more likely the cause of secondary than primary amenorrhea. If a girl has been keeping track of her periods on a calendar, she can easily identify the date of her last menstrual period, and from there calculate how many weeks pregnant she is. This is important for her to know when considering her options: to continue the pregnancy with prenatal care, or to terminate the pregnancy. (See chapter 8.)

Stress or depression is another frequently encountered explanation for missed periods. A girl's reproductive hormonal system is very sensitive to changes in her life. A girl who has suffered the death or departure of a loved one, her parents' separation or divorce, or another traumatic event might find that her periods have subsided for a while . . . as if her very system is in sympathy with her need for a time-out to assimilate and recuperate from these changes.

This may be the case even for life changes that are not necessarily bad but still require her to adjust to a new situation. Moving to a new town and going off to college or away to camp for the summer may be welcomed events, but they still involve getting used to a new situation and place and to making new friends. Travel abroad, especially when the time zone changes dramatically, can also interrupt the monthly cycle, but usually only briefly.

An *acute illness* that seemingly has nothing to do with the reproductive system—such as mononucleosis, hepatitis, pneumonia, or a severe flu—can nevertheless contribute to its temporary shutdown.

Polycystic ovary syndrome (PCOS), or hyperandrogenic amenorrhea, is a relatively common condition affecting adolescent girls (although often not diagnosed until adulthood) caused by mildly high levels of androgens. Androgen hormones (the most well-known is testosterone) are normally produced in the ovaries and adrenal glands of girls in low amounts, and in the testicles and adrenals of boys in much higher amounts. Some girls, for reasons not well understood yet by medical science, produce somewhat higher amounts of androgens than are considered within the normal range for a female—although much lower amounts than are made by a male. These higher androgen levels are responsible for the development of acne, hirsutism (excessive growth of body hair, usually on the face, breasts, and abdomen), and decreased regularity and frequency of menstrual periods.

Most girls with PCOS had a normal age of onset of their periods, and regular periods for a few years followed by fewer periods over time (a period every few months) or eventually no periods. Their ovaries usually contain many small cysts (therefore, the name of this syndrome) and ovulation might not occur regularly. When a woman with PCOS wants to become pregnant, gentle hormonal treatment helps her succeed.

The manifestations of PCOS are quite variable. Many girls/women are obese, but some are thin. Some but not all girls/women have acne and/or hirsutism, and some have acne and hirsutism but regular periods. Especially if the girl is obese, there is a risk of developing Type 2 diabetes mellitus. In this situation, weight loss generally lowers the risk. A similar, rarer condition, congenital adrenal hyperplasia, originates in the adrenal gland and is often not diagnosed until adolescence, when the symptom of secondary amenorrhea prompts an evaluation.

The diagnosis of PCOS should be suspected in a girl with one or several of the findings noted above. Simple blood tests are confirmatory. The treatment recommended for most adolescents is birth control pills containing both estrogen and progesterone. The Pill suppresses the excessive production of the androgens, thereby reducing the acne and hirsutism, and regularizing menstrual periods.

If a girl misses a period, the first question she should ask herself is "Could I be pregnant?" and the second question is "What else is going on in my life right now?" When she sees her health care provider, she should discuss her missing periods in the context of her activities, state of mind, and overall physical condition.

THE FEMALE ATHLETE TRIAD

The female athlete triad is a syndrome identified in 1992 by the American College of Sports Medicine (ACSM). Very active female athletes and dancers often struggle to maintain the extremely lean physique favored by their art or sport. The triad consists of three consequences of their quest for thinness: disordered eating, amenorrhea, and osteopenia or osteoporosis (see below).

These young women tend to be participating in art forms or sports that value or require low weight for effective or aesthetically pleasing performance. Form-fitting, revealing clothing shows off their disciplined bodies, their bones sleekly rippled with muscle.

The classic build for the classical ballerina is tall and thin, with a small head and long, expressive limbs. Gymnasts are girlishly slight, unencumbered by curves as they contort their bodies or tumble in space. Long-distance runners have a characteristically all-muscle look; their mileage melts body fat—and estrogen along with it. Swimmers, cross-country skiers, skaters, cheerleaders, and competitors in track events wear unforgivingly skintight or midriff- and leg-baring clothing. Jockeys, wrestlers, and other athletes must weigh in at or under the required weight or risk being disqualified.

Many girls therefore feel that they must defeat the urge to eat. Along with a girl's satisfaction in artistic or athletic achievement comes the worry that the weight gain of puberty or of just eating normally will sabotage her efforts. She has worked very hard to attain her level of skill. It would be so unfair, she thinks, to risk excess pounds that could render her less competitive or capable.

She'll Feel It in Her Bones

When a competitive dancer or athlete aggressively pursues low body fat, she suppresses her estrogen level. Not only does this make her menstrual periods stop, she also develops osteoporosis or osteopenia.

Osteoporosis, the more serious of the two, is a metabolic bone disease. Bones normally maintain a cycle of breaking down and building up, two complementary activities that keep bones strong and dense. Osteoporosis results when bone breakdown exceeds bone buildup. The outcome is fragile bones that can fracture from falls or other trauma that normal bones would easily withstand. Osteopenia is a less-severe form of bone loss—but if not caught and reversed in time, it can lead to osteoporosis.

Adolescence is the prime time for building strong bones. Most of a woman's bone mass peaks by age 30. After that age, her gradually declining estrogen level slowly but surely causes her bones to lose mass and strength. This is why women are advised to take active steps to protect their bone mass, such as doing weight-bearing exercise and taking calcium and vitamin D supplements. Estrogen replacement therapy (ERT) may be prescribed for postmenopausal women, but ERT for amenorrheic adolescents with low weight or low body fat has not been shown to be particularly helpful to bones as long as these two factors and poor nutrition persist.

Girls with amenorrhea due to low estrogen should be taking a calcium and vitamin D supplement (approximately 1,200 milligrams of calcium per day) but also working hard on improving their nutritional state and weight as soon as possible.

Preserving bone density is critical. The younger the girl and the shorter the time she is amenorrheic, the greater the likelihood of reversing her osteopenia/osteoporosis and her emerging into adulthood with healthy, strong bones. In some instances, doctors may prescribe a medication like Fosamax or a nasal spray like Neocalcin that support bone rebuilding. However, nearly all research on such drugs has been on postmenopausal women rather than adolescents. Treatment of osteopenia and osteoporosis in adolescents is still an evolving science.

Trapped in the Triad

The American College of Sports Medicine notes that the triad "is often denied, not recognized, and underreported."[5] The ACSM recommends that anyone with one characteristic of the triad should be evaluated for the others. Thus, a physically active adolescent who has stopped menstruating should have a bone density test. It will reveal how her bone mass compares with the expected bone mass of someone her age. A girl who has lost a great deal of weight might not always confide in her parents that she is no longer menstruating—indeed, she might even think it is a good thing. But parents should talk with her health provider about their concerns.

A girl who has put her heart and soul into dance or sport might not welcome interventions that will require her to gain weight. Like the anorexic and bulimic adolescents described in chapter 10, she is heavily invested in maintaining her thinness. Even if she acknowledges the toll on her health, she might insist that it is worth it. She might point out that a dancer or athlete has only so many years before she is out of her prime, out of the game. So why jeopardize her chances by gaining weight? Her bone density is not something she can see and is a problem she might easily deny. Her denial might persist unless or until she gets injured. She needs to be made aware that bone weakness can lead to fractures that will prevent her from dancing or competing.

She also needs to be assured that medical attention will be sensitive to her concerns. No one is trying to make her a pudgy ballerina. But there are ways to be healthy and effective at the same time. The ACSM advocates for more realistic standards and health-informed coaching to help adolescents withstand the pressures to become too thin.

Meanwhile, it is also important to assess the degree to which a girl attaches her self-esteem to her dance or athletic performance. Does she feel that she is only worthwhile if she wins? The aim of reversing eating disorders, amenorrhea, and osteoporosis is not only to improve her health now, but for life. She should be supported in her art or sport, but also encouraged to explore other interests and relationships. As she knows all too well, youth is fleeting. Investing in her health now—and affirming her value as a person who is going to be around for a long time—are critical for her long-term outlook. (For more on eating disorders, see chapter 10.)

DYSFUNCTIONAL UTERINE BLEEDING

Most girls have irregular and unpredictable menstrual cycles during the first year or two after the onset of periods. The frequency, the heaviness, and the length of flow may vary from period to period. Although this state of affairs can be exasperating at times, it is not abnormal. In fact, many girls seem never to have perfectly regular classic twenty-eight-day cycles, although the number of days and amount of flow seem to settle into a pattern as the girls mature.

It is not at all uncommon for a girl to have mostly typical periods and then once in a while (sometimes with travel or stress) experience spotting or bleeding between periods. This is called *dysfunctional uterine bleeding* (DUB). It is caused by an interruption in the normal cycling of estrogen and progesterone, or in the younger adolescent is due to an immature production of these hormones, which leaves the lining of the uterus in an "unstable" state.

DUB typically is not accompanied by the usual symptoms of cramps and bloating, and except for the bleeding the girl doesn't "feel" like she has her period. DUB is not something to worry about, especially during the early years of menstruation, unless the bleeding is exceptionally heavy and/or prolonged (or on-again, off-again) for more than ten to fourteen days. Although DUB is usually simply a sign of stress or immaturity of hormone production, there are a few other causes, such as thyroid disorder, mild bleeding disorder, a sexually transmitted infection such as chlamydia, a miscarriage, or rarely a genital tumor.

If the amount of bleeding is so significant that it results in anemia (low blood count), dizziness, or enormous frustration, then it should be treated with progesterone alone or with birth control pills for several cycles until the system settles down. The use of such hormones usually stabilizes the lining of the uterus and shuts off the relentless flow. Rarely, hospitalization is needed to achieve the same result with intravenous estrogen treatment.

VAGINAL HYGIENE AND HEALTH

Drugstores are full of products that perpetuate the notion that female genitalia are inherently displeasing. Douches, feminine hygiene sprays, and deodorant tampons are sold as ways to counteract supposedly unappealing vaginal odors. The irony is that these products are likely to irritate the vagina or diminish healthy bacteria in the vaginal tract. The irritation might make it more likely that problems will arise—in which case, women will turn to these products more!

An allergic reaction to these products can cause vaginal or vulvar pain and redness, which should go away when use of the spray or other product is discontinued.

The vagina cleans itself through its fluids. The basics of hygiene are simple.

- Avoid feminine hygiene sprays and similar products.
- Avoid douches, whether they are homemade (usually vinegar and water) or store-bought. Douches disrupt the vagina's natural acidic pH balance, causing it to become more alkaline, which increases the risk of bacterial vaginosis and yeast infections (described later in this chapter). Douching might also lead to pelvic inflammatory disease and ectopic pregnancy. The vagina

does a good job of cleansing itself, and the disadvantages of douching far outweigh any momentary "clean feeling" a girl might have.

- Keep the vulva clean by taking a shower, bath, or sponge bath every day. Warm water cleansing with a soft cloth or just your hand is preferable to scrubbing this sensitive area with a strong soap.
- Wear cotton underwear or at least underwear with a cotton shield at the crotch. Avoid wearing tight underwear, panty hose, or snug-fitting pants for long periods of time; they promote a moist environment in which odor-causing bacteria and yeast like to grow.
- After using the toilet, always wipe from front to back (from the vaginal/urethral area back toward the rectum).
- If an unpleasant odor or unusual discharge occurs, consult a doctor to see if it might be a sign of vaginitis (see page 130) or a sexually transmitted disease (see chapter 8).

VAGINAL DISCHARGE: SIGNS OF PUBERTY AND OVULATION

About two years before girls get their periods, they begin to have a clear, white, or yellow-white vaginal discharge. Many girls, and also some mothers, worry that the wet feeling and the crusty yellowish substance that spots their panties are signs of infection. Girls need to know that this is normal, not a sign of anything wrong. Vaginal discharge, also called vaginal fluids or secretions, is another sign (in addition to breast buds) that the ovaries are beginning to produce estrogen. The discharge keeps the vagina moist and clean. One way to think about this is to realize that vaginal discharge is produced by glands something like the glands in our mouths that make saliva. The mouth has a throat that swallows the saliva (and prevents drooling), whereas the vagina does not, so the discharge comes out onto the vulva and panties.

Once mature menstrual cycles are established, the appearance and texture of vaginal fluids change during the month, providing interesting and important clues to what is happening in the reproductive system. Following a period the consistency of cervical mucus is clear, thin, and watery. At the time of ovulation it becomes goopy, like raw egg white, and is called *spinbarkeit*. This German word describes the thick, tenacious, slippery quality of this discharge, which can be pulled apart like a piece of taffy. Spinbarkeit discharge favors the movement of sperm and helps them swim. After ovulation, discharge tends to be white and pasty.

A woman can learn to observe these changes to help her determine when she is most and least fertile. The sympto-thermal method of contraception combines three fertility awareness strategies: observing and recording these changes in cervical mucus, taking and recording daily morning temperatures (body temperature increases by 0.4 to 0.8 degrees on the day a woman ovulates), and recording menstrual cycles on a calendar to help predict future ones and the most likely timing of ovulation (two weeks before the period). This low-tech approach to contraception has its appeal but can be difficult to implement effectively and is not recommended as a contraceptive technique for adolescents.[6]

VULVOVAGINITIS

Vulvovaginitis is an inflammation of the mucous membranes of and around the vulva and vagina. It may be caused by infection with common bacteria (which normally reside inside the vagina and rectum, such as strep, staph, or *E. coli*), yeast (*Candida*), *Trichomonas*, or *Gardnerella*. Symptoms include:

- Pain.
- Itching.
- Redness.
- Foul-smelling vaginal discharge.
- Unusual color (green, gray) and texture of discharge.

These infections may or may not be sexually transmitted. (For a description of sexually transmitted diseases, see chapter 8.) However, if a girl is sexually active, treating her partner may be indicated to prevent them from passing the infection back and forth. They should abstain from intercourse while they are being treated for an infection to avoid even further irritation or chance of reinfection and should use a condom (which they should be doing always) when intercourse resumes.

Bacterial Vaginitis

This condition (also called *nonspecific vaginitis*) is seen in younger children as well as adolescents, and is often related to poor hygiene or sometimes a foreign body in the vagina. Thorough cleansing between the labia and the thighs might be particularly difficult for an obese adolescent and requires special attention to be sure that sweat and vaginal fluids are removed daily. A forgotten tampon in an adolescent or sometimes a small object inserted into the vagina by a younger child is likely to result in a foul discharge and redness. Treatment is directed at the specific bacteria found (and, of course, removal of any foreign body), but most important is attention to prevention by improved hygiene, looser fitting clothing, and use of cotton panties.

Yeast Infection

This cause of vulvovaginitis is common, not serious, but highly annoying. Most cases are caused by *Candida albicans* and typically include intense itching, redness of the vulva and vagina, and burning of the skin—especially during urination. It often produces a distinctive vaginal discharge that is odorless but curdlike, often described as being similar to cottage cheese. Yeast and bacteria normally reside quietly in the vagina, causing no problem. However, predisposing factors result in the overgrowth of yeast and its dramatic symptoms. Such factors include recent treatment with antibiotics; excessive sweating or dampness in the area due to tight clothing, wet bathing suits, or poor hygiene; having sex; diabetes; and the higher vaginal pH in the week prior to menstruation.

Mild infections often go away without any treatment (a warm bath with Aveeno powder is soothing), especially when a period intervenes and a lower vaginal pH then suppresses the yeast. If symptoms worsen, various over-the-counter creams and suppositories (such as Monistat and Gyne-Lotrimin) are available. It is probably best if a doctor confirms the first infection, because similar symptoms might be caused by something else.

Gardnerella Vaginalis

A small bacterium called *Gardnerella vaginalis* is the usual causative agent of bacterial vaginosis, an infection caused by the overgrowth of this bacteria that replaces the normal vaginal flora. A thin grayish discharge with a foul "fishy" odor and sometimes mild itching or burning are characteristic. The diagnosis is made after examination of the vaginal fluid under a microscope, and treatment with an antibiotic (oral or vaginal cream) should result in quick resolution of the symptoms. This is not a sexually transmitted disease, and the partner need not be treated unless the infection recurs.

Trichomoniasis

"Trich" is a sexually transmitted disease caused by the microscopic protozoa *Trichomonas vaginalis*. Its characteristic discharge is gray-green, frothy, and malodorous, but the symptoms of burning on urination, vaginal itching and irritation, and spotting after intercourse might be more prominent to the sufferer. Diagnosis is made by examination of the discharge under a microscope with the finding of characteristic "trich" swimming around. Usual treatment is with a single dose of the antibiotic metronidazole (Flagyl) for the girl and her partner. This antibiotic can cause abdominal pain and vomiting and should never be taken by a pregnant woman or someone who might be pregnant, so treatment may be postponed until a girl gets her next period. Use of metronidazole and alcohol around the same time can cause serious vomiting and malaise.

URINARY TRACT (BLADDER AND KIDNEY) INFECTIONS

The urinary tract consists of four structures involved in the process of clearing waste from the body.

The *kidneys*, located within the abdomen at the level of the mid-back, filter waste products and excess water from the bloodstream to make urine.

The *ureters*, two narrow tubes several inches long, carry the urine from the kidneys to the bladder.

The *bladder*, a muscular, balloonlike organ, holds the urine until it fills to a point when the urge to urinate is felt, its sphincter relaxes, and urine is released.

The *urethra*, a very short tube (about 1 inch) carries the urine out of the body from the lower portion of the bladder and exits from a fold of skin just above the vaginal opening. Every day a person releases about one and a half quarts of urine, or more or less depending on the quantity of fluid he or she drinks.

Common Infections—Especially Among Women

Urinary tract infections are the second most common type of infection (after respiratory tract infections).[7] About one of every five women will have a urinary tract infection (UTI) during her lifetime, and many women have more than one.

Women's vulnerability to UTI is largely due to an anatomical injustice. A woman's urethra is only one fifth as long as a man's. This means that although urine has only a short distance to travel out of the body, bacteria likewise have only a short distance to travel *into* the body. Bacteria, originating on the nearby skin or inside the vagina or rectum, can work their way up the urethra, first to the bladder, and then to the kidneys. At each step of the way they can cause increasingly serious problems.

Why Urinary Tract Infections Occur

Unlike skin, vaginal fluids, or stool, urine is sterile. This means it should not contain any bacteria. In fact, it has antibacterial properties that would help to keep the urinary tract relatively trouble-free but for three little problems: location, location, location. The urethra is one of three openings of a woman's body that are very close together. Its proximity to the anus and vagina expose it to bacteria that can cause infections.

The anus is the major source of bacteria, primarily *Escherichia coli (E. coli)*. That is why it is so important for a girl to learn to wipe from front to back after urinating. To wipe in the other direction could spread bacteria from the anus to the urethra, and then up into the urinary tract. Little girls are particularly susceptible to UTIs for this reason. Bigger girls—adolescents and adults—often experience their first UTI with sexual activity, especially after intercourse, when bacteria from the vagina and anus can spread to the urethra.

Most of the time, urine passing out of the urethra will clear the bacteria and no infection occurs. Sometimes an infection remains inside only the urethra (*urethritis*), most often it moves up into the bladder (*cystitis*), and occasionally it spreads all the way up to the kidneys (*pyelonephritis*). Any of these three levels of infection may be referred to as a "UTI."

Urethritis (or "acute urethral syndrome") is felt as a burning sensation inside the urethra, especially during urination. It often comes on within a few hours after having sex and might clear on its own after a day or two without any treatment. In addition to irritation from intercourse, the urethral opening may become inflamed from soaps, deodorants, or douches. More serious and persistent is urethritis caused by the sexually transmitted infections *Chlamydia trachomatis* or *Neisseria gonorrhea*.

The most common kind of UTI is cystitis, an infection inside the bladder. *Honeymoon cystitis* is the term given to a urinary tract infection that came about after ardent lovemaking by a previously virginal newlywed. Cystitis causes burning on urination (especially at the end of the stream) and a frequent urge to urinate even when the bladder has just been emptied. In addition, there can be lower abdominal pain, awakening in the middle of the night with an urge to urinate, cloudy foul-smelling urine, or blood in the urine. Typically, a woman with cystitis does not have a fever or feel otherwise sick.

The most serious UTI is pyelonephritis, an infection in the kidney itself. Pyelonephritis can be a complication of an untreated cystitis, with bacteria traveling up the ureters from the bladder to the kidney(s), or it can develop without any sign that cystitis has occurred. In either case, the person with pyelonephritis feels ill and often has a high fever, back pain (in the mid-back region at the level of the kidneys), nausea, and vomiting. Untreated pyelonephritis can cause severe damage to the kidney(s).

Seek Help Promptly

It is important to treat a UTI as soon as possible because it is likely to be quite uncomfortable (especially cystitis) or progress and make you quite sick (pyelonephritis). A UTI is easily diagnosed because symptoms tend to be specific and simple office procedures suffice. The diagnosis is based on a characteristic urine analysis (containing white blood cells and often red blood cells) and is confirmed by a urine culture grown overnight.

Treatment of the infection is an appropriate antibiotic taken for about five to seven days for cystitis and ten to fourteen days for pyelonephritis. With pyelonephritis, hospitalization sometimes is needed to provide intravenous fluids and medication.

It can be helpful to take a urinary anesthetic called pyridium (available over-the-counter as Uristat or Azo-pyridium) for a few hours to relieve the burning and pressure to urinate frequently until you get to the doctor. Pyridium turns the urine a bright Day-Glo yellow-orange color but does not interfere with making an accurate diagnosis.

Drinking lots of fluids (such as acidic juices like cranberry and grapefruit) helps to dilute the urine, relieve some burning, and clear the infection. A heating pad over the bladder or back may also feel good.

An adolescent girl with recurrent UTIs should be evaluated for any structural abnormality of her urinary system that might be increasing her risk of acquiring infection.

How to Prevent Urinary Tract Infections or Recurrence

- Drink plenty of water (at least eight glasses a day) to keep kidneys and bladder flushed out. Cranberry juice or vitamin C might help by acidifying urine, which can create an environment less hospitable to bacterial growth.
- Obey the urge to urinate; don't "hold it in." By emptying the bladder regularly any bacteria won't be given the chance to proliferate.
- Observe the color of your urine. It should be very pale yellow or nearly clear. Dark urine indicates that you haven't been drinking enough water.
- After using the toilet, always wipe from front to back.
- Take showers instead of baths.
- Urinate and wash the genital area both before and *after* sexual intercourse.
- Do not use feminine hygiene sprays or douches.

BREAST CONCERNS AND DISORDERS

One adolescent hopes her breasts will be voluptuous. She wants to borrow her older sister's yellow angora sweater and round it out like a movie star. After all, people say she resembles the actress Drew Barrymore. In Woody Allen's Everyone Says I Love You, *Drew's nipples showed right through her dress, but she didn't seem embarrassed at all.*

Another girl prays for small breasts that won't get in her way when she does gymnastics. Big breasts would throw off her balance on the balance beam. Anyway, who ever heard of a busty gymnast?

A third girl frets that she is not developing fast enough. She stands

*sideways in front of the mirror, frustrated that her rib cage protrudes far-
ther than her breasts. While everybody else is busy stocking up on colorful
bras at the Victoria's Secret sale, all she needs for "support" is a word of
encouragement:* "Be patient. You're developing just fine. In a year or two
you'll catch up." *A year or two! That's forever.*

*A fourth girl hates her large, heavy breasts. They pull on her shoulders
and make her back hurt. Boys make lewd comments about them, so she
has taken to wearing oversized shirts and slumping to disguise their size.
She would love to take modern dance class, but her school requires
dancers to wear leotards. No way is she going to march out there and display her cleavage (not to mention her slightly bulging tummy).*

Breasts are certainly a focus of attention for adolescent girls. With excitement or apprehension, they are on the lookout for breast development. They are
appalled to discover things no one ever mentioned, like nipple hairs or stretch
marks or breasts that do not match. Often they will not talk about these concerns with their parents or anybody else, but stew silently in their shame.

If they are lucky, they will learn from parents, their doctor, a sexuality education class, a friend, a book, or a website that these things are normal. Unlike
a Barbie doll's perky and perfectly symmetrical, nippleless breasts, a human
girl's breasts are as idiosyncratically special as she is.

As breasts take form during puberty, girls may need more information about
some of the changes they are experiencing.

- *Breast soreness* is normal, especially (but not exclusively) before a
  period. Some girls' breasts swell before their periods, causing bras to
  feel too tight. It might help to buy a bra in a larger size to wear at this
  time. Often breast tenderness is simply a kind of "growing pain" due to
  hormonal stimulation, and will subside when puberty wanes.

- *Uncertainty about bra size* is notorious among adult women and especially confusing for girls who are just learning and whose size may be
  changing rapidly. Wearing a bra that is too tight can cause skin redness
  and discomfort. Wearing one that is too loose can cause breast soreness
  in a girl with large breasts who needs firm support. Underwire bras
  that fit properly can offer superior support, but those that do not fit
  well can cause discomfort from wires poking into ribs. Even if she is
  shy, a girl might find it worthwhile to go to a department store or lin-
  gerie shop that specializes in fitting bras. An expert fitter can teach her

how to measure bra size and help her find a sports bra and other bras that provide the support she needs.

Bra fit is especially important to girls with "jogger's nipples," which result from persistent rubbing of the nipples by an overriding bra or other fabric, usually during running or other vigorous exercise. Symptoms include chafing, redness, even a blood-tinged discharge from the nipples. Wearing a properly fitting sports bra and protecting the nipples with Vaseline and a thin Band-Aid when out running can prevent this abrasive injury to the nipples.

• *Areola hair around the nipples* is common among girls of Mediterranean, Latin, and other ethnic groups. Most girls accept these hairs without any concern, but others attempt to pluck them or remove them with creams or wax intended for other parts of the body such as legs. These techniques can result in skin infections. Breast hair removal is best approached with the help of an electrologist or dermatologist. A girl should never use a depilatory on her areolae.

• *Stretch marks* are thin, pinkish red lines that might appear on growing breasts as the overriding skin is stretched. This typically occurs in fair-skinned girls during early adolescence, at times of weight gain, or after starting on the birth control pill. Once the breasts (or other parts of the body) stop growing, the stretch marks begin to fade, and they will eventually disappear over several months or a year or two.

• *Breast asymmetry,* to some degree, is the rule rather than the exception. One breast may bud later than the other or grow more slowly. Sometimes the slower breast catches up with the faster one, but at other times a mild asymmetry remains even after both breasts have reached maturity. In fact, most women's breasts are at least slightly different in size. Usually the disparity is subtle. If the difference is significant and noticeable in some outfits, a girl may opt to wear cotton or foam rubber padding in one cup of her bra. If she is very unhappy, she may choose to consult with a plastic surgeon about reduction and/or augmentation procedures that can be done after her breasts are fully developed.

Rarely, a girl is misdiagnosed with breast asymmetry when the problem is really an unevenness of her chest wall caused by scoliosis (described in chapter 4) or other skeletal or muscular irregularity. Also rare is asymmetry caused by a giant fibroadenoma, a large benign solid tumor located in one of the breasts.

- *Concern about breast size* leads some girls who want larger breasts to be susceptible to ads for creams or exercise gadgets that promise to increase breast size. These girls should save their money. Breast size is determined by genetics, and creams won't work. Firming the pectoral muscles will not make the breasts larger, but it can create a more toned appearance that makes breasts seem more prominent. However, it is more economical and just as (or more) effective to tone with free weights or by doing push-ups. At least that way girls will not be contributing to the coffers of marketers who are trying to profit from the insecurity of vulnerable young consumers.

- *Breast hyperplasia* is especially large breasts. Other terms are *macromastia, gigantomastia,* or *virginal breast hypertrophy* (to distinguish it from breast enlargement during pregnancy). Large breasts may simply run in the family. Or they may enlarge further in an already large-breasted girl taking oral contraceptives. In this case, a pill containing less estrogen should be considered and should help.

    Breast reduction surgery may be explored and considered once breast development is complete. Some young women choose surgery to relieve back pain caused by the heavy breasts, while others choose surgery for cosmetic reasons. Most girls and women who have had this procedure are very pleased with the outcome. Some say it has changed their lives, all for the better.

- *Breast hypoplasia* is failure of one or both breasts to develop at all, or to develop only a minimal amount of breast tissue around the nipple and areola. Like breast hyperplasia, very small breasts may simply reflect family history, but if hypoplasia is extreme or only on one side it may present a more significant challenge. If lack of development is bilateral and accompanied by failure to menstruate (amenorrhea) it may indicate an eating disorder, endocrine or chromosomal abnormality, or other medical condition. One-sided breast hypoplasia is more likely due to a congenital abnormality.

- *Concern about the ability someday to breast-feed* worries some girls. An otherwise healthy girl with very small breasts might incorrectly think that she will be too small-breasted to nurse a child. In fact, a woman with small breasts is likely to breast-feed just as successfully as a larger-breasted woman, because milk ducts have no relationship to breast size. A girl may draw some comfort from the wonderful story of Jade, a character in Pearl S. Buck's novel *Dragon Seed*, who had a similar concern. Jade had disguised herself as a man in order to pass through enemy lands, then had a child:

> This Jade had in these hard months grown almost as strong as a man and her slender body was hard and all the softness in her face was gone. Anywhere she might have passed for a young man if one did not take notice of her little bosom, which for all its smallness yet nourished the child well. What she ate seemed to go to the child and not to her . . . the milk flowed out of her so rich and full that the child had to gulp to take it in, and out of the other breast it flowed, too, there was so much.[8]

Women who have had breast reduction surgery for breast hyperplasia, or augmentation surgery with an implant, might experience difficulty breast-feeding, a consideration that is discussed with the surgeon and factored in before surgery is done.

Inverted nipples are not an impediment to breast-feeding and can be drawn out through manipulative exercises.

- *Polythelia* is the presence of an extra, usually tiny "supernumerary" nipple, usually located on the breast or chest wall, and seen on about five percent of people. They rarely cause problems but can be removed surgically if desired.

- *Fibrocystic changes and breast lumps* may be cause for alarm in an adolescent girl or her parent. Happily, breast cancer is extremely rare in teenagers, and alarm and worry are not warranted. Nonetheless, you should consult with your doctor to find out more about the lump or lumps. Breast texture varies. Some women have very smooth breast tissue; others have naturally lumpy breasts. The all-over lumpiness (fibrocystic changes) of some girls' breast tissue is not a disease but rather a normal reaction to hormonal stimulation, and can also feel sore and swollen, especially during the week or two before menstruation. Decreasing intake of caffeinated beverages might help to decrease these changes and their discomfort.

  Two types of isolated breast lumps are encountered regularly by teens. The most common solid lump is called a fibroadenoma, and a fluid-filled lump is called a cyst. If a teenage girl discovers such a lump, often about the size of a pea or a grape, her doctor might simply check it again in about a month, after her next period. Cysts often go away on their own, whereas a fibroadenoma will remain or even grow slightly. A sonogram of the breast lump can definitively distinguish a solid lump from a fluid-filled lump. Solid lumps are generally removed, in order to make absolutely sure they are benign and also because they tend to grow. A cyst can be left alone and will soon resolve, or if it is painful the fluid can easily be removed through a thin needle aspiration.

• Different types of *nipple discharge* are occasionally encountered by teenage girls. The galactorrhea (a thin, milky discharge from the nipples) of pregnancy is the most likely cause, but galactorrhea can also occur in a girl who has never been pregnant.

   Galactorrhea is stimulated by increased levels of the hormone prolactin, which is produced in the pituitary gland. Higher prolactin levels may result from a variety of factors besides pregnancy, including emotional stress, stimulation of the nipples, various medications (such as birth control pills and psychiatric drugs), some medical illnesses, or a central nervous system (brain) disease, most commonly a prolactin-secreting tumor of the pituitary gland. Such a tumor is not malignant, and management is surgical if the tumor is larger than one centimeter, but more often medical (with the drug bromocriptine) since most of these tumors are very tiny. Galactorrhea should always be evaluated by a doctor.

   Excessive breast manipulation by a girl or her sexual partner might result in a clear, yellowish, watery discharge from the nipples. A similar discharge tinged with blood might be due to "jogger's nipple," described on page 136. Occasionally a young adolescent will notice a watery, light brownish discharge from a tiny bump on the areola, not from the nipple. This totally benign condition is thought to come from a tiny areola gland, usually stops after a week or two, and rarely recurs.

BREAST SELF-EXAM

Although it is extremely unlikely that an adolescent girl will discover breast cancer, she might want to learn how to do a monthly breast self-exam (BSE). It is meaningful for a girl to start getting familiar with her own breasts; as an expert in her own anatomy, she will be the one best equipped to identify any problems early when she matures and the risk of cancer becomes more real. On the other hand, many girls are not ready to focus on learning and doing BSE until late adolescence or early young adulthood. Although her doctor should examine her breasts at each annual checkup throughout adolescence, formal teaching of BSE can wait until about age 18. It's an easy thing to do in the shower or in bed, and takes only about a minute. The best time to do BSE is during the week following a menstrual period, when breasts are softer and less tender and lumpy than just before a period.

Visual Inspection

The first step is simply for a girl to look at her breasts in a mirror. Although this might seem obvious, there is a difference between an everyday glance in a mirror versus a more purposeful and lingering gaze. With her hands pressed inward on her waist and then up behind her head, she should look at both front and side views. Does she see any changes? Dimples in the nipple or breast? Protrusion? Changes in texture or color of the skin?

Palpating (Feeling) the Breasts

This most important part of the exam can be performed either lying down or standing up, using the right hand to examine the left breast and vice versa. Breast tissue actually extends beyond the apparent edges of the breasts, all the way up to the clavicle bones, into the underarms, and around to the sternum (breastbone). Our fingertips are very sensitive feelers and should be pressed both gently and firmly in a methodical pattern everywhere there is breast tissue. This may be in the form of a spiral that emanates outward from the nipples or in-and-out like the spokes of a wheel. What is being looked for is a specific lump that stands out from the surrounding breast tissue (which may be lumpy) and feels something like a raisin, lima bean, pea, or grape. Different parts of a normal breast feel different, and it takes time for a girl or woman to learn what is normal for her and to distinguish a true lump from simply breast tissue or underlying ribs or other chest wall structures. What's most important is that a teenager be aware that she should not panic if she finds a lump, that cancer is rare at her age, but that any lump should be checked out by her doctor. Because adolescence and young adulthood are low-risk times for breast cancer, it is an excellent time to learn BSE without having to feel scared.

HER FIRST GYNECOLOGIC EXAM

A teenage girl of any age should have her first gynecologic examination if she has had sexual intercourse (even once) or if she has a gynecologic problem (such as certain menstrual disorders, unusual vaginal discharge, or unexplained lower abdominal pain). If she has reached age 18 and none of these criteria apply, then now (or within the next year or two) would be an appropriate time to consider having this exam.

A gynecologic exam, performed patiently and with gentle hands, should not be a painful or unpleasant experience, although there might be mild discomfort for about a minute. It is especially important that the first exam be "successful" in this way, so that future exams are not dreaded. The first gynecologic exam is a milestone in a girl's life, and it is normal for her to be apprehensive. However, even for a virgin the exam should not be painted as a very big deal. Nonetheless, some virginal girls of 18 or 19 just don't feel ready yet, and they should not be made to feel pressured into it. They will likely feel ready soon.

Primarily, the exam is an opportunity to confirm good health, identify any problems, and in a sexually active girl screen for sexually transmitted diseases and pregnancy. It is also a chance for the teen to learn more about her body, both by experiencing the exam and by talking with her health care provider, who will answer any questions she might have.

Various types of health providers are experienced in doing gynecologic examinations and would be appropriate to do an adolescent's exam. Some pediatricians and family doctors, all gynecologists and midwives, some nurse practitioners, and nearly all adolescent medicine specialists are qualified to do the exam. The most important thing is to choose a health professional with whom the teenager will be at ease, preferably someone she knows, who welcomes an

---

THE FIRST GYNECOLOGIC EXAM: WHAT TO EXPECT

The examination itself takes only a minute or two.

External. With the girl lying on her back, knees bent up and spread apart, the examiner first visually inspects the external genitalia region, including the pubic, vulva, and anal areas, looking for any bumps or rashes.

Internal. Next a speculum is inserted into the vagina to view the cervix and vaginal walls for any lesions or unusual discharge.

Tests. A Pap smear (to test for cancerous or other abnormal cervical cells) and culture specimens (for chlamydia and gonorrhea, if sexual activity has ever occurred) are obtained by gently rubbing the cervical opening with a tiny brush and swab.

Check of Internal Organs. Finally, the speculum is removed and the examiner's gloved forefinger of one hand is inserted into the vagina while the other hand gently presses on the lower belly to feel the uterus and ovaries to check their size and shape. Sometimes a gloved finger may also be placed in the rectum (doesn't hurt; feels like having a small bowel movement) to get a better feel of the pelvic organs.

opportunity to work with adolescents and will be available to counsel the teen and answer her questions.

BODY IMAGE: HELP YOUR DAUGHTER ACCEPT HERSELF

As girls' bodies change they often feel increased pressure to conform to society's current standards of attractiveness. Many adolescent girls are notable for their critical eyes—and for turning that criticism against themselves.

Some girls play a harsh game: "If you could change one part of your body, what would it be? What's your favorite part of your body? Your least favorite?" A fly on a wall in a school bathroom or in a store fitting room would get an ear-ful of scathing self-reviews. Some girls assess their bodies top to toe, enumerating their flaws part by part. If it's not one thing, it's another:

My chin is weak. (Or: *My chin sticks out.*)

My tummy bulges. (Or: *I have no curves.*)

My thighs are flabby. (Or: *My legs are like sticks.*)

My toes are ugly. (Or: *It's so unfair, my toes are my only good part, and most of the time nobody sees them!*)

My boobs are too big. (Or: *I'm so flat-chested.*)

Many girls who are merciless with themselves would not tolerate someone picking apart their best friend that way. But they don't understand that they need to be their own best friend. They do not need to be "perfect." While most girls eventually mature into self-acceptance, others are forever stuck in the dis-content of adolescent self-centeredness.

Frequently girls learn brutal self-talk from overhearing their mothers, aunts, or older sisters blame and shame themselves: *I'm so fat! I've gained an ounce! I was so bad today, I ate a brownie.* Such comments teach girls that weight is a valid measure of self-worth—and food is a potent enemy.

Food should be about nourishment and enjoyment. But for too many girls, food is about tension . . . or release. Life becomes a food fight, a struggle with cravings, shoulds and should nots, calorie charts, funny mirrors, and skinny Spandex dresses that are as unforgiving as the queen in *Alice in Wonderland*. "Off with her head!" shouted the queen. "Off with the pounds!" screams the stretchy little dress. Skimpy little tops, low-slung jeans, and other bare-to-there fashions give a girl nowhere to hide.

Body image and eating disorders are discussed further in chapter 10. But it is important to keep them in mind as you reflect on your daughter's develop-ment.

HEALTH-PARTNERING TIPS FOR PARENTS

- Encourage your daughter to learn about and take pride in her body.
- Be an "askable parent," and raise health issues on your own if your daughter does not.
- Provide your daughter with pamphlets or books about health issues, so she can learn about things she might be reluctant to discuss with you. (See the bibliography and "Books for Teens.")
- Enlist other family members to talk with your daughter if you are uncomfortable. If you are a single dad, for example, you might want to ask a female relative to discuss with your daughter such matters as pad or tampon use, sexuality, and breast self-exams. (However, many dads are comfortable doing so themselves.)
- Make sure your daughter knows how important it is to seek prompt treatment for discomfort or pain in the lower abdomen, kidney area, or urinary tract.
- Long before puberty actually begins, start to talk with your daughter (at about age seven or eight) about some of the changes she can expect to see first: little breast buds and fine pubic hairs. She may or may not choose to show them to you when they occur. Some girls are very private about their earliest signs of puberty.
- Talk about menstruation as a positive event coming in her life. Assure her that her first period will come several years *after* breasts and pubic hair, so she need not worry that it will come out of the blue.
- If about two years have passed since the onset of breast buds, then remind your daughter that her first period may be coming soon. She should be prepared with a sanitary pad in her bookbag in case she gets her first period in school. Also find out who at school can help her at that time (such as a school nurse) if needed. If she is going off to camp over the summer, she should go prepared with a supply of pads.
- Remind your daughter that there is a wide range of normal ages for the onset of puberty. Understand and support her anxiety about this, especially if puberty for her comes earlier or later than for most of her peers.
- Help your daughter find a doctor or other health professional who can help her deal with any routine or other gynecologic problems or concerns— someone who will listen, answer all her questions, provide sensitive counsel, and if needed, do a gentle gynecologic exam.
- There is no greater gift you can give your daughter than the mercy of self-acceptance, the permission to be imperfect, and the reassurance that all she needs to do is simply be herself.

SIX: Health Issues for Your Son

Adolescent boys struggle with the push-pull between boyhood and manhood. They have a lot on their minds, and not only sex—although some men recall their teen years as a blur of masturbation interrupted by school, sports, and massive meals. Some boys wonder whether they "measure up" to manhood. Are they growing tall enough, fast enough? Are their genitals in the normal (or greater) range? Seeking to capitalize on that concern, some marketers bombard boys with E-mail ads for bogus penis enlargement methods. That these companies make money off boys' fears shows that many boys do not know that genes, not machines or creams, determine penis size. Boys also need to know that size is far less important in lovemaking than feelings, sensitivity, and communication with a partner.

If genital size can't be changed, maybe muscles can. Magazines promise readers that they can attain the awesome muscle definition displayed by the model on the cover. A magazine does not mention that the model spent countless hours in a gym, hardly realistic or attainable for most busy teenagers. Boys who try to push themselves ahead of the pack by using steroids can suffer devastating side effects.

Your son needs you to provide a perspective at home that can counterbalance the hype. Let him know that there is a whole range of "normal" in boys' growth and size and development. This chapter describes the process of puberty and the many changes a boy can expect in how he looks and feels.

This chapter also covers a number of penile, scrotal, and other medical concerns. By alerting your son to symptoms to look out for, you can help save him from life-altering injury or fatal disease.

Your discussions can also set a tone of openness, helping him to avoid the embarrassment that can be the greatest deterrent to early, most effective treatment.

WHEN DOES PUBERTY BEGIN?

It would be nice if all boys could enter puberty at the same time, lining up like runners, setting off in unison at the sound of the starting gun. Some would reach maturity faster, but at least all would feel that they were in sync with their peers. Yet nature is not so kind.

Some boys get a head start. As early as 9 or 10 they are already adding inches to their height, developing pubic hair, and noticing that their penis and scrotum have begun to grow, while most of their friends still look like little kids. The average age at which boys enter puberty is 12, but it is normal for puberty to begin as late as age 14 or 15.

A boy who begins puberty earlier is not always happy about looking different from his friends. It's not necessarily fun to tower over peers, to be the one whose voice cracks first. During adolescence, most boys would rather blend into the crowd than be the first or the last to show physical changes.

The later starter is frustrated to find not a hair on his groin, no need for new jeans at the start of the school year. Meanwhile, he finds himself looking up at girls who are growing faster than the boys around them. Girls begin puberty on average two years earlier than boys (at an average age of 10). This disparity in onset of maturation makes the late-blooming boy feel even more conspicuous.

His growth spurt will come, but maybe not until age 16 or 17. Parents can offer reassurance and understanding, and a doctor can make sure he is normal and encourage him to be patient. By 14, when the early developer might be nearly finished growing, the late developing boy might just be starting to grow at an accelerated rate. He can expect to continue growing into his early twenties.

It can be helpful for a boy to get some insight into family growth patterns. When did his dad or Uncle Stan begin to grow? How tall were they at his age? Learning that they, too, got tall early or had to wait to grow can put his own growth pattern into perspective.

But what if family history does not match his experience or is not available? The universal message is that growth patterns are as distinctive as people—and that a man can live a happy and healthy life at any height.

TANNER STAGES FOR BOYS, AND RELATED CHANGES

Given the great range of "normal," how does a doctor assess a boy's development? In addition to measuring height and weight (see chapter 2), a doctor evaluates the progress of sexual maturation using the Tanner stages, a method of identifying five phases of growth developed in the early 1960s by Dr. James. M. Tanner, a physician at the University of London. The Tanner stages for boys pertain only to scrotal/testicular and penile development and pubic hair growth. But coinciding with these are additional changes in a boy's hormones, growth, musculature, voice, and skin.

Tanner Stage 1 (prepubertal): Before puberty begins, a boy has no pubic hair, and his penis and testicles have not yet begun to mature.

Other Features: Boys at this stage of development still look and sound child-like, even if they are "teenagers" chronologically.

Tanner Stage 2 (early puberty): The first sign of puberty is enlargement of the testicles and, a few months later, the growth of scattered fine and straight strands of pubic hair at the base of the penis. The penis may begin to grow slightly, but the testicles take the lead. The skin on the scrotum may deepen in color or become more textured.

Other Changes: A boy is growing taller but not yet at an accelerated rate. His body is still not "filling out," but the area around the nipples, the areola, gets darker and a bit larger.

Tanner Stage 3 (mid-puberty): The testicles continue to grow larger and the penis begins to lengthen and thicken. Pubic hair becomes thicker and curlier in a triangular area above the pubic bone.

Other Changes: Height continues to increase at a steady rate, and the body begins to fill out into a more adult silhouette, with shoulders broadening. The larynx grows, causing the voice to deepen.

Tanner Stage 4 (preadult stage): The penis and testicles continue to grow and mature, looking more like a man's genitalia than a boy's. The glans (head of the penis) changes in contour, becoming larger and wider, and the scrotum darkens further. Pubic hair surpasses its previous boundaries, becoming bushier and coarser but still not extending past the groin.

Other Changes: The testicles begin to produce sperm. The voice continues to deepen. More hair grows in the underarms and on the face. The most rapid rate of growth in height (the "growth spurt") occurs between Tanner stages 4 and 5.

Tanner Stage 5 (adult development): The penis and scrotum have achieved their adult size and maturity. Pubic hair now extends onto the inner thighs.

Other Changes: The boy continues to head rapidly toward attainment of his full adult height. He might have chest or darkening body hair, or these might grow later. His voice is now fully changed.

HOW THE MALE BODY WORKS

Adolescent boys sometimes wonder why they need to know the details of how their reproductive system works. One reason is that knowledge of how sperm

Male Genitalia

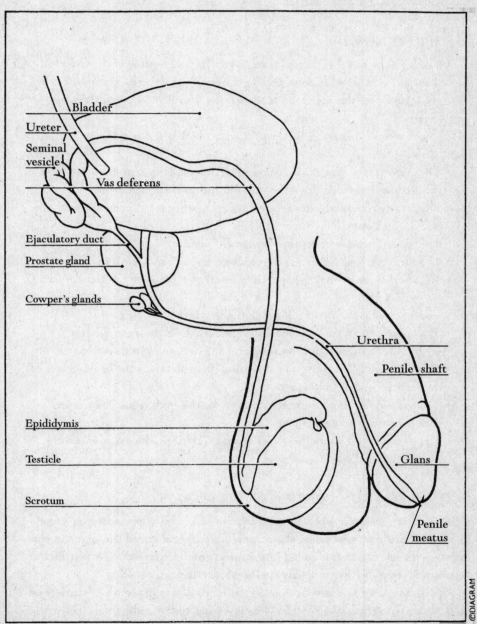

Bladder

Ureter

Seminal vesicle

Vas deferens

Ejaculatory duct

Prostate gland

Cowper's glands

Urethra

Penile shaft

Epididymis

Testicle

Glans

Scrotum

Penile meatus

©DIAGRAM

and preseminal fluid are produced, stored, and travel helps them understand how pregnancy can be caused or prevented. It also explains genital sensations and observations boys commonly experience, as well as anomalies for which they should seek a doctor's advice.

THE MALE GENITALIA

- The *pubic area* is the triangular region at the very bottom of the abdomen that lies over the pubic bone. During the course of puberty, pubic hair will gradually cover this area, and in some males it will grow upward toward the navel.
- The *penile meatus* is the opening through which urine or semen exits the penis.
- The *urethra* is the tube that runs through the penis and carries urine from the bladder and sperm from the testicles and ends at the meatus.
- The *foreskin* covers the lower portion of the penis; it has been removed in a circumcised male.
- The *glans* is the lower portion (tip) of the penis.
- The *corona* is a raised line of tissue along the back surface of the glans.
- The *shaft* is the main portion of the penis that is between the glans and the abdominal wall.
- The *scrotum* is the sac of thick skin that holds the testicles.
- The *testicles* (two), also called the testes, are the male organs located within the scrotum that produce sperm and hormones (testosterone).
- The *epididymis* is a collection of tubules that runs along the back surface of the testicles and collects sperm.
- The *vas deferens* is a tube that extends from the epididymis into the urethra carrying sperm and semen.
- The *prostate* and *seminal vesicles* are glands that produce semen and are located inside the lower abdomen.

WHY THE SCROTUM CONTRACTS AND RELAXES

Sperm are manufactured in the testicles, the two almond-shaped organs inside the scrotum (also called the *scrotal sac*). Sperm travel through the epididymis, a long tube that is coiled into a spiral and hugs the testicles within the scrotum. The epididymis is where sperm mature and are stored.

Sperm are very sensitive to temperature. That is why, in cold weather or cold water, the scrotum moves the testicles closer to the body, snug against the groin to keep sperm from getting too cold. In hot weather, warm water, or when body temperature is higher due to a fever, the scrotum is looser. This lets the testicles dangle farther away from the body so that air can circulate around them and keep sperm a few degrees cooler than the rest of the body.

TWO PERILS OF TIGHT JEANS

Fertility specialists have noted that men who wear tight briefs or jeans might have lower sperm production because their testicles' temperature is often too high. In some instances, when men have switched to loose boxers, thus restoring the scrotum's natural ability to regulate the testicles' temperature, their sperm production increased, improving fertility. Wearing tight pants is not a method of birth control, of course. But your son should be aware of the physiological changes that wearing tight clothing might cause. (It can also lead to "jock itch," described later in this chapter.)

EXPLAINING ERECTIONS

During sexual excitement blood flow to the penis increases, causing an erection. Ejaculation may or may not follow.

It is common for adolescent boys to have erections that occur for no discernible reason, often at very inconvenient and embarrassing times. (A math teacher calls a guy to the chalkboard at the very moment when he desperately needs to stay seated!) "I looked at the clock during class, calculating whether my erection would go down in the three minutes before the bell rang, or if I'd have to get up and carry my books in front of my crotch to hide my erection," said one young man. "I thought about banking, Santa Claus, even my grandmother—anything to try to make my erection go away."

Oversize T-shirts and pants may disguise the "hard-on" if a guy is lucky, or he may just hope that no one notices.

WET DREAMS

During sleep boys may experience penile erections several times per night. Whether from spontaneous surges of testosterone or in response to a sexually stimulating dream, a boy may awake some nights to discover the sticky surprise of semen on his body and bed sheets. This ejaculation during sleep is called a "wet dream" or a "nocturnal emission." A wet dream is the body's way of releasing sperm that the testicles have manufactured and stored.

It is important that your son knows to expect wet dreams. Discuss them as a positive thing. A wet dream shows that his body is maturing normally and his hormones and genitals are in good working order. Many boys are embarrassed and don't know what, if anything, to do about the newly stained sheets. In a matter-of-fact way, just tell your son he can either wash the sheets himself (what a great time to get your son to do his own laundry, if he doesn't already) or toss them in with the other laundry.

The Myth of "Blue Balls"

Poor, miserable wretch, balked in your amorousness! What tortures are yours! Ah! You fill me with pity. Could any man's back and loins stand such a strain. He stands stiff and rigid and there's never a wench to help him!

—Aristophanes, *Lysistrata*

From ancient Greece to the present day, men must contend with the male equivalent of being all dressed up with nowhere to go. Men who are sexually excited but do not ejaculate may end up with testicles that ache for several hours (after which the ache subsides, with no ill effects). After making out with his girlfriend, many a young man will protest that if they stop before he ejaculates, he will be in terrible pain from "blue balls." He may indeed believe that this discomfort can be harmful to him, or he may be using this ploy as a pressuring tactic. More important, he is not in any lasting danger if ejaculation does not occur.

RETROGRADE EJACULATION

Although lack of ejaculation, as described above, is not harmful, there may be a problem if an adolescent wants to prevent ejaculation (such as while masturbating) and puts his hand or an object over the end of his penis to stop the flow of semen—for example, to keep it from staining his clothes. The resulting backflow of semen through the urethra into his bladder is called "retrograde ejaculation." This may cause no more than a temporary clouding of his urine (now mixed with semen) or the semen may enter the prostate gland, causing inflammation of the gland (prostatitis) and pain at the base of the penis or in the testicles. Prostatitis may require treatment with antibiotics. Most important, boys should refrain from blocking ejaculation, but if this were to occur, they must get over any embarrassment and let their doctor know what happened.

If a boy is concerned about being in a situation again where his pants could be stained, he could take precautions like carrying handkerchiefs or spare clothing. Better to be prepared with practical solutions than to risk another infection.

HEMATOSPERMIA

After masturbation or sexual intercourse, a young man may notice that his semen is reddish, indicating the presence of blood. This condition, hematospermia, may be alarming but is usually harmless and results from the breakage of a small blood vessel that leaks into semen on its route from the epididymis to the urethra. It should be checked by a doctor to rule out a urinary tract or sexually transmitted infection, urethritis, or prostatitis. Most likely, in a few days the semen will be back to normal.

THE ROLE OF PRESEMINAL FLUID

Semen, the fluid that carries sperm out of the body during an ejaculation, is comprised of liquids from several glands: the seminal vesicles, the prostate, and the Cowper's gland (also called the *bulbourethral gland*). The Cowper's gland not only contributes to seminal fluid, it also produces preseminal fluid, a clear fluid that moves through the urethra to cleanse it of urine when a man becomes sexually excited and appears at the tip of the penis during an erection and prior to ejaculation.

Preseminal fluid is important because urine can be acidic, and acid can kill sperm. Preseminal fluid (also called *precum*) contains sperm. There have been instances of virgins who became pregnant because sperm deposited by contact with preseminal fluid swam up the vagina. For the same reason, ejaculation on the vulva, the area just outside the vagina, may result in a pregnancy.

Preseminal fluid can also transmit a sexually transmitted disease (STD). So to prevent pregnancy or an STD, it is important to wear a condom throughout sexual contact and avoid exchange of preseminal fluid, semen, or vaginal fluids.

TESTICULAR CANCER AND THE IMPORTANCE OF SELF-EXAMS

Your son's doctor should teach him to perform testicular self-examination, and you should strongly encourage him to perform it once a month. Testicular cancer, although rare, is the type of cancer most common in men ages 15 to 35, and is the leading cause of death from cancer for men in this age group.[1]

The good news is that testicular cancer has one of the highest cure rates of all types of cancer. When caught early the cure rate is 95 to 99 percent. If the cancer has spread to other parts of the body, the rate drops to about 50 percent.

Adolescent boys and men should do a testicular self-exam at least once a month. By doing the self-exam regularly, a boy can get to know the normal feel of his testicles and adjacent structures and be more sensitive to any changes. He will learn to distinguish between the relative smoothness of the testicles and the bumpiness of the epididymis. Everyone's body is different. By starting early and examining himself regularly, a boy will appreciate what is normal for *him* and be better able to detect and seek a doctor's advice on anything new.

Testicular Self-Exam

- *Examine testicles once a month.* To make it easier to remember, you may want to do a self-exam on the first day of every month.
- *Conduct self-exam during a hot bath or shower,* when the scrotum is relaxed, allowing you to feel testicles more easily.
- *Palpate (feel) every part of the testicle,* using the thumb and fingers. It is normal for one testicle (usually the left one) to hang lower or be heavier than the other. Knowing what is normal for *you* makes it easier for you to detect any changes.
- *Check for:*
  » a hard lump.
  » unusual heaviness (one testicle suddenly becomes heavier or higher).
  » change in texture or size.
  » pain or discomfort.
- *Ask a doctor to check any abnormalities as soon as possible.*

Boys who have or had an undescended testicle (see below) are at higher risk for developing testicular cancer, and should take extra care to perform regular self-exams.

SCROTAL DISORDERS

AN ESSENTIAL MESSAGE FOR YOUR SON

If you have any pain, discomfort, or irregularity in your testicles, have a doctor check it out immediately. Do not feel embarrassed about seeking help. Delay in getting medical attention could result in infertility, loss of a testicle, severe illness, or death.

Your son would think nothing of asking for help with a broken arm, a sprained ankle, or stomach pain. But he might feel shy about giving his more "private" parts the same attention. *His genitals, like the rest of his body, need to be a no-embarrassment zone.* Otherwise, as described on page 153, he could risk infertility (from torsion or sexually transmitted diseases), severe illness, or death (testicular or other cancer).

TESTICULAR TORSION

If your son experiences testicular pain, it is extremely important for him to get medical attention immediately—and to understand why. If testicular torsion is the cause of that pain, your son could be in imminent danger of losing a testicle.

Each testicle is attached to the scrotum by a spermatic cord, a tube of tissue that contains a section of the vas deferens, a spermatic artery, and two spermatic veins. Torsion occurs when the spermatic cord twists, yanking the testicle from its normal position and usually causing sudden pain. The sharp pain (often accompanied by nausea and vomiting) may spread throughout the groin, and perhaps into the abdomen, before localizing in the scrotum, which may appear red and swollen. Occasionally there may be no pain, but the affected testicle is pulled out of its normal position by the twisted cord. Some boys report past brief episodes of scrotal pain over the previous few weeks that abated spontaneously. Torsion is most common among males ages 12 to 18, and may occur during physical activity, sometimes following trauma to the testicle, or spontaneously, even during sleep.

Whatever the cause, *testicular torsion is always an emergency*. It is essential to get medical treatment to untwist and tack down the cord and testicle immediately. If the condition is corrected within six hours, full recovery can be expected. However, the effectiveness of the surgery to save the testicle declines over time. If the condition is not corrected within twenty-four hours, the twisted-off blood supply to the testicle results in death of testicular tissue and loss of the testicle's ability to make sperm.

Alert your son to the possibility of torsion. Tell him never to believe that testicular pain is something that can be "waited out." The pain of torsion may indeed subside, but by then the testicle could be dead. Quick action is necessary to save the testicle.

Warning Signs of Testicular Torsion

- Most common among males 12 to 18.
- May occur during or after physical activity, testicular trauma, or sleep.
- Pain:
  - » may be sudden and sharp, felt in groin, abdomen, and/or scrotum, *or*
  - » may come and go, *or*
  - » may be absent, but the testicle is pulled out of normal position.
  - » may be accompanied by nausea and vomiting.
- Red, swollen scrotum.

- Torsion is *always an emergency.*
- Most effectively treated within six hours.
- Delay in treatment can cause infertility or loss of a testicle.

EPIDIDYMITIS

Epididymitis is inflammation and swelling of the epididymis, the tubelike structure adjacent to the testicle. Males who have been sexually active or who have a history of urinary tract abnormality and infections are at risk. Inflammation is caused by bacteria that are sexually transmitted such as chlamydia and gonorrhea, or organisms arising from the urinary tract.

Warning Signs of Epididymitis

- Gradual or sudden painful swelling of the epididymis and sometimes also the testicle.
- Discharge from the urethra.
- Dysuria (pain while urinating).
- Pus in the urine.
- Fever.

Epididymitis is diagnosed by findings on physical examination and also tests of the urine and any urethral pus, looking for white blood cells and specific bacteria, indicating either an STD or urinary infection. If an STD is found, it is important to inform the sexual partner(s) to be tested as well. Chlamydia and gonorrhea are often asymptomatic in females. Even though having epididymitis is a painful experience, at least it provides an STD alert for one's partner(s) to be treated, which will prevent reinfection.

Epididymitis is treated with antibiotics, bed rest, and support of the scrotum on a towel or pillow, which helps alleviate pain and reduce swelling.

ORCHITIS

Orchitis is inflammation of the testicles, usually caused by a virus or following a case of epididymitis. With the widespread use of mumps vaccine (usually combined with measles and rubella as MMR) the incidence of orchitis has become less frequent. Thirty percent of males who get mumps develop orchitis, and about one third of cases result in testicular atrophy and infertility. Bed rest and scrotal support on a pillow can relieve the pain. Unlike epididymitis, orchitis does not respond to antibiotics, but it does resolve after a week or two.

VARICOCELE

A varicocele is an abnormal enlargement of the veins emerging from the testicle. A varicocele first appears early in puberty and is present in 10 to 15 percent of adolescent and young adult males, and in 90 percent of cases is located adjacent to the left testicle.

Since most varicoceles do not cause discomfort, a varicocele is usually first discovered during a physician's examination. The varicocele may be large and easily visible (appearing like a bluish "bag of worms" pushing out the wall of the scrotum), or not visible but easily felt by the examiner's fingers, or detectable only upon Valsalva maneuver by the patient (pressing downward with his pelvic muscles).

Sometimes a varicocele causes achiness or a boy feels a mushy lump inside the left side of the scrotum. These veins seem less prominent when a boy is lying down, because when he sits or stands gravity is more likely to pool blood in the veins.

Varicoceles are unlikely to cause problems in adolescence, but all varicoceles should be checked out by a doctor. The main concern is the preservation of the size of the affected testicle and the fertility (sperm production) of both testicles. In some instances surgery will be recommended.

INGUINAL HERNIA

While a male fetus is developing, the testicles are not in the scrotum but are tucked into a pouchlike space within the body. Just before birth, or in the weeks or months after birth, the testicles exit that space through a passage called the inguinal canal, go through an opening called the internal ring, and descend into the scrotum. The internal ring usually closes completely and permanently. But in some boys, it stays fully or partly open. If fully open, the internal ring may allow part of the intestine to slip through. This condition is called an inguinal hernia, and it appears as a soft bulge in the groin.

If the hernia is untreated, the pressure of the intestine may cause the opening to stretch even more, and more of the intestine may droop through it. Strangulation of the trapped portion of intestine is one danger, since loss of blood flow may cause that part to die. Inguinal hernias must be corrected through surgery to nudge the intestine out of the opening and back into place and to sew the opening closed so the hernia cannot recur.

HYDROCELE

A hydrocele is a collection of fluid in the scrotum. As with a hernia, a partial opening in the internal ring allows the condition to occur. The opening is not large enough for the intestine to pass into it, so it does not cause a hernia. But it is large enough to allow fluid to accumulate in the membranes surrounding the testicle.

A hydrocele may cause an uncomfortable feeling of fullness or heaviness but usually is asymptomatic. A hydrocele may be smaller in the morning, because fluid has drained overnight, and larger by the end of the day, when fluid has collected again. If large, a hydrocele may cause the testicle to appear to bulge, which can be embarrassing for the adolescent. While most hydroceles do not require treatment, one may need to be surgically repaired if it causes significant discomfort or if the testicle appears excessively large.

SPERMATOCELE

A spermatocele is another type of fluid-filled "lump" adjacent to the top portion of the testicle near the epididymis. Unlike a hydrocele, it rarely causes problems or needs treatment, and can be left alone once diagnosed by a physician.

TRAUMA

Some parents first consider the possibility of testicular trauma when their sons join Little League. The coach requires them to buy their son his first jockstrap and the hard plastic athletic cup that fits inside it. Some coaches line up the players before each game and walk down the line, knocking at the boys' crotches to make sure they are wearing the cup. The rule: If you don't wear the cup, you can't play the game. It is an early and important lesson on the importance of protecting testicles from harm.

The need for protection doesn't end with Little League. Tell your son to wear an athletic cup and supporter when he plays baseball, lacrosse, or any other team or pickup sport, or when he engages in any vigorous activity that could put him at risk, such as horseback riding. He should periodically check the fit to make sure the equipment is neither too large nor too small. Correct fit is essential for protection from genital injury.

If an adolescent is hit or kicked in his genitals, whether during sports or in a fight, he is likely to experience not only pain but to also feel sweaty, dizzy, and nauseated. If injuries are minor, these sensations and pain usually subside in less than an hour. However, it is necessary to see a doctor to rule out torsion (see page 153) or testicular rupture, which occurs when the testicle is crushed by an object or when the impact of a blow slams the testicle against the pubic bone. The impact may cause blood to seep into the scrotal sac.

When to See a Doctor After Testicular Trauma

See a doctor if:

- Pain lasts an hour or more.
- There is substantial swelling.
- The testicles or surrounding area is discolored.
- A testicle was punctured or crushed.
- There is vomiting or abdominal pain.
- There is any concern about the injury.

CRYPTORCHIDISM

A cryptorchid testicle is one that has not descended into the scrotum by the time of birth. The incidence of cryptorchidism is approximately 4 percent in full-term infants, and higher among premature infants. During gestation, testicles reside inside the lower abdomen. In most full-term infants born with one or both testicles not inside the scrotum, the testicles will spontaneously descend into the scrotum by six weeks, or among premature infant boys, by the age of three months. When testicles do not descend by the age of one year, surgery should be done to bring the testicles down into the scrotum. This procedure is done not only in order for the child to appear normal but also to protect future fertility, to lower the risk of testicular cancer, and to permit adequate examination of the testicles for early detection of testicular cancer.

What does this have to do with adolescence? Males with a history of undescended testicles have a higher incidence of infertility and are about twenty times more likely to develop testicular cancer than boys born with both testicles in the scrotum, even if the corrective surgery was done early in life. Boys with a history of one or both undescended testicles must be made aware of it and be especially urged to perform monthly testicular self-exams. In fact, both testicles are at increased risk of developing cancer, even if only one was undescended at birth. If an undescended testicle is diagnosed after puberty, testicle removal is recommended because it can no longer produce sperm and is at high risk for cancer.

TESTICULAR IMPLANT

A boy may wish to consider having a testicular implant placed into his scrotum to replace a testicle removed due to cryptorchidism, disease, or trauma.

Many men who have a testicle removed compare their situation with that of women who have a breast removed: A body part that represented part of their sexuality is gone. Just as some women want breast reconstruction or implants, and others do not, men also differ.

Some men want a prosthesis so they won't feel or appear so different from before. They think a prosthesis will help them feel more normal and less self-conscious with a sexual partner.

Men who do not want an implant often say that although the testicle was removed, their sexuality certainly was not. They prefer that their sexual partner accept them as they are, and do not feel self-conscious about appearing different. Indeed, some men say that having a single testicle does not make a significant difference in their appearance.

The technology is still evolving, with implants offering greater or lesser degrees of "real thing" feel, while newer models that might feel more natural linger in the Food and Drug Administration's lengthy approval process. The travails many women have had with adverse side effects of certain types of breast implants have made some men hesitate to go that route themselves. Furthermore, not every man who gets a prosthesis likes it. One man disliked the "spongy feel" of his implant. Another said his prosthesis was harder than a normal testicle. But some men are pleased with their implants.

The Testicular Cancer Resource Center does not recommend getting an implant "for cosmetic reasons," but acknowledges that the decision is very personal and provides information on its website (see "Resources").

Even if you think your son is not concerned about looking or feeling different after losing a testicle, or has not yet become sexually active, you or his doctor could initiate a discussion or arrange a consultation with a urologist who is experienced with testicular implants. It may seem like an awkward concept to introduce, but your son may be relieved to have this topic addressed and should know that implants are an option.

UNDERDEVELOPED TESTICLES

By age 14, testicular growth and development should be apparent. Failure of the testicles to grow during puberty may indicate a chromosomal abnormality such as Klinefelter's syndrome, in which a male has two X and one Y chromosomes (XXY) instead of the normal XY. Another possibility is that puberty was never triggered due to a hormonal deficiency originating in the hypothalamus or the pituitary gland. Testicular failure resulting from mumps, orchitis, or some other cause may also result in small testicles.

A boy with Klinefelter's syndrome usually has little or no facial and body hair, enlargement of his breasts (gynecomastia, see page 162), a tall and non-muscular physique, sometimes learning or behavioral difficulties, and a low sperm count. A boy with a hypothalamic-pituitary problem or testicular failure is more likely to resemble a prepubertal child of around age 10 or 11 in size and body shape. Precise diagnosis by an endocrinologist of which disorder exists is necessary in order to prescribe the most appropriate treatment.

PENILE HYGIENE AND DISEASE PREVENTION

CLEANING UNDER THE FORESKIN

Uncircumcised males must be aware of the importance of cleaning the penis properly. This is done by gently pulling the foreskin back toward the penile shaft, exposing the glans (head of the penis), washing the glans with warm water, and drying it thoroughly before replacing the foreskin.

If the glans is not kept clean and dry, a malodorous secretion called smegma may collect under the foreskin.

PHIMOSIS AND PARAPHIMOSIS

Cleaning under the foreskin is done not only for hygiene but because it also helps keep the foreskin supple and easily movable, thus preventing a few annoying problems. Phimosis is a condition in which the foreskin is attached so tightly and with so small an opening that it is difficult or impossible to slide it back off the glans. Phimosis may cause discomfort during urination or sexual activity and is surgically corrected by circumcision.

A condition called paraphimosis results if the retracted foreskin cannot easily be slid forward to cover the glans due to local swelling. Application of cold compresses and lubricating gels may aid in sliding the foreskin back into place. Circumcision will prevent a recurrence of this painful situation.

BALANITIS

Balanitis is an inflammation or infection of the glans of the penis, seen mainly in uncircumcised males, and often associated with phimosis. The inflammation may simply be an "irritation" or allergic reaction to spermicide or other substance, or infection with candida, a type of yeast that flourishes in moist environments, or infection with bacteria or a virus that may be sexually transmitted.

Symptoms of Balanitis

- Redness.
- Swelling.
- Itching.
- Burning.
- Discharge from under the foreskin.

A doctor will prescribe an appropriate cream, ointment, or antibiotic that is specific to the underlying cause of the balanitis. Most important, the adolescent must respond to balanitis by using improved and consistent hygiene in this area of his body.

TINEA CRURIS ("JOCK ITCH")

One unpleasant consequence of overly tight clothing is *tinea cruris,* more commonly known as "jock itch," a fungal skin infection that erupts in the moist creases of the genitals and inner thighs. The infection may cause the skin to turn red, itch, burn, crack, or peel. Applying an antifungal cream twice a day for up to several weeks, as well as keeping the area clean and dry (loose underwear and clothing helps), will cure the infection. Laundering clothing between wearings to destroy any fungus on them will prevent recurrences of infection.

PENILE DISORDERS

PINK PEARLY PAPULES

About 15 percent of males have pink pearly papules on the penis.[2] They are tiny benign bumps arranged in a row or in several parallel rows at the corona of the penis, the ridge at the bottom of the glans (head of the penis). Their name describes them well; they look like small pearls. They are harmless and do not need to be treated. However, self-diagnosis is never a good idea. Have a doctor take a look and confirm that they are indeed pink pearly papules and not the painless warts associated with the sexually transmitted disease HPV (human papilloma virus).

HYPOSPADIAS AND EPISPADIAS

Hypospadias and epispadias are abnormalities of fetal development in which the urethra does not extend to the center tip of the glans, but exits somewhere along the underside (hypospadias) or top (epispadias) of the penile shaft. Associated with this misplacement of the urethral opening is often a curving of the penile shaft. Except in the mildest cases, when these conditions may not be noticed until adolescence (especially at the time of erections), most boys will receive surgical correction during early childhood. Adolescents with hypospadias or epispadias may suffer from having a penis that looks "different" and that poses challenges when urinating or making love. These structural and functional difficulties range from nearly imperceptible in a boy with a slight curve and a urethral opening close to the glans to much more severe malformation and disability. Adolescents may find it helpful to access a chat room through the Hypospadias Association website or to explore, with their parents, the possibility of reconstructive surgery.[3]

PRIAPISM

Priapism is a persistent and painful erection caused by an excessive inflow of blood into the arteries of the penis and sluggish outflow of blood through the penile veins. Priapism should not be confused with normal, spontaneous, and long-lasting erections, which may be prolonged but are not painful.

Priapism occurs in adolescents with sickle cell anemia, and is uncommonly associated with other conditions including urethritis, trauma, or malignancy. Treatment should always involve a physician and includes ice packs and pain management, and on occasion surgical care.

IMPOTENCE

As embarrassed as boys can be by frequent, spontaneous erections, sexually active adolescents can be just as troubled about impotence, the inability to have or sustain an erection. Anxiety about sexual performance or insecurity within a relationship may cause a young man to lose an erection. Loss of momentum— for example, interrupting sex play to put on a condom—may also be a factor. For this reason, some young people avoid condoms, instead of realizing that condom use needs to be built into foreplay and regarded as part of the couple's sexual relationship. (And privately practicing putting on a condom prepares a young man for action when he is actually with his partner.) Alcohol or marijuana may loosen inhibitions but can also inhibit sexual performance, keeping a boy from getting or staying fully erect.

Many adolescent boys would have a hard time discussing a concern about impotence with a parent, and for most boys the problem improves with time. If the problem does not resolve, he should ask his doctor for advice. Specialists in adolescent medicine are especially attuned to the need to ask boys if they are sexually active and if everything is working okay.

Besides alcohol and recreational drugs, various medications (most especially antidepressants and high blood pressure meds) may interfere with libido and sexual functioning. Various medical, spinal cord, or surgical conditions may also be factors to consider.

URETHRITIS

Urethritis is an inflammation of the urethra, the tube that carries urine or semen through the penis.

Symptoms of Urethritis

- Painful burning sensation on urination.
- Discharge of mucus or pus from the urethral meatus (the opening at the end of the penis).

The infections that cause urethritis are predominantly sexually transmitted, most commonly chlamydia and gonorrhea, less commonly herpes, trichomonas, ureaplasma, or mycoplasma. Painful burning on urination may be due to a urinary tract infection, but this diagnosis is rare in a healthy adolescent boy who has no abnormality of his urinary system.

Urethritis caused by any of the infectious agents listed above is easily treated with antibiotics, especially if diagnosed early. Untreated urethritis can spread and cause epididymitis, or a disseminated form of gonorrhea characterized by arthritis and dermatitis. If urethritis occurs, it should be a wake-up call to the adolescent to inform his sexual partner(s) to be checked out by a doctor and treated, and in the future to always and correctly use a latex condom or abstain from sex to prevent a recurrence. (Also see the discussion of sexually transmitted diseases in chapter 8.)

GYNECOMASTIA

Gynecomastia is the presence of any breast tissue in a male that can be seen or felt. Mild gynecomastia (less than 4 centimeters in diameter) is very common, occurring in as many as 70 percent of boys, typically during the mid stages (Tanner 3–4) of pubertal development. A small lump of tissue appears under the nipple and areola (the darker area of skin surrounding the nipple) of one or both breasts, and is often tender. The lump may stay around for several months or, rarely, up to two to three years. Most often the tissue enlargement is apparent only to the boy himself, but sometimes the breast tissue grows to resemble female breasts that visibly protrude beneath a T-shirt. This situation can be disturbing or even devastating to any boy, especially at this vulnerable stage of his development, when body image and self-esteem are often fragile.

It is not known for certain why many but not all boys develop gynecomastia. It is thought to result perhaps from a temporary hormonal imbalance that occurs during these mid stages of development. A mild and temporary presence of breast tissue is almost always the case in a healthy boy, taking no medications, whose pubertal development is normal. Less commonly, gynecomastia may result from the ingestion of certain medications or recreational drugs, malnutrition, a chronic illness, a hormonal or genetic disorder (for example, Klinefelter's syndrome, described on page 158), or a tumor.

Although for the great majority of boys, gynecomastia is related to the unpredictable hormonal hijinks of puberty, its presence can compound a boy's lack of confidence or worries about sexual identity. Gynecomastia can be devastating to a boy who wants more than anything to appear manly. Reassure him that the growth of breast tissue does not indicate anything about his virility. It may comfort him to know that for most affected males, also in the middle stages of puberty (Tanner stages 3–4), gynecomastia subsides within six to twelve months. Boys who have more severe breast enlargement, or persistence of breast tissue beyond the expected time frame of six months to two years, or simply feel too upset by its presence, may consult with a plastic surgeon to discuss surgical intervention, the most reliable and safest form of treatment.

HEALTH-PARTNERING TIPS FOR PARENTS

- *Eradicate embarrassment.* Encourage candid discussion of all sorts of health issues, including reproductive health. Tell your son that if he ever has any pain or discomfort in his testicles or penis, or any question about how they look, he needs to speak up immediately. Don't let embarrassment lead to a delay in treatment—and possibly serious consequences.
- *Encourage testicular self-exam.* "Know thyself" is time-honored advice, and should refer to knowing not only one's mind and soul but one's body, too.
- *Be aware of your child's rate of development.* If your child does not seem to be maturing, ask him about it. (Again, this requires a no-embarrassment policy.) Is he noticing any changes, such as pubic hair growth? Consult your child's doctor if you suspect any problems.
- *Be sympathetic to voice changes.* If your son is worried about his voice cracking or squeaking, reassure him that this is normal and won't last. If he must do public speaking (such as on a debate team, for his bar mitzvah, or for a school report), remind him that everyone goes through voice change. If his voice cracks, he should just smile and continue with his speech.
- *Be alert for signs of steroid use.* Some boys use steroids to appear more muscular or enhance athletic performance. Steroids are dangerous. Warn your son of the dangers, and watch for and inform your son's doctor of excessive signs of masculinization that seem to be out of sync with your son's age and rate of development, such as rapid "bulking up" of muscles, deepening of voice, or hairiness.
- *Speak directly to your son and his doctor.* Be sure the doctor is examining your son's genitals and breasts, teaching him and encouraging testicular self-exam, informing him of symptoms of testicular torsion and other disorders, discussing aspects of sexual functioning and safe sexual practices, and encouraging your son to speak up about any questions or concerns—even if they are embarrassing.

SEVEN: Coping with Chronic Health Problems

In *Living with Diabetes,* Nicole Johnson, who went on to become Miss America 1999, recalls being hospitalized at age 19 and receiving a diagnosis of diabetes:

> Control over my life was completely stripped away along with my shoes and clothing. I was put in bed and people began fussing over me. A bracelet was put on my wrist, like a handcuff declaring me a prisoner for a crime I hadn't committed. I resented the nurses and doctors who were taking care of me. I felt that they were the ones stealing my life, as if their presence caused the disease. I knew deep inside that it wasn't their fault, of course . . . I felt manacled to this thing called diabetes . . .[1]

Much as they like to be appreciated as individuals, most adolescents ardently want to blend in with their peers. But adolescents with chronic health problems face reminders every day that they are "different." Indeed, improved medical treatments and technologies have extended life, and mainstream inclusion in school and other activities is normal now for many adolescents who not that long ago would likely have died or lived extremely curtailed lives. In this chapter we will discuss how chronic diseases affect adolescents' lives and describe the most common ones.

CHRONIC HEALTH PROBLEMS DIFFER

It is useful to understand and acknowledge that all chronic health problems are not alike. Their differences pose different kinds of challenges for the teenagers trying to successfully cope and for their parents trying to appropriately help them.

Some are congenital (since birth). Others strike suddenly later in childhood or during adolescence. A child born with spina bifida and lower limb paralysis has always had to incorporate the disability into his life. An injured champion skier with a similar disability must deal with a sudden tragic loss.

Some affect the individual's appearance as with a physical handicap or deformity or by stunting height, weight, and pubertal development, which may occur if the illness presents before or during the early adolescent years. Other illnesses are hidden from view. A ten-year-old with severe inflammatory bowel disease (such as Crohn's disease) may not enter puberty until age 16 and looks much younger than he is, whereas a teen with epilepsy looks totally healthy and her actual age.

Some illnesses can effectively be controlled by an individual's compliant use of medications and other treatments, while other illnesses seem to have "a mind of their own" and wax and wane or progress no matter what the teenager does to take good care of himself. A teen with diabetes or asthma can substantially control the illness and how he feels. A teen with lupus or rheumatoid arthritis must learn to endure flare-ups even when she takes "perfect" care of herself. And a 20-year-old with cystic fibrosis or sickle cell disease must face the prospect of a shortened life span despite great strides in the medical treatment of these diseases.

Some very serious illnesses go away while others simply never get better or worse. Many teens with cancer are cured and can put the problem behind themselves forever, except for lingering worry about long-term effects of their treatments. A mentally retarded teen learns to accept her fate and live within the bounds of her disability.

HEALTH COPING SKILLS

Learning to live with a chronic health problem requires an evolving set of skills. The adolescent

- Must learn or take greater responsibility for self-care and medical management strategies.
- Must cultivate emotional fortitude, in order to stay hopeful and withstand other people's lack of knowledge or empathy.
- Must come to terms with the condition, in order to visualize and pursue goals that can be achieved within any limitations the condition may impose.

These are demanding competencies to ask of an adolescent—but in fact, adolescents ask these things of themselves. They may pass many anguished nights, resenting their illness or despairing of finding a place for themselves in a world geared to the able-bodied and able-minded. But with the support and faith of their family, health care providers, and friends, these adolescents can become more resilient, independent, and optimistic adults than many of their peers.

In addition to developing these health-related skills, young people with chronic health problems are by no means exempt from the three fundamental tasks of adolescence that were described in chapter 1, nor do they want to be. In this way, they share a powerful common denominator with their healthier peers. The themes of independence, sexuality, and planning for the future weave through these adolescents' lives. In this chapter we will review the tasks within the context of chronic health problems, and identify ways that parents can support their adolescent through this process.

Adolescent Task #1
TO GAIN INDEPENDENCE

*To Feel Capable of Approaching Life's Challenges,
Based on a Personal Belief System of Values and Priorities*

To an adolescent, nothing is more desirable (and scary) than independence. What a powerful feeling, to be in control of your own life—nobody telling you what to do with your time, your body, your friends. *(But, hey, don't abandon me here!)*

Some adolescents can control their own health, and do not feel significantly hampered by their conditions. Josh, age 15, for example, is resolutely cheery as he discusses his asthma.

I was diagnosed with asthma when I was about 3. My mom has it, but my dad and brother don't. With my medicines, my asthma has always been completely under control. I mean, I've never been in serious danger. Asthma has never stopped me from anything I wanted to do—except maybe long-distance running or sprinting full out during a basketball game. My breathing gets too short. I have to stop and lock my hands behind my head, or hold them up in the air and walk. Or I put hands on my knees and bend over for a few seconds. That gets the adrenaline going somehow. You'd think that I'd feel a lull. Instead, taking the break gets me going again.

My friends have grown faster than I have. My doctor said asthma does not stunt growth but makes you grow later in life. He said I have a very good chance to be six feet tall. I'm 15 and I'm just starting to get taller. Finally! The problem is not that I'm that short. It's just that for some reason I hang out with tall friends.

Josh's parents can count on him to carry and use his medications properly, and not to push himself too hard.

In contrast, Lowell, also 15, has a more serious case of asthma, but has yet to learn how to cope with it. While Josh is almost blasé about his asthma, Lowell is ashamed. In the gym, he would rather slouch against the wall and struggle to catch his breath than admit to the teacher that he has asthma. His school, responding to the city's asthma epidemic, sent home flyers that explained how parents could request permission for children with asthma to use inhalers in school. Lowell threw his flyer away.

"I don't want guys pointing at me as the guy with the disease," says Lowell. "Forget it. I'll be okay."

Yet his frequent absences from school make it hard for Lowell to keep up with his schoolwork.

Perhaps what Lowell was missing, but Josh got in ample supply, was the kind of health support that went beyond delivering diagnosis and medications, and addressed the emotional impact of having the disease.

Levels of Help from a Medical Support Team

The essence of educating adolescents about their health is not simply to deliver the facts but to help these young patients assimilate the information—literally, "learn to live with it." This involves encouraging adolescents to develop constructive attitudes and practice effective health-management skills.

One person may not be able to provide help on all of these levels, even if that person is an esteemed specialist. It helps to think of having a medical support team. Parents are part of the team. A team may include a nurse, therapist, social worker, nutritionist, support group, or other individuals to help support, teach, and listen to the adolescent.

Rare is the adolescent who simply acquiesces and says, "Okay, tell me what to do and I'll do it." Adolescents often deny their illness, resist treatment, or are inconsistent. Sometimes "good patients" lapse, tired of toeing the line. An adolescent's support team can help identify and address lapses quickly and strengthen his or her capacity for self-care.

Encourage your adolescent to communicate directly with the doctor and other members of the team. Suggest that your adolescent write down concerns or questions, then bring the list to medical appointments and jot down the answers, either alone or with your help. Keeping the questions in a single notebook will provide a cumulative record that the adolescent can review as needed. Eventually, you will be proud to slip more and more into the background as your adolescent takes a more assertive role.

Support Groups and Mentors

Some doctors, hospitals, and organizations can introduce adolescents to others with the same health problem. The adolescent may join a support group with other teens or be referred to an adult "mentor" who passes on some good advice and listens with an "I've been there" sagacity. Groups or mentors make adolescents feel less alone and better equipped to anticipate and handle the challenges that are bound to come along.

For example, adolescents sometimes need some tips simply on how to explain their condition to their friends. It helps to learn how others with the disease talk about it. They don't have to reinvent the wheel, but are prepared with a ready-made, proven explanation.

> *Jocelyn, 14, attended a support group for adolescents with asthma. The group leader mentioned a simple way to help people understand asthma. Not long thereafter, Jocelyn had an opportunity to put the tip into action. After missing school for a few days with an asthma attack, she was sitting in the school cafeteria with friends.*
>
> *"What does asthma feel like?" one girl asked.*
>
> *Jocelyn remembered her support group.*
>
> *"Pinch your straw," she told her friend, "then try to drink your milk."*
>
> *With her fingers compressing the plastic straw, her friend had to struggle to get a single sip.*
>
> *"That's how it feels when I try to breathe," said Jocelyn. "I have to fight for air."*

Baby Steps Add Up

Parents and health care providers must tread a careful line between their desire to protect and adolescents' increasing desire to protect themselves.

Especially if an adolescent's health problem began at birth or during early childhood, everyone in the family is used to the parents being in very careful charge. Indeed, that system was probably comforting to the child, who felt well taken care of.

Nowadays, however, the adolescent's gratitude seems to be in short supply. Still too young and self-centered to appreciate the parents' sacrifices, the adolescent is focusing only on the parents' strictures. But parents can only relax and relinquish control when they feel convinced that their adolescent is ready to take it on—and is mindful of the possible consequences of messing up.

On the other hand, just how perfect does the adolescent need to be? Clarify just how much leeway there may be with various aspects of the adolescent's self-care. Does she always need to give herself a shot at 10 P.M.—or on the night of a party, can she put it off until she comes home at midnight?

In partnership with your adolescent and the doctor, make a plan that clarifies how your teen can begin to take over more aspects of his or her care. Start small. As the adolescent demonstrates responsibility, gradually cede control.

The Urge to Rebel

A chronic illness might feel like a constant test—and an adolescent some-times cannot resist testing it right back. A diabetic teen, for example, fed up with always having to test blood sugar and inject insulin, might erupt in frus-tration one day and conduct an experiment: *What would happen if I just stopped?* Or rebel: *I'm tired of people telling me what I have to do.* Or indulge in a little magical thinking: *Maybe all this insulin I've been taking has turned things around—or has masked the fact that I don't need it any more!*

These interior monologues occur when adolescents' emotional immaturity collides with their intellect. They know the medical facts they have to live with. But they don't like those realities. Even if this game of pretend is haz-ardous, it is too tempting to resist:

Scott played a dangerous game of chicken with his own disease. In his freshman year of college, he was on his own for the first time. He stayed up late, pigged out on desserts, and got way off schedule with his insulin injections. It was as if he were flirting with his own body, dodging his system's threatened breakdowns by jumping in just in time with a glass of orange juice or a decent meal when his glucose strips indicated he was taking things too far.

During sophomore year Scott fell in love with Brenda. She thought it was kind of cool to watch him inject himself with insulin every morning, but otherwise never gave much thought to his diabetes. Why should she? It was his business, and he was on top of it—she thought.

One night, Scott collapsed. Brenda stayed at the hospital all night to make sure he was okay. When he was out of danger, she finally let out her feelings—and they were not tender.

"What is wrong with you? Do you expect me to simply stand by, won-dering if this is going to happen again? I am not going to be your mommy. Either you act like a man and take care of yourself or we're through."

It was a pivotal moment for Scott. For the first time, he realized that neglecting his health was not some rakish expression of rebellion, but that it burdened and upset the people he cared about.

Independence of Mind

"Independence" is not just about controlling an illness the best one can by following a doctor's advice and parents' admonitions. It's also about making personal choices and being in the driver's seat, not the backseat, when consult-ing with others or thinking on one's own about how to live your life. All teens have to work on achieving such an independence of mind, but a teen with a chronic illness or handicap and that teen's parents will have to work even harder to overcome a pattern of dependency and protectiveness that began many years before.

Even in early adolescence, teens with chronic health problems should begin spending time alone with their doctor or other members of their health team. Conferencing about how things are going and treatments should be directed primarily to the maturing adolescent, with parents listening a little bit in the background, and not the other way around. The teen should be given the first opportunity to ask any questions, and then comes the parents' turn. After all, *the teen* is the patient. Prescriptions and next appointment cards should be handed to the teen first. With such approaches, doctors and other health professionals begin to chart a new relationship with the teen that fosters independence, and in turn enhances the teen's taking responsibility for his or her own care.

Jane had been seizure-free on medications for three years and was now eligible by state law to learn to drive and get her license. Her parents offered to drive her anywhere she needed to go. Her mom and dad even alternated working shorter days at their jobs to accommodate Jane after school in case she needed them to take her somewhere.

Mom kept saying, "Don't worry about getting your license. We are happy to drive you."

Dad firmly agreed. "We probably should wait at least another year to see what happens with your seizures," he said.

Jane felt both frightened and exhilarated by the thought of driving on her own. After months of silence on the subject, she announced one day that she had gotten her permit and planned to begin driving lessons.

Sometimes a teen has to assert not only a need, but also a right, to disagree with his or her parents.

Harold had struggled since age 14 with a rare form of cancer that carried an uncertain prognosis. Over the past four years, he enjoyed months of relative good health alternating with months of heightened debilitation. Early on, his parents hadn't told him the whole story. At first his treatments went smoothly and he felt pretty well and optimistic. In the second year the illness worsened and treatments became more difficult to endure, but repeatedly he pulled through.

Now his doctors were offering an experimental treatment that could bring about a cure or could fail miserably. Harold's parents, above all, didn't want to lose him. Harold, above all, wanted an opportunity to get on with his life. Against their wishes, but with their blessings, he mustered the independence of mind to decide to chance the experimental treatment.

Taking insulin regularly and using an asthma inhaler are easy compared with having to think through and make decisions, sometimes with life-and-death implications, which may even go against parents' wishes or best judgment. It is equally tough and excruciating for parents to "let go" and let their adolescent do what he or she needs to do.

For both teens and their parents, the Serenity Prayer provides comfort and guidance: "Grant me the serenity to accept the things I cannot change, courage to change the things I can, and the wisdom to know the difference."

Adolescent Task #2
TO CLARIFY SEXUAL IDENTITY

*To Feel Comfortable in a Mature Body and
in Establishing Close and Intimate Relationships*

Sexuality is a universal element of the human experience. Adolescents with health problems and disabilities have the same longing as their peers to love and be loved, to touch and be touched, to experience intimacy.

They want to wear fashionable clothing. They want to keep up with popular music, movies, and TV shows. They want to receive compliments on their hair or manicure, their pretty eyes or their charming smile. They want to be invited to parties, to a movie, to a basketball game. They want to be desired.

Inextricably bound up with sexual feelings is body image, a sense of one's own attractiveness based on one's own feelings and on other people's reactions. It is difficult enough to figure out how to handle sexual feelings, and even healthy adolescents agonize about whether other people like the way they look. All people want to be loved for who they are, warts and all. But adolescents with chronic health problems may worry that their "warts" are more than most partners are willing to handle.

In some instances, an adolescent's health issue proves to be a nonissue: *I don't care that you have a heart problem. I like being with you.* But other adolescents may need to prepare in advance for the stressful but urgent process of finding a partner.

Parents and other members of their medical support team can help the adolescent be prepared by discussing such issues as how to:

- Select partners who are more likely to be receptive to the news.
- Explain the disease and its symptoms, treatments, and limitations.
- Cope with rejection.
- Muster the faith that someday the right person will come along—someone who lovingly accepts that health problems are part of the package.

An adolescent can find it immeasurably encouraging to hear about a support group member or an adult mentor who is in a good relationship: *Yes, it is possible to find love—here's the evidence. Keep looking, you'll find love, too.*

An Unseen Disease

What if I have a seizure in school? I'd be so embarrassed!

What if I have an asthma attack—will he know what to do?

You should have seen her face when she came over and saw my insulin syringes on my dresser.

She seemed disappointed that I can't join a team.

You can't tell by looking at people whether they have epilepsy, asthma, diabetes, or congenital heart disease. But having them can still shake adolescents' sexual self-confidence, especially if they feel they must conceal their disease. It is stressful to keep such a secret, to worry about being "found out."

An adolescent may fear that a prospective partner might be turned off, fearful of "catching something," or unwilling to invest emotional energy in a person with iffy long-term health prospects.

So disclosing the health condition is just the beginning. The adolescent may also need to be an educator, a salesperson, and a spin doctor, putting the best face on things and dispelling myths.

No, you can't catch asthma.

Yes, my diabetes is under control.

Yes, I occasionally have a seizure, but I am getting all A's.

No, my cardiologist says I can't go on long bike rides, but we can take long walks or go to the movies.

A support group can be invaluable here, as adolescents share how they have coped with people on the "outside" who needed to be initiated into their world.

The Naked Truth

What if she hugs me and feels the bulge of my ostomy pouch?

I always wear crewneck or turtleneck shirts because of the big ugly scars on my chest from surgery. What will happen when my shirt comes off?

Will he be able to look at the stump of my amputated leg?

With clothes on, it's easy to "pass" as normal. But at some point an adolescent may need to tell someone what will be revealed when the clothes come off.

Prospective partners can't be counted on to react with grace and tact. The worst-case scenario is not only the brutal insult, but also the averted eyes, the quick exit, the phone calls that suddenly stop. So an adolescent with "something to hide" may want to bide his or her time indefinitely. It's like feeling stuck in the middle of a seesaw. One moment, the eagerness to take a relationship to the next level has the upper hand. Then it is pushed down by the pressure to stay within the safety zone of the status quo.

But at some point, relationships come down to this: *We either move forward or we move on.* Due to the adolescent's own urges or a partner's insistence on going further, kissing and fully clothed touching will not be enough. The moment may come when there's nowhere to hide.

Even adults are notoriously backward when it comes to talking about sensitive sexual issues. The media certainly don't help when they portray partners coupling wordlessly, without uttering a single caveat about using condoms (or first getting to know each other better).

So these adolescents have to master sexual ground that daunts people older (though not necessarily wiser) than they are. Either on their own, or with some deft and sensitive coaching from a support group or a member of their medical team, they need to come up with some opening lines:

I'm really attracted to you. But I'm a little self-conscious about something, and we need to talk about it.

We're so honest with each other. That means a lot to me, and I respect you. So I need you to know that if we become intimate, I will understand if it takes you a while to get used to the way I look.

I really want us to feel comfortable together. I hope you'll ask me any questions you may have about my health, or anything you're concerned about.

These statements, of course, are only the beginning. Throughout a relationship, an adolescent with a chronic health problem may need to take the initiative in keeping lines of communication open. This may include explaining a relapse, a new treatment, or even mood swings or other side effects of a medication.

Visibly Different

Paradoxically, an adolescent with an easily visible health condition may have it easier than one whose problem is hidden. Visibly affected teens don't have to endure the suspense of wondering how someone will receive their secret news. For these adolescents, "what you see is what you get."

But there will still be some explaining to do:

- *Welcome to Barrier Land.* Able-bodied folks often have no clue about navigating a world that still has a lot to learn about being "handicapped accessible." It can be a real eye-opener to discover that a particular movie theater's ramp is practically useless because there's no cut in the curb to give access to it.

- *"I never heard of that disease."* It's the story behind the story: why an adolescent looks or acts a certain way. He limps because juvenile rheumatoid arthritis caused one leg to grow longer than the other. She is so tall because she has Marfan's syndrome. He blurts out obscenities when stressed because he has Tourette's syndrome. The only way she will reach five feet tall is by wearing high heels, because she has growth hormone deficiency. He still looks so young because cystic fibrosis causes pubertal delay. She has an eyelid that droops because she had a brain stem tumor that affected her facial muscles.

- *Medications save lives and play tricks.* An adolescent being treated for lupus has to take a steroid medication that causes severe acne and a chubby torso. Another adolescent has lost all her hair from having chemotherapy for cancer.

Adolescents should not have to feel that they must divulge their life or medical stories. They have as much of a right to privacy as anyone else. But they should also be aware of the upside of openness. The more comfortable they are talking about their conditions, the more comfortable they will make other people feel.

Many able-bodied people pair up with disabled ones, or people with one disability pair off with someone with a different disability. To these couples, what counts most is love and trust, good times, sexual chemistry, companionship, and mutual interests.

Mature Body, Childlike Mind

Mentally retarded adolescents are likely to have sexual curiosity and desires that are just as lively as those of other adolescents. It is especially important that they receive the sexuality education they need to assure their emotional and sexual protection.

Not all programs for mentally retarded teens do an exemplary job with this. Some deny the need. Others give sexuality education short shrift or do not gear it to the adolescents' ability to learn. For example, some teachers and parents may discuss abstinence but not clearly define it. Euphemisms don't work with literal-minded young people. Telling a girl to "keep her clothes on" may not necessarily translate, in her mind, to "do not have sexual intercourse." She might think that having sex is okay if she just pushes her panties aside. Be clear. Tell girls, "Do not let anyone put his penis or anything else into your vagina." Tell both boys and girls: "Do not let anyone put his penis or anything else into your mouth or anus."

Similarly, it is not enough to say "Use a condom." Mentally retarded adolescents need to see and feel a condom and practice putting it on an anatomically correct model. As with other skills, they can learn the steps of correct condom use with plenty of repetition and practice. Mentally retarded girls may need birth control; the Pill or Depo-Provera might work quite well. (See chapter 8 for more about birth control.)

Mentally retarded adolescents are often especially susceptible to sexual abuse, often by older teens who callously exploit their disability. Flattered by attention or lured into unsafe situations, mentally retarded adolescents may suffer physical and emotional harm, get pregnant, or contract a disease. Whether or not the school's program addresses abuse prevention adequately, parents need to discuss it, too. Together with your adolescent, regularly role-play "risk scenarios" and talk about safety. Doing so not only helps prepare your adolescent for greater independence, it also increases the likelihood that he or she will tell you if something goes wrong.

Adolescent Task #3
TO EXPLORE SOCIETAL ROLE AND SELF-IMAGE

*To Feel Clarity of Direction to Assume Mature Roles
Based on Interests, Talents, and Opportunities*

Tomorrow waits, an open expanse, like a blank page awaiting a pen. A page can hold only so much; choices must be made. Chronic health problems differ in the degree to which they limit or dictate an adolescent's choices in how to live now and how to plan for the future. Pivotal to the adolescent's prospects are his or her adjustment to the demands of the disease, emotional stability, access to support, and ability to explore what *can* be without being embittered by what cannot.

Chronic health problems may occupy a limited space in an adolescent's daily life or play a significant role. When adolescents are forced to bow to the demands of their disease, their success in swerving around obstacles and finding satisfying alternatives is greatly affected by their attitude.

Just Another Set of Habits

Joanne, a diabetic adolescent, is so used to glucose testing and insulin injections that they have become as routine as washing her hair in the morning or watering the plants on her windowsill. A sociable girl who loves playing the piano, Joanne smoothly incorporates her disease into her life.

"Diabetes doesn't stop me from doing whatever I want," she says. "When I'm out with my friends, I've learned to pass up the chocolate cake without feeling like I'm the odd one out. In fact, I have learned so much about nutrition that I am collecting yummy recipes for a cookbook for diabetics."

Kurt, who has a relatively mild case of asthma, keeps a mental checklist of do's and don'ts: *Carry an inhaler, vacuum dust regularly, pet pets rarely, check lung function with a peak-flow meter to detect early signs of a potential asthma attack, and use treatment accordingly.* He considers himself a normal teen with an extra layer of things to which he has to pay attention. Sure, he would like to be able to compete in track and field. But he has channeled that interest into covering sports for the school newspaper.

Accommodations and Alternatives

Alvin always must take into account the factors that can exacerbate his chronic eczema and many allergies. He is something of a clotheshorse but confines himself to cotton and other natural fabrics that are kinder to his skin. He has developed a killer barbecue sauce but probably won't pursue a career as a chef. The constant handwashing, let alone being exposed to a wide variety of foods, could end up making his life miserable. He loves photography but cannot tolerate darkroom chemicals. Switching to a digital camera took care of that problem.

Brynna has rheumatoid arthritis. Some days she feels pretty good, and some days she feels awful, and she can't tell until she wakes up in the morning what kind of day it will be. So when she makes plans with friends, she has to "educate" them, explaining that she will not be able to confirm arrangements until the day of the event.

It can be a frustrating experience to have to make every plan a tentative one—but Brynna has figured out two ways to cope with the situation. First, she has learned not to waste energy lamenting her disease; it helps to accept that some days will be tough. Second, she and a couple of her closest friends deliberately "save" some videos for those times when plans have had to be canceled. Brynna has watched so many videos, in fact, that her friends call her to ask for recommendations. Brynna wants to combine her interest in film and writing to become a freelance movie reviewer. This career would give her the flexibility to work when she is well and take off when she is not.

Alvin's and Brynna's attitudes help them cope. As Martin E. P. Seligman, Ph.D., wrote in *Learned Optimism,* "Optimism and pessimism affect health itself, almost as clearly as do physical factors."[2]

Translating Disability into Passion

Until a few years ago, Olivia could see as well as anyone. Then she began losing peripheral vision and was diagnosed with retinitis pigmentosa. Her field of vision is narrowing rapidly, and she knows she may someday be totally blind.

Olivia is not giving up without a fight. She has avidly explored technological advancements for the visually impaired, and has decided to make it her life mission to advocate for research and programs for the blind. While some adolescents yearn for more "mainstream" lives, Olivia feels that her disease has revealed her calling, giving her a purpose in life.

Other adolescents have channeled their health problems into careers as nurses, doctors, researchers, teachers, therapists, and lobbyists. Patient activists have argued successfully for bigger budgets and improved programs for people with AIDS, breast cancer, and other diseases.

IN THE SHADOWS: DEPRESSION AND UNSAFE BEHAVIORS

The adolescents described above have not exactly embraced their diseases, but they have found ways to live with them. However, many adolescents wrestle terribly with their illnesses, often feeling knocked down and unable to struggle to their feet. They often fall into depression, substance abuse, unsafe sex, and other risk-taking behaviors.

Depression

Depression is a hazard that often comes with the territory of chronic illness. While plenty of attention may be paid to an adolescent's physical disability, her bleak state of mind may go untreated. Yet her depression is inextricably linked with her overall state of health. A depressed adolescent may neglect the three basics of health described in chapter 3—nutrition, exercise, and sleep. She may feel such a sense of hopelessness that she sabotages her own medical care, skipping doses of medicine or failing to keep appointments. Depression may make an adolescent suicidal, and any comments the adolescent may make about wanting to end it all or give up hope must be taken very seriously.

It is essential to recognize that depression is not an inevitable, inescapable, or untreatable response to a chronic health condition. If your adolescent shows symptoms of possible depression, including lack of appetite or overeating, getting too much or too little sleep, request a referral for a psychiatric evaluation in addition to exploring medical explanations. Depression is a treatable disease. Medication and/or psychotherapy may help lift an adolescent from hopelessness. (See chapter 11, "Your Teen's Mental Health.")

Substance Abuse

To some adolescents with chronic health problems, alcohol or other drug use may almost seem like a logical way to respond to their difficulties. In our society, after all, many people—with *and* without chronic health problems—"self-medicate" in response to pain, distress, isolation, and a bitter awareness of their own mortality.

Some adolescents with chronic health problems smoke, even those who have lung disorders such as cystic fibrosis and asthma. Others drink or experiment with the range of drugs described in chapter 9. Adolescents whose health is already precarious, such as those with cardiac disease, may be at even higher risk of death from stimulants such as cocaine or amphetamines. Adolescents also may risk taking drugs that will interact with their medications, with devastating results.

How terribly ironic that some adolescents who have every reason to take extra-good care of their health instead choose to defiantly test it further by using drugs. Furthermore, with all the medical attention adolescents can get, clinicians might overlook signs of substance abuse.

Risk-Taking Sexual Behavior

Like substance abuse, unsafe sex and other risky behaviors can grow out of an adolescent's desire to "act out" rage about health problems. Adolescents may turn to promiscuous or unsafe sex to seek validation of their attractiveness, to escape real-world troubles, or to rebel against the compliant-child, good-patient personas in which they have often been cast during countless doctor's appointments and hospital visits.

Emotional stress, low self-esteem, sexually transmitted diseases, and unwanted pregnancy will only further complicate their lives and compromise their health. Counseling on safer sex and healthy decision making must be part of their overall care plan.

Poor Compliance with Health Care

Some adolescents express their morbid resentment of their diseases by defying their doctor's advice, skipping or abandoning medications, or spurning treatment. It is heartbreaking to see a kidney transplant recipient throw away his chance at life through reckless disregard of medical advice—or to see teenagers with diabetes, asthma, or seizures not take medications that can truly control their diseases.

Health care providers should be sensitive to their adolescent patients' overall state of mind, paying extra attention to providing support and supervision as needed. Parents who see or suspect that their adolescent is disregarding or flouting medical advice may request a psychiatric evaluation, and perhaps request help in collaborating with the adolescent on a plan to improve compliance. It is important to keep in mind that the teenager with a chronic health problem is first and foremost a teenager, and to remember to look for assistance to find situations that focus on helping the *whole adolescent* achieve his potential and not simply on enhancing compliance with treatment of the disease. Various approaches—including individual psychotherapy, behavioral strategies, and group therapy (with teens with the same disease or with teens experiencing other problems but not chronically ill)—can be enormously relieving and helpful for the adolescent struggling with his feelings.

Family Stress

Tension in a family may or may not predate an adolescent's diagnosis with a chronic health problem. But ongoing family discord can markedly affect an adolescent's behavior and outlook. Just as a supportive family can help an adolescent through rough times, a dysfunctional family can plunge an adolescent further into despair, rebellion, and recklessness.

An adolescent's chronic illness affects all members of a family. Emotional and financial stress and the need to provide or arrange constant or occasional care can strain marriages. Parents may feel guilty for passing on defective chromosomes. They may feel despondent that they cannot afford the best possible care or facilities—or may strain their bank accounts to the detriment of other family members' needs.

Siblings may resent the ill adolescent's claims on attention, even as they feel guilty for having such feelings. They may wonder why they escaped with their own health, and might experience "survivor guilt." They may feel cut loose as parents leave them to fend for themselves, or feel indignant that they must do chores and adhere to certain rules, while in their judgment the overindulged adolescent with the health problem seemingly gets a free ride.

Many families have found marital counseling or family therapy indispensable for helping them cope with these and many other issues. Positive family support is one of the most crucial elements to adolescents' ability to cope with their health—but no one said it was easy.

EXPLORING THE POSSIBLE

Every individual has a different answer to the question of what makes life meaningful. Adolescents with chronic health problems must formulate an answer that can co-exist with the demands of their disease. Whether or not it is "fair," they must develop the knack of thriving within any health-imposed limits. They must identify talents and professions and living situations that work for them within the context in which they must live.

An adolescent with Down's syndrome, unlike her siblings, may not be able to have her own apartment. But she may be able to move into a group home.

And a young man with a rare form of cancer may settle near the university best known for researching it—and still maintain his business of handcrafting mandolins.

"UnpredictAbility"

Such illnesses as inflammatory bowel disease and lupus inflict a certain measure of unwanted suspense on adolescents, for they never know when they will experience a flare-up of symptoms and need to be hospitalized. For these adolescents perhaps a new expression can be coined: unpredictAbility, the skill of coping with the unforeseen. This skill involves devising contingency plans, cultivating hope, and rolling with the punches.

Able-bodied people do not have to live like this. They blithely make long-term plans, unaware of what a luxury that may seem to a person who lives with a constant fear of disease recurrence.

Yet perhaps they will never taste the intense appreciation of each day of good health and the gifts of life held by those with an illness.

HEALTH-PARTNERING TIPS FOR PARENTS

- *Assemble the best possible medical support team.* In addition to top-notch physicians, check out organizations in your community that offer medical information, support groups, and other programs for adolescents with chronic health problems and their families.
- *Encourage your adolescent to become educated about both illness and options.* Understanding how certain treatments or medications work can help your adolescent stay on track. Reading a book such as *The Road Back: Living with a Physical Disability*[3] can empower your adolescent to

explore new ways of coping with a disability, making new friends, and making constructive plans for the future (see "Books for Teens" in Resources section).

- *Keep track of the "three basics."* As discussed in chapter 3, nutrition, exercise, and sleep are important for all adolescents and should be considered integral to your child's overall health care plan.
- *Support your adolescent's independence at school.* Adolescents with chronic health problems can often self-administer medication, plan their own schedule, participate in extracurricular activities, and obtain other needed services in school. However, not all school administrators, teachers, and counselors are knowledgeable about the scope of services that are possible, available, or indeed required by law for students with illnesses and disabilities. If your child's school is unreceptive to your adolescent's requests, explore the matter further (contact the school district office).
- *Expect and acknowledge that your adolescent will have sexual and romantic desires.* Be available to listen.
- *Make sure your adolescent is well-informed about abstinence, safer sex, and the risks of alcohol and other drug use.* Discuss these topics and obtain educational materials.
- *Encourage your adolescent to express his or her feelings and ideas.* In addition to joining a support group, your adolescent may find it useful to keep a journal, check out Internet support sites, or see a therapist for individual or group counseling.
- *Assist your adolescent in beginning to explore paths for higher education, summer jobs, or career planning,* even if it means moving away from home.
- *Remember the healing power of the arts.* Music, theater, art, and dance can add a great deal to your adolescent's life, whether he or she is a participant or an observer.
- *Always remember that your child first and foremost is an adolescent who strives for the same goals as all teens and wants to grow up to be a contributing member of society.* Help your adolescent achieve full potential, now and in the future, by limiting the amount of space the illness is allowed to occupy, and focusing on his or her individuality and strengths.

Following are descriptions of six chronic illnesses that are some of the most common among adolescents. Each presents challenges for teens, who must cope with the confluence of managing an illness and mastering developmental tasks.

ARTHRITIS

The word *arthritis* means "inflammation of a joint, such as the ankle, knee, hip, finger, wrist, elbow, shoulder, and spine." Inflammation of a joint includes the signs and symptoms of swelling, redness, warmth, and pain, especially on movement of the joint.

Various distinct diseases beginning in childhood or adolescence include arthritis as a primary symptom. Some of the most common include juvenile rheumatoid arthritis (JRA), rheumatoid arthritis, spondyloarthropathies (including psoriatic arthritis, ankylosing spondylitis, and others), systemic lupus erythematosus, dermatomyositis, and others. Because there are so many disorders associated with arthritis, no single course and outcome can be described. Juvenile rheumatoid arthritis often resolves during adolescence, spondyloarthropathies tend to remain mild and easily controlled with antiinflammatory medications, and other disorders may progressively worsen. Many of these disorders affect other systems of the body besides joints, such as the skin, bowel, kidneys, and eyes.

Treatments are variably successful and may have debilitating side effects. Teenagers with arthritis may be minimally compromised and able to perform in dance and sports while experiencing tolerable pain or discomfort. Other teens are disabled or disfigured by their arthritis, or other symptoms of their illness, and must learn to manage their lives within the limitations of their disease, which may wax and wane.

ASTHMA

Asthma is the most prevalent chronic illness among children and adolescents, responsible for more doctor visits and days missed from school than any other chronic health problem of young people. Sometimes asthma can begin in the teen years, although most adolescents with asthma have had the disease since early childhood. For most of them the symptoms of asthma have become milder over time, but some teens suffer daily from shortness of breath, wheezing, cough (sometimes with mucus), chest tightness, and fatigue. Although asthma treatments have improved dramatically in recent years, more teens than ever experience symptoms of this illness, and for unknown reasons fatality rates have risen.

The symptoms of asthma are caused by several factors that obstruct the airway (the bronchial tree) of individuals with this illness. As air rich in oxygen is breathed in (inspired) it travels through a system of open tubes (bronchi and tiny bronchioles). Deep inside the lungs, oxygen diffuses into the bloodstream and carbon dioxide diffuses out of the blood into the airway, and is then expired (breathed out) into the air. Symptoms of asthma are caused by three mechanisms that contribute to airway obstruction: narrowing of the airway tubes by a reactive constriction (tightening) of the bronchi and bronchioles, swelling of the airway lining, and mucus production within the airway (both caused by inflammation). These events inevitably make inspiration and expiration more difficult and result in the shortness of breath, chest tightness, wheeze, and cough that characterize an asthma attack.

The airway constriction and inflammation may be set into motion by a number of triggers, which vary among individuals. Most commonly, asthma is triggered by substances to which the teen is allergic, such as dust mites, pollen, molds, cats or dogs, medications, or irritants such as tobacco smoke or other pollutants. Viral respiratory illnesses, emotional upset, exposure to extremes in weather, exercise, and other triggers commonly interact or alone may set off mild, moderate, or severe symptoms.

Although asthma can be a scary and debilitating disease, it can also be managed effectively. With the help of the doctor or health care team, an action plan is developed to deal with whatever level of severity of asthma a teen has. Some teens wheeze, cough, or feel tight only occasionally, and are prescribed an inhaler to use at such times. The inhaler contains medication (such as albuterol) that relieves airway constriction and inflammation. Other teens will need to use inhaled and/or oral medication(s) on a daily basis to try to prevent or diminish symptoms.

By testing their lung function several times per day with a simple device called a peak-flow meter, teens can learn to adjust medication dosages to meet their changing needs. The use of daily inhaled steroids has resulted in a marked lessening of symptoms and a lowered need for additional medications for many adolescents. The key point is that most teens with asthma, with the advice and support of parents and health providers, can effectively learn to manage their disease and live full and active lives. Many teens find it inspiring that a number of Olympic athletes have asthma.

CANCER

To receive a diagnosis of cancer is a shock at any age. For an adolescent, fully capable of understanding the implications, yet developmentally at a stage of life full of strength and anticipation, it is crushing. No adolescent can ever prepare for such a sudden change of fortune, and the ordeals of treatment and uncertainty that lie ahead. Of all potentially fatal illnesses that may strike during adolescence, cancer is the most common. At a time in life when a teen is naturally growing bigger and stronger and becoming increasingly independent from parents, caught up with peers, and oriented toward future planning, cancer puts on the brakes and demands an about-face.

The good news is that most teens with cancer get better, first in remission and then with a cure. They are able to get back on track and resume their lives fully, having been through a rigorous and stressful detour that likely hastened their maturity as it interfered with their fun. Some teens with cancer, whether diagnosed earlier in childhood or only recently, are not as fortunate, but often muster a courage and hope and involvement in their teenage life that inspires awe and admiration in their family and friends.

The types of malignancies that most frequently begin during the adolescent years are leukemia, Hodgkin's disease, brain tumors, bone and other sarcomas, thyroid, female genital tract, and testicular cancers (see "Testicular Self-Exam," chapter 6).

Treatment regimens depend upon the type of cancer and its stage (level of spread) at the time of diagnosis. Most types of cancer are treated with one, two, or three modalities, including chemotherapy, radiation, and surgery. The side effects from chemotherapy and radiation and the potential disfigurement from surgery are hurdles that teens with cancer and their close family and friends somehow must handle. Many roller-coaster emotions inevitably intervene, including sadness, anger, guilt, fear, relief, and joy. All teens with cancer and their families need a capable health care team and the emotional support derived from their community, self-help groups of individuals with similar concerns, caring organizations, and each other.

DIABETES MELLITUS

Early adolescence is often the time when insulin-dependent diabetes mellitus (IDDM, also known as Type I diabetes) is first diagnosed, although onset in early childhood or later in adolescence also occurs. Individuals with this most serious form of diabetes produce an insufficient amount of insulin, a hormone. Insulin is required for glucose (sugar) to move from the blood into cells, where metabolism takes place. Insulin deficiency leads to abnormally high levels of glucose in the blood and inadequate supplies of glucose in the cells.

Early symptoms leading to diagnosis include weight loss despite good appetite, increased thirst despite a large intake of fluid (with increased urination), blurry vision, and fatigue.

The treatment of IDDM is both simple and complex. Injectable insulin corrects the deficiency, but determining the correct dosage schedule and motivating the adolescent to test blood sugars and inject insulin several times per day, as well as to conform to recommendations regarding diet and exercise, can be daunting for all involved. The goals of treatment are to prevent the unpleasant or serious immediate and long-term medical complications of the illness, to maintain normal growth (weight, height, and pubertal development), and to help the adolescent learn to integrate the management of the illness into a normal daily routine, which will be necessary for the rest of his or her life.

Most adolescents with IDDM, with the support of their family and health care team, are able to achieve these goals and lead full and happy lives during and long beyond the teenage years. Gradually taking on the responsibility of managing the insulin and other aspects of care parallels the adolescent's increasing desire for independence and control over his or her life. Adolescents with IDDM are able to participate fully in academic, athletic, social, and other age-appropriate pursuits. They must, however, be sure to eat regularly and healthily, avoid alcohol (which can cause hypoglycemia), monitor and manage their blood sugar, and comply with other recommendations of their health care team.

EPILEPSY (SEIZURE DISORDERS)

Adolescents with epilepsy may have had childhood-onset seizures or onset during adolescence. Childhood-onset seizures often resolve before or during adolescence. A seizure is a disturbance in function of the brain that leads to a transient, usually recurrent and uncontrollable, episode. Seizures vary greatly in their appearance, ranging from a brief blank stare with eye blinking or jerking of a hand with consciousness intact to loss of consciousness with symmetrical jerking movements of all four limbs; frequency of occurrence; and ease of controlling them with antiepileptic drugs. A seizure disorder may be an isolated medical problem or associated with other neurologic or medical disabilities.

For the otherwise healthy and intellectually normal adolescent, the greatest challenge of having a seizure disorder may be social and psychological. Although most teens achieve good or complete control of their seizures with medication, the fear (and potential embarrassment) of an unexpected occurrence, the need to take drugs with possible side effects, and the restrictions on driving and a few other activities (such as scuba diving or mountain climbing) until full and prolonged control has been achieved are difficult burdens. Seizures may be precipitated by sleep deprivation or the use of alcohol or drugs, thus requiring extra vigilance and discipline by the adolescent.

A majority of adolescents with seizures will eventually be seizure-free off medication, and be able to lead fully independent lives and to participate in all activities they choose.

INFLAMMATORY BOWEL DISEASE (IBD)

The inflammatory bowel diseases Crohn's disease and ulcerative colitis often begin around early adolescence. They are the most common serious intestinal disorders in adolescents, and often profoundly affect their growth, development, and quality of life.

The conditions' precise cause(s) are not known. Crohn's disease may affect any part of the intestinal tract from the mouth to the anus; ulcerative colitis is limited to the large intestine (the colon). The symptoms, however, may be quite similar, with diarrhea (often bloody) and abdominal pain heading the list. Many teens with IBD find it difficult to eat enough food, and lose weight at a time when marked weight gain should be occurring. As a result they neither grow in height nor experience pubertal change when expected. The disease may blunt appetite, but teens also may avoid eating in order to avert pain and embarrassing diarrhea. Many adolescents with IBD tend to look much younger than their actual age, and for those with serious disease, life is further complicated and compromised by fatigue and feeling poorly. Adolescents with unstable IBD often lack the energy and desire to participate in activities with their peers.

Treatment consists of antiinflammatory medications, immunosuppressive agents, antibiotics, cautious use of antidiarrheal drugs, and selective surgery. Eventually adolescents with IBD reach a normal adult height and complete their pubertal development. Although often delayed, menstruation begins in the girls. Even the most compliant patient can experience recurrences of the disease following periods of control. Although planning for the future at times seems bleak or tricky, most adults with IBD live full and productive lives, in many instances with their IBD mostly in remission.

EIGHT: Risks and Realities of Teen Sexuality

Sexuality is an integral part of human life. It carries the awesome potential to create new life. It can foster intimacy and bonding as well as shared pleasure in our relationships . . . Yet when exercised irresponsibly it can also have negative aspects such as sexually transmitted diseases—including HIV/AIDS—unintended pregnancy, and coercive or violent behavior.

—The Surgeon General's Call to Action to Promote Sexual Health and Responsible Sexual Behavior, June 2001[1]

When adolescent girls begin to look like women, and boys like men, parents often have mixed feelings: pride, because these are normal changes and signs of healthy development; and concern, because although these newly minted bodies look all grown up, the hearts and minds within don't have a matching maturity. The situation has tricky timing written all over it, as hormones activate sexual desires that adolescents are often ill-equipped to handle.

Ready or not, many adolescents are following through with the urges they feel. According to the U.S. Centers for Disease Control and Prevention's Youth Risk Behavior Surveillance System (YRBS), a biennial survey of representative groups of high school students in grades nine to twelve:

- Half of all adolescents surveyed have had sexual intercourse (8 percent before age 13) and 16 percent of these adolescents have had four or more sex partners.
- About 6 percent reported having been pregnant or having caused pregnancy.
- When currently sexually active students were asked about their last sexual intercourse, 58 percent reported using a condom, 16 percent reported that they or their partner used birth control pills, and 25 percent reported having intercourse after using alcohol or drugs.
- Slightly more than 90 percent of students reported that they had received instruction in school about HIV infection or AIDS.[2]

These statistics just begin to show how high the stakes are. Although the vast majority of students surveyed had HIV/AIDS instruction, many fewer actually used condoms. So although they probably learned that HIV, the virus that causes AIDS, can be transmitted during sexual intercourse, their failure to use condoms shows that they did not take that information personally.

The great challenge of sex education is to persuade young people to translate knowledge into action. Sexuality educators—and that includes parents—need to find ways to help adolescents perceive disease and unwanted pregnancy not as abstractions that occur to "other people" but as real consequences that could happen to *them* if they do not avoid or reduce their risks.

A SEXUALIZED CULTURE

Some parents wonder whether talking about sex may put ideas in their kids' heads. Chances are, those ideas are already there. Sexual themes weave through TV sitcoms and radio talk shows, movies and music, magazines and books. This is a "sex sells" society. Advertisers stitch sexual references through come-ons for almost any product one can think of—shampoos and radial tires, soft drinks and blue jeans, boating supplies and breakfast cereals. Fashions dip and skimp, and bejeweled navels wink like impudent third eyes. In an effort to steer pubescent readers along the "fine line between 'Ooh la la' and 'Oh my God,' " *Teen Vogue* advises that a "tiny sliver of tummy (and *tiny* is the operative word here) can appear alluring . . . but when major cleavage is involved, the look goes from flirty to downright flashy."[3]

It's a festival of skin out there, it's sexsurround, it's outside your front door and inside your computer. As *Yahoo!* magazine pointed out, "Never before has a society been exposed to so much graphic material and sexual interaction, all a few clicks away, 24 hours a day, available to kids and adults alike. We are the first postcensorship generation."[4]

Parents can limit TV, monitor Internet use, rule out salacious films and raunchy rap, and urge their kids to hang out with kids of like-minded parents. But parents can't censor the world at large. The older adolescents are, the more they see, hear, and learn about things parents may wish they didn't. Parents have no control over the conversations their kids have and overhear at school, over the magazines they see at newsstands, or over the videos or websites they see at the home of a kid whose parents trust him to be the kind of a kid he's not.

But parents *can* control their own words and actions, and these can be surprisingly effective counterweights to all those other messages.

THE IMPORTANCE OF PARENTS' VOICES

Open communication and accurate information from parents increases the chance that teens will postpone sex and will use appropriate methods of birth control once they begin.

—*American Academy of Child and Adolescent Psychiatry*[5]

One-shot talks about sexual decision making are not enough. Parents and adolescents need ongoing dialogue about the importance of making thoughtful, informed, and responsible decisions. When adolescents are faced with a choice, a temptation, or a dare, they may recall those conversations and think twice: *Mom would be so disappointed in me*, or *Dad would be so upset if he found out*, or *I don't want to let them down*. The parents are not physically there at that moment, but their words are, and they are powerful.

Even adolescents who turn away from parents' attempts to talk about sexuality do register the fact that their parents are expressing love and concern. Deep down (sometimes *way* deep down) they welcome parents' efforts even while seemingly renouncing them.

Articulating values does not guarantee that adolescents will abide by them. But it does at least assure that they are not operating in a moral vacuum. It is the absence of adult leadership that puts young people at greatest risk—not the presence of adults who say things kids don't want to hear.

SEXUALITY: AN INTEGRAL PART OF LIFE

Within the context of a loving relationship, sex is one of the great benefits of being alive. Sexual intimacy within love gathers around a couple the feeling of a wonderful private world and gives them a heightened sense that life is good.

But sexual intimacy with a person with whom there isn't that close connection can leave a person feeling lessened, empty, disaffected, or blasé.

Talk with your adolescents about what a good relationship is and how they want to be treated and to treat others. Talk about how friendships and dating relationships should enhance their ability to enjoy life, make them feel proud of themselves and the people they spend time with, and support them in their goals.

TALKING BACK:
TEN THINGS TEENS WANT PARENTS
TO KNOW ABOUT TEEN PREGNANCY

The National Campaign to Prevent Teenage Pregnancy (NCPTP) conducted interviews with teens throughout the country on the roles parents should take in helping their kids avoid pregnancy. In its brochure "Talking Back: Ten Things Teens Want Parents to Know About Teen Pregnancy," the NCPTP reports that "young people do want to hear from parents and other adults about sex, love, and relationships. They say they appreciate—even crave—advice, direction, and support from adults who care about them. But sometimes, they suggest, adults need to change *how* they offer their guidance. As the following list shows, adolescents want real communication, not lectures and not threats."[6]

1. Show us why teen pregnancy is such a bad idea. For instance, let us hear directly from teen mothers and fathers about how hard it has been for them. Even though most of us don't want to get pregnant, sometimes we need real-life examples to help motivate us.

2. Talk to us honestly about love, sex, and relationships. Just because we're young doesn't mean that we can't fall in love or be deeply interested in sex. These feelings are very real and powerful to us. Help us to handle the feelings in a safe way—without getting hurt or hurting others.

3. Telling us not to have sex is not enough. Explain why you feel that way, and ask us what we think. Tell us how you felt as a teen. Listen to us and take our opinions seriously. And no lectures, please.

4. Whether we're having sex or not, we need to be prepared. We need to know how to avoid pregnancy and sexually transmitted diseases.

5. If we ask you about sex or birth control, don't assume we are already having sex. We may just be curious, or we may just want to talk with someone we trust. And don't think giving us information about sex and birth control will encourage us to have sex.

6. Pay attention to us before we get into trouble. Programs for teen moms and teen fathers are great, but we all need encour-

agement, attention, and support. Reward us for doing the right thing—even when it seems like no big thing. Don't shower us with attention only when there is a baby involved.

7. Sometimes, all it takes not to have sex is not to have the opportunity. If you can't be home with us after school, make sure we have something to do that we really like, where there are other kids and some adults who are comfortable with kids our age. Often we have sex because there's not much else to do. Don't leave us alone so much.

8. We really care what you think, even if we don't always act like it. When we don't end up doing exactly what you tell us to, don't think that you've failed to reach us.

9. Show us what good, responsible relationships look like. We're as influenced by what you do as by what you say. If you demonstrate sharing, communication, and responsibility in your own relationships, we will be more likely to follow your example.

10. We hate "The Talk" as much as you do. Instead, start talking with us about sex and responsibility when we're young, and keep the conversation going as we grow older.

This list is reprinted with permission from NCPTP, www.teenpregnancy.org/back_talk.htm.

ADOLESCENTS' SEXUALITY ISSUES

One of the central tasks of adolescence is clarifying sexual identity. Following are some of the common questions adolescents have (whether spoken aloud or not), some issues to consider, and some ways parents might choose to respond.

GENDER IDENTITY

What does it mean to be female or male?

Do I buy into society's definitions, or am I inclined to challenge them?

How do my family, friends, and community define male and female roles?

Are they roles with which I'm comfortable?

Do I think others see me as a "real girl" or a "real guy"?

How free do I feel to explore nontraditional roles?

Traditional pink-for-girls and blue-for-boys baby clothes testify to the importance our culture places on at-a-glance differentiation of the sexes. In recent decades there has been growing awareness that sex stereotyping can harm both boys and girls. Yet many families and cultures still have different expectations of boys and girls, and treat them accordingly.

There is a broad spectrum of gender roles in this country. At one end are families whose gender expectations have been cultural mainstays for generations. At the other end are families who challenge the validity of virtually any gender role and emphasize individual choice. In between are families who, consciously or not, feel that there are some things a boy just shouldn't do, some ways a girl just shouldn't be.

Adolescents who feel that they don't fit into gender expectations may have lower self-esteem. They may wonder if they are "real men" or "real women." They may question their sexual orientation (see page 199), since homophobic slurs often attach to nontraditional people.

A Parent's Perspective

Consider whether there are differences in the ways that you treat your sons and daughters. Do you allow or encourage all of your children to cry, pursue independence, play on sports teams, express an interest in fashion, speak up, do housework, fix the car, excel in math, paint a still life, ride a skateboard, take a bus alone to visit relatives in another city, date or ask someone out on a date, learn to cut hair, go fishing, cook meals? Many successful people attribute their growth to parents who encouraged their interests, hobbies, and ambitions even when they seemed unconventional.

Some parents expect a daughter to remain a virgin and a son to gain sexual experience before settling down. What happens if your daughter does proceed to have sex? Will she think that you'll be so disappointed or angry that she won't feel able to talk with you? What if your son decides to wait for sex until he falls in love and is in a serious relationship? Will he feel that you question his masculinity?

Consider how you can best help your children grow up to think for themselves while remaining close with you. Think long and hard before denying an adolescent's goals because they aren't "manly" or "womanly." Try to affirm your children's individuality so they don't feel the need to "prove" their gender or feel rejected for being different.

SEXUALITY AND DECISION MAKING

How do I want to handle the sexual feelings I have?

Do I want to take things slow and focus on other aspects of my life?

Or maybe I can't wait to start experiencing how it feels to kiss, to touch and be touched.

Do I want to downplay sex?

What limits do I want to set?

What am I eager or willing to do?

Do I want to abstain from sexual intercourse until marriage, or until college, or until high school, or until eighth grade, or for the rest of my life, or until tomorrow?

The sexual drive and the drive to connect with other people are fundamental to life. Some adolescents form satisfying, loving, and responsible sexual relationships. But others discover that sexual relationships can lead to distressing complications: sexually transmitted diseases, unwanted pregnancy, emotional upheaval, heartache, and emptiness. Sexual relationships can distract or derail adolescents from achievement of academic, athletic, artistic, and other goals.

Adolescents may decide to have sex for a mind-boggling multitude of reasons:

- To express affection or love.
- To satisfy curiosity or desire.
- To relieve sexual tension.
- To feel grown up and independent.
- To feel filled up and not alone.
- To do what they feel is expected of them.
- To attract or keep a boyfriend or girlfriend.
- To generate excitement.
- To stave off boredom.
- To have something to do.
- To satisfy their need to be touched.
- To deepen or lock in a relationship.
- To give in to the demands of a pushy or abusive partner.
- To have something to boast about.
- To reassure themselves that they are attractive and desirable.
- To party.

- To do what they think everyone else is doing.
- To defy the rules.
- To keep from being left out.
- To rush to adulthood.
- To have a baby.
- To explore who they are.

A Parent's Perspective

Contemplating these reasons, it is apparent that sex can serve many needs and mean many things to adolescents. Decisions about sexuality are not made in a vacuum; they aren't necessarily decisions about "sex," but are about adolescents' emotional and social needs and how the rest of life is going.

For parents, therefore, providing guidance about sexual decision making covers a broad range of areas.

Forming Healthy Relationships

Talk with your children about what kinds of relationships they want and how to assess the relationships they have. Does a friendship or romance seem to open up the world, provide exciting new possibilities, offer support and caring and openness? Or does it gradually shrink the world due to the other person's possessiveness, jealousy, limited interests, negative outlook, or low feelings of self-worth?

Having sex too soon can have the unintended effect of stunting a relationship. Using sex to keep or attract someone is sure to backfire. Teens are likely to be happier if they focus on friendships and get to know each other outside of a sexual context.

Timing

Let your children know what your values are. If you want them to postpone sex, say so. If you accept (enthusiastically or not) that they are sexually active, let them know that your first priority is not judging them but assuring that they stay healthy and happy. Talk with them about protection. And let them know that every single day is a clean slate and every decision is new.

Many adolescents feel that once they have had sex they no longer have the right to decline it, as if sex were a river and they are on the far bank, never to return "home" again to feeling they have the right to decide what they do with their own body. People can lose their virginity only once, but they have unlimited opportunities to decide what to do next.

Staying Busy

An adolescent with little to do may turn to sex to fill the void. Show a strong interest in your child's life. Spend time together as a family; encourage varied interests. Provide opportunities to learn about and explore new possibilities. Scout around for a summer job at a day camp, community pool, deli counter, library, or park. Pick up on your child's love of music and offer guitar lessons. Take part in community service activities, such as tutoring or neighborhood clean-up or serving food at a soup kitchen.

Find ways to help your adolescent discover his or her capacity to succeed in study or work or creativity or service to others. An adolescent with a strong sense of purpose is less likely to want a baby now, or to get so wrapped up in a sexual relationship that there is little time for anything else.

Living a Well-Rounded Life

Sexuality decisions attain their rightful place when they become one component in an overall context of life planning. Teens who have plentiful support, goals, and a variety of challenging and rewarding activities are less likely to engage in sexual risk-taking that could compromise their dreams.

Some of the most successful pregnancy prevention programs appear to the casual observer to mimic academic enhancement and recreation programs. For example, a renowned Children's Aid Society pregnancy prevention program, developed by Dr. Michael Carrera, includes comprehensive family living and sex education, as well as primary, reproductive, and mental health care. But in keeping with its philosophy of considering young people to be "at promise," not "at risk," the program also offers counseling; a job club with paid work, assistance with opening a bank account, and financial and career planning; homework help, tutoring, SAT preparation, and assistance with college applications; and arts and sports programs. An evaluation showed that "the risk of pregnancy in the program group was less than half of that risk in the control group."[7]

No wonder, then, that when Donna Shalala, former Secretary of Health and Human Services, gave a speech honoring Dr. Carrera's program, she cited Eleanor Roosevelt: "The future belongs to those who believe in the beauty of their dreams."[8]

Parents can refer to this model in helping their own teens prevent pregnancy by asking themselves: *Does my child . . .*

- Have regular checkups with a provider who will address his or her reproductive health care needs?
- Have mental health services, if needed, and someone to talk to about stress and problems?

- Know the gratification of earning, saving, and managing money?
- Have the necessary support to perform to his or her potential in school?
- Have outlets for creative expression?
- Participate in sports or other exercise?

MASTURBATION

Is masturbation okay?

Is it something to be ashamed of?

Do other people do it?

What would other people think if they found out that I masturbate?

In *Growing Up Feeling Good,* an advice book for teens, here's how author Ellen Rosenberg discussed masturbation:

> *Because your genitals are special, very personal, private areas of your body, the "tingly when touched" feelings that can be felt in the genitals are also thought of as personal, private feelings . . . Girls or boys (adults, too) may purposely touch the sensitive areas of their genitals just so they can feel those feelings.*[9]

This is a nonjudgmental, straightforward definition. Masturbation is natural, it feels good, it's private—and it is very, very prevalent.

Masturbation provides an outlet for adolescents to express sexual feelings, vent sexual tensions, and explore the various textures of touch. Some call it a form of safe sex. There's no way to get pregnant or contract a sexually transmitted disease when one is all alone. And masturbation may be just the alternative adolescents need to help them abstain from sexual activities for which they are not ready. In other words, masturbation can be empowering.

Yet masturbation is rarely discussed in such positive terms, and many young people are anxious about it. In an article on adolescent boys, the *Journal of Sexual Research* reported:

> *Rather than being perceived as a normal sexual outlet, masturbation may be seen as a tacit admission of not having "real" sex . . . Masturbation is also associated with feelings of guilt and anxiety among teens . . . It is the rare parent who openly discusses masturbation with their adolescent son and touts it as an appropriate and normal sexual outlet. For adolescent boys, partnered sexual experience may be seen as a marker of*

achievement or adequacy, and of a transition to adult status, whereas masturbation may be viewed as a secret substitute for preferred partner activity.[10]

Some religions and cultures frown on masturbation. Some parents are concerned that it can become obsessive. Anything can, of course, but this is rarely a problem. Some parents are concerned that adolescents who masturbate may eventually turn to "mutual masturbation" (doing it in front of or with a partner), which may lead to other forms of sexual activity. In this way of thinking, masturbation is incompatible with abstinence and self-control.

A Parent's Perspective

Most adolescents will, at some point, masturbate. The medical fact is that it is highly unlikely to harm them and far more likely to be not only harmless but also helpful. As a means of self-soothing as well as sexual stimulation, masturbation may provide comfort, release, and self-knowledge that can contribute to reduced stress and to future sexual happiness with a partner.

SEXUAL LIMIT SETTING

How far do I want to go?

What happens after the first kiss?

What does my partner expect of me?

How sexually experienced are other people—and what are they doing?

Do I have to have sexual intercourse if I'm not ready?

What am I really ready for?

Here's what happens in the movies: Boy meets girl. They gaze into each other's eyes. They kiss. Then—*whoosh!*—in the next frame they're in bed, making passionate, acrobatic love.

Hey, movie producers have to keep the action going. They have a high stake in making a film sizzle into a lucrative R rating. Anyway, showing all the steps of courtship between smooching and stripping would make the movie too long. But adolescents need to know there's no need to hurry—no rush to lose virginity, or even their shirt. Holding hands is cool. Hugging is great. Kissing—now, that's an activity a couple can hang out with for a long time. Ready to move on? Think about it and decide.

There are an infinite number of points along the line from eye gazing to intercourse, and adolescents need to know they have a right to be in control of where along that line they decide to position themselves.

Some sexuality educators advocate discussing "outercourse" as a valid alternative to intercourse. Outercourse is nonpenetrative sexual contact; that is, sexual expression excluding oral, anal, or vaginal intercourse. For a couple who want to progress beyond clothes-on touch but stop short of intercourse, outercourse deepens intimacy but enables young people to avoid disease and pregnancy.

Oral sex is far more prevalent among younger adolescents than it used to be. Some call it "hooking up" and don't consider it to be the same as "having sex." Some adolescents have anal sex as a way to remain "virgins" and avoid pregnancy. They choose not to think of anal sex as "real sex." But oral and anal sex are intimate sexual acts and also present a risk of acquiring a sexually transmitted disease.

Whether an adolescent draws the line at petting or at partially clothed exploration or at oral sex, there is always a risk that a partner who wants more will leave and find someone else. But it is even more likely that a partner will accept the boundaries an adolescent sets.

Sometimes a young woman allows herself to go further than she really wants to because she doesn't know how to verbalize her limits, and perhaps isn't clear in her own mind about what her limits are. The situation snowballs as her date exploits her ambiguity and forces her to have sexual intercourse. This does *not* mean she was responsible for being raped, but it does mean that her own confusion may have contributed to her vulnerability to rape. Yet often a girl is, in fact, forcibly date raped against her clear protests or when she is so drunk that she is unable to protest.

Young people empower themselves by deciding on their sexual limits, articulating them, and not permitting themselves to be in a situation where those limits could be crossed. Such risky situations involve drinking or using drugs, or being in the company of people who are, or being alone with a date at home when parents are out.

A Parent's Perspective

The concept of deciding in advance what one is and is not willing to do is new, radical, and very empowering to most adolescents. And talking about it with a partner is a fabulous skill that can make both people feel more comfortable, and often very relieved. Let those actors on the screen get swept away. Encourage your adolescent to consider his or her values, protect health, determine how sexually involved he or she does or does not want to be, and then say so.

The question should not be "What does my partner expect of me?" but rather "What do I want to tell my partner that he or she can expect from me?"

If you can, talk with your teen in specific ways about how to articulate limits. For example:

I really love kissing you, but I'm not ready for anything else now.

Touching you feels so good, but we have to keep our clothes on.

Let's get to know each other better before we go any further.

Granted, not all teens will be receptive to such discussions with their parents. But you can introduce the idea of limit setting in nonsexual contexts, too. If your child doesn't seem to know what to say in a challenging situation, role-playing may really help. So pose some hypothetical situations: What would you say if someone wanted to cheat off you on a test? Or if someone pressured you to try drugs at a party? Or if someone wanted you to get into a car even though the driver had been drinking?

Practicing such situations with you in advance may give your child confidence, let you brainstorm together—and perhaps give you an opportunity to ease into a discussion of sexual pressures and how to deal with them.

SEXUAL ORIENTATION

Am I straight, gay, bisexual, or transgender?

How sure am I of this answer?

Do I want the answer to be different?

Is my sexual orientation apparent to other people?

To whom can I talk about my sexual feelings?

Between 2 to 10 percent of males and 1 to 3 percent of females are estimated to be homosexual.[11] It is also common for adolescents to be confused about what their sexual identity is.

Being gay or lesbian is no longer viewed as a mental disorder but as an integral component of one's identity. That's why many homosexuals reject the term "sexual preference." Being gay is not something one chooses or "prefers." It is simply who one *is*.

Except that it's not so simple, because many people won't let it be. In many cultures and neighborhoods, in high schools and the U.S. military, in social and work settings, stigma about homosexuality clouds the lives of gay and lesbian adolescents. These young people often feel that they must hide their real selves, lest they be subjected to teasing, ridicule, or assault. Some pursue opposite-sex relationships to test whether they really are homosexual, or to hide who they really are.

Many gay and lesbian adolescents experience enormous stress or depression about having to conceal their homosexuality, endure taunts, or brave the reactions of people when they "come out." A significant number of gay, lesbian, bisexual, or questioning adolescents attempt or commit suicide as a result of this stress, according to the American Academy of Child and Adolescent Psychiatry (AACAP).[12]

Among the most stressful experiences in a homosexual child's life is coming out to parents. Will the parents affirm their unconditional love or express shame or sorrow? Will everything change? Will relationships from "before" survive this revelation?

A Parent's Perspective

Parents' support goes a long way toward helping homosexual teens feel safe within the family, giving them confidence that they have a solid home base. Teens long for their parents' unconditional love: *I love you and want you to be happy. Whether you're straight or gay, or you're not even sure yet, I'm here for you.*

But what if you feel that homosexuality is wrong? You can maintain your own beliefs without chasing your child away. You can still love your child even if you are disappointed or disapproving.

You may find it helpful to talk with other parents in this situation for insight into how their own relationships with their children have evolved. One organization you may want to check out is PFLAG, which stands for Parents, Families, and Friends of Lesbian, Gay, Bisexual, and Transgendered Persons. Founded in the early 1970s by parents whose son was beaten at a gay rights march, the organization seeks to "celebrate diversity and envision a society that embraces everyone, including those of diverse sexual orientations and gender identities."[13]

Be alert to any problems your child may be facing in school based on his or her sexual orientation. Is your child being teased, discriminated against, or ostracized? The organization GLSEN, the Gay, Lesbian, and Straight Education Network, a national network of parents, students, educators, and others, works to end discrimination related to sexual orientation and gender identity/expression in schools from kindergarten through grade twelve.[14]

Even if there is no discernible discrimination, some gay, lesbian, bisexual, or questioning youth have high stress levels or self-consciousness that may prevent real engagement with school.

Encourage your child to go to counseling or support groups, not to be "converted" to heterosexuality but to express feelings and learn to cope with being homosexual in a heterosexual-dominated world. The AACAP cautions that "therapy directed specifically at changing homosexual orientation is not recommended and may be harmful for an unwilling teen. It may create more confusion and anxiety by reinforcing the negative thoughts and emotions with which the youngster is already struggling." [15]

SEXUALLY TRANSMITTED DISEASES

Could I get a sexually transmitted disease?

How would I know if I got an STD?

How can I keep from getting one?

What should I do if I think I have an STD?

If I have an STD, whom should I tell?

Can I count on my partner to tell me if he or she is infected?

How should I tell my partner that I have an STD?

Sexually transmitted diseases are epidemic in this country and pose a threat to the health, fertility, and lives of sexually active adolescents.

According to the American Social Health Association:

- Two-thirds of all STDs occur in people twenty-five years of age or younger.
- One in four new STD infections occurs in a teenager.
- At least 15 percent of all infertile American women are infertile because of tubal damage caused by pelvic inflammatory disease resulting from an untreated STD. [16]

Myths about STDs feed into adolescents' denial of risk. They include:

Myth: HIV and other STDs don't affect teens from nice neighborhoods.
Fact: Viruses and bacteria don't read zip code maps. Anyone is vulnerable.

Myth: You can tell by looking at someone if he/she is infected with an STD.
Fact: It's unlikely that a clothed person with an STD will look any different from anyone else. In some instances, a herpes blister, genital wart, or chancre sore on or near the genitals or anus may be apparent—but only to an adolescent who knows what they look like. And who actually looks. Many teens are too shy or inexperienced to know how to visually inspect a partner, or

they have sex in the dark and don't get the chance. Even if they do see or feel something unusual, they may be too shy, intimidated, polite, or inexperienced to say, "I see something that looks like a rash, what's going on here?" Or "That looks like it could be an STD—you should get it checked out." If the partner protests, "I'm fine, don't worry about it," prepare your teen with exit words: "Sorry, I'm not comfortable about this" or "I've changed my mind. I don't feel like having sex right now" or "I just feel better about waiting." If the partner persists, your teen should plead a sudden headache, stomachache, or intestinal upset—anything to get out. No one should ever insist on having sex if the other partner is not willing.

Myth: I can't get infected the first time I have sex.
Fact: There's no grace period. Viruses and bacteria don't believe in beginner's luck.

Myth: I'll know if I have symptoms of an STD.
Fact: Many STDs have no symptoms, and girls are less likely to have symptoms than boys are. With an STD like chlamydia, for example, the disease can progress without a girl's ever knowing it. Years later, when she tries to have a baby, she'll discover that scar tissue from the disease blocked her fallopian tubes.

Myth: My partner will tell me if he or she has an STD.
Fact: If only all partners *could* be counted on. That's why some states have partner notification laws—precisely because many people never tell, for a variety of reasons. They might not know they are infected, because some STDs may have no signs or symptoms. They don't know how to tell. They're afraid of the reaction. They've moved away or moved on, lost the phone number, procrastinated too long, just don't care, or don't realize why sharing the information is so important. They were lucky enough to have symptoms that signaled them to seek care. They may just assume their partners had the same luck. And, rare but real, there are a few angry people who are so bitter about having HIV or another STD that they deliberately want to infect others, too.

Myth: Condoms will protect me from all STDs.
Fact: Condoms offer protection against such STDs as HIV and gonorrhea. However, human papilloma virus (HPV), for example, can pass from an infected partner through cells on skin not covered by the condom. And a condom must be used correctly. If it slips off or tears, it does not protect.

Myth: I'm on the Pill. I can't get an STD.

Fact: Birth control pills, diaphragms, IUDs, and other contraceptives don't protect against STDs. It's important to use a condom *and* another contraceptive method.

Myth: My doctor will be able to tell if I have an STD during my annual checkup.

Fact: STDs can only be diagnosed through specific tests, and many doctors, unaware that their adolescent patients are sexually active, neither ask nor test. Adolescents must learn to be alert medical consumers and ask for what they need. Adolescents need to also be aware of the possibility of false negative tests, which fail to diagnose an infection that is in fact present in themselves or a partner.

Since the advent of the AIDS epidemic, many schools offer HIV/AIDS instruction. Indeed, at the beginning of this chapter it is noted that 90 percent of high school students say they have received such instruction. But that doesn't mean they have learned about all the other STDs. HIV receives unique attention because it can be fatal and because instruction may be specially funded and mandated.

But there is an entire constellation of STDs, many of them dimmed by HIV's harsh glare but possessing tragic consequences themselves. HPV (human papilloma virus) can lead to cervical cancer. Chlamydia and gonorrhea can result in pelvic inflammatory disease (infection of and around the fallopian tubes), which can cause infertility. Herpes can cause death to a newborn who is delivered vaginally during an outbreak, not to mention the painful recurrences that can occur throughout life in both males and females.

Syphilis that is untreated can lead to sterility, mental illness, and death—all consequences that can be avoided through timely diagnosis and treatment with penicillin or other antibiotics.

Countless young people know of someone with HIV, but they don't hear enough about the STDs that are actually more prevalent, even rampant, among teens, like HPV and chlamydia and herpes. So teens are not as mindful of the risks or as vigilant in looking out for symptoms or getting tested. Having sex (vaginal intercourse as well as oral and anal sex) always carries some risk of acquiring an STD, but the risk can be reduced dramatically by using condoms and limiting the number of lifetime partners one has.

A Parent's Perspective

Sexually transmitted diseases are nothing to be shy about. Urge your sexually active teen to ask the doctor about HIV/STD testing and to be alert to any indication that something may not be quite right. Young people who have one or more of the following STD symptoms should stop having sex, see a doctor, and ask their partner(s) to be tested, too.

STD Symptoms

- Pain, stinging, or burning sensation during urination.
- Increased frequency of urination.
- Pelvic (lower abdominal) pain, during intercourse or not.
- Upper abdominal pain, especially on the right side near the liver.
- Bumps, lesions, rashes, sores, blisters, warts, raised lines, redness, or any other skin changes on or near the genitals, anus, or mouth.
- Genital or anal itching or pain.
- Rash on the body or unexplained bruises (lesions from Kaposi's sarcoma, a rare form of cancer, are a symptom of AIDS).
- Fever, chills, aches, pain.
- Yellowing skin.
- Unusual vaginal or penile discharge or unpleasant odor.
- Change in flow or frequency of menstrual periods.
- Bleeding between menstrual periods.
- Night sweats.
- Unintended weight loss.
- Diarrhea.

Talk to your teen about the fact that the more partners a person has, the greater the odds of getting an STD. It is best to have as few sexual partners in one's life as possible. Having very few partners can be achieved by not ever having casual sex, and reserving sex for only important, loving, and ongoing relationships.

There is also a strong association between use of alcohol and drugs and STD infection. Teens who are high are less likely to take precautions. Getting drunk or stoned is practically a setup for casual sex or date rape. It is not unusual for an adolescent to confide in a doctor that she was so drunk she didn't even know if she had sex. If she did, it was surely without a condom.

Learning about a partner's past sexual history may be helpful, but may also provide a false sense of security. People may say they never had an STD—but may not know that their previous partner did. People may say they were "tested" but be vague about the details. They may not have been tested for every STD, including HIV, for which they have been at risk. Some STDs are nearly impossible to screen for, such as certain types of HPV in a male. And some people lie, or misrepresent, or don't quite tell the whole truth and nothing but the truth. So interviewing a partner can't be counted on as a protective device. It certainly should be done, but it is no substitute for a condom.

Some Sexually Transmitted Diseases Your Teen Must Know About

Although human immunodeficiency virus (HIV), which causes AIDS (acquired immune deficiency syndrome), is by far the *most serious* STD, teens are *most likely to acquire* human papilloma virus (HPV), herpes simplex virus (herpes), and the bacterial infections chlamydia and gonorrhea. Trichomonas and pubic lice are also common but of relatively minor consequence.

HUMAN IMMUNODEFICIENCY VIRUS (HIV) is the pathogen that causes AIDS (acquired immune deficiency syndrome) by impairing the body's immune system. HIV can be transmitted through activities that result in an infected person's semen (or preseminal fluid), vaginal fluids, blood, or breast milk getting into another person's body. These risk activities include oral, vaginal, or anal sexual intercourse; and sharing needles and other paraphernalia for drug injection, piercing, or tattooing. The virus can also be transmitted from woman to child during pregnancy or breast-feeding, and through blood transfusion, although the chances of this are quite low since blood banks started testing blood for HIV in 1985. According to the Centers for Disease Control and Prevention (CDC), people under age twenty-five account for at least half of all new HIV infections, most transmitted sexually.[17]

There can be a substantial gap—ten or more years—between infection with HIV and the appearance of AIDS symptoms. Therefore, most people with HIV do not know they have it, and can unwittingly transmit it to others. Young people who believe they might have been exposed to the virus should seriously consider getting tested, since the earlier the infection is detected the sooner they can receive treatments that may delay onset of disease. If infected, they should also take steps to avoid infecting others, and inform prospective sexual partners of their HIV status.

An HIV-infected person is considered to have AIDS when he or she develops one of the opportunistic infections associated with an impaired immune system, or when a blood test indicates that the person's CD-4 (immune) cell count is very low, as defined by the CDC.

Although there is no cure, there are medications that can suppress (but not eradicate) HIV and delay the onset of AIDS. Many people have enjoyed years of health as a result of these medications, although not everyone is able to tolerate the complicated treatment regimens and the attendant side effects. Because of the complexity of the disease, AIDS educators often state that the best treatment is prevention: abstinence from risk behaviors or consistent and correct use of latex condoms.

HUMAN PAPILLOMA VIRUS (HPV) is in actuality a large family of viruses, including those that cause the common warts that grow on fingers or toes. These, of course, are not sexually transmitted. Other types of HPV, which *are* sexually transmitted, cause genital warts or Pap smear abnormalities that, if left untreated, could develop into cervical cancer.

Genital warts are small, painless, irregular bumps (resembling tiny pieces of cauliflower) located on the skin in the genital region of males and females. They are diagnosed by their characteristic appearance or by biopsy. A patient can remove the warts by applying Podofilox solution or gel or Aldara (Imiquimod) cream, both of which require a doctor's prescription, careful directions, and follow-up. If the genital warts are numerous, large, or in hard-to-reach locations, treatment by a physician is preferred. Doctors might apply liquid nitrogen, podophyllin resin, or bichloro- or trichloroacetic acid; or use surgical excision or curetage; interferon injection; or laser surgery.

When HPV causes abnormal cells (called dysplasia) on the cervix, their presence is unknown to the female until, as part of her gynecologic examination, a Pap smear is done and the report comes back indicating the finding of characteristic HPV effects. Males infected with the types of HPV that cause Pap smear abnormalities in their partners generally have no visible signs. For this reason, it is nearly impossible to screen males for HPV. Males are unaware they have the infection (unless genital warts are present), female partners are unsuspecting, and HPV has become rampant among teens and on college campuses. Condoms do not always protect against transmission of HPV; indeed, HPV may be present in the cells of skin that a condom does not cover.

If a Pap test indicates the presence of HPV and dysplasia, a procedure called colposcopy (a gynecologic examination through a magnifying lens) may be recommended in order to take a closer look and possibly biopsy any areas that appear abnormal. Whether or not colposcopy is done, the Pap smear should be repeated more frequently (every three to six months) for a year or two to monitor for possible progression to a more serious precancerous form of dysplasia. Sometimes HPV infections and the dysplasia heal on their own without any treatment. If this does not occur, treatment of the cervix with laser or loop electrosurgical excision procedure (LEEP) would likely be advised.

HERPES SIMPLEX VIRUS (HSV, "HERPES") is one of the most dreaded STDs because of the severe pain associated with its sores and its unpredictable recurrences. A tingling sensation on the skin precedes the outbreak of vesicles (tiny blisters), often sprouting in a cluster, which after a few days rupture to form a painful ulcer. Oral herpes generally appears on an edge of the lip, and genital herpes on the labia, the vestibule to the vagina, or inside the vagina or on the cervix, on the penis, or in the anal area.

Local burning of the herpes sores can be intense, and is exacerbated by urination. A herpes attack may be associated with feeling somewhat ill and feverish and with swollen, tender lymph glands in the region. Oral herpes can be spread to the genital region by oral sex (and vice versa), so even virgins can transmit herpes sexually.

The first bout of herpes is usually the most severe (lasting ten to twenty days). Recurrences may occur never, infrequently, or several times per year. Diagnosis is by culture. Treatment is directed toward relieving local symptoms (painkillers, sitz baths, topical anesthetic gels) and shortening the attack with antiviral medications such as Zovirax (acyclovir) and Valtrex (valacyclovir). In the event of a recurrence, medications should be taken at the first sign of tingling. Ask the doctor for a course of medication that can be kept handy at home.

CHLAMYDIA and GONORRHEA are bacterial STDs with similar symptoms and have the highest occurrence rates among adolescents. Although gonorrhea may be better known, chlamydia is, in fact, about four times as common among teens. Transmission of both bacteria is by sexual intercourse and can be prevented by condom use.

In males, chlamydia or gonorrhea causes urethritis, an inflammation of the urethra, the tube that carries urine and semen out of the body. Symptoms of urethritis are burning on urination and a puslike discharge from the penis. Infection may spread beyond the urethra and result in more complicated genital infections (such as epididymitis, see chapter 6) or dissemination to more distant parts of the body.

In females, chlamydia or gonorrhea initially infects the cervix, causing cervicitis and the symptoms of puslike vaginal discharge, pain on intercourse, and bleeding between periods. Infection may spread beyond the cervix through the uterus into the fallopian tubes, causing pelvic inflammatory disease (PID), which can result in infertility or ectopic pregnancy.

Although infection with chlamydia or gonorrhea can produce quite dramatic symptoms, both STDs can be completely asymptomatic in an unsuspecting male or female or their partner. Diagnosis is made by culture or DNA techniques. Treatment is with antibiotics.

TRICHOMONAS is a protozoa that is sexually transmitted and causes a characteristic vaginitis in females. Symptoms include a malodorous, bubbly, yellowish gray discharge accompanied by vulvar irritation, burning on urination, and sometimes pain during intercourse.

Males with trichomonas generally have no symptoms but may have burning on urination and urethral discharge.

Diagnosis is made by microscopic examination of discharge or urine that shows the motile protozoa. Treatment is with the antibiotic metronidazole. Abstain from drinking alcohol for twenty-four hours after taking the medication to avoid unpleasant side effects. (See chapter 5 for further discussion of other causes of vaginitis.)

PUBIC LICE ("CRABS") are parasites and most characteristically cause itching in the region of the pubic hairs in both males and females. Diagnosis is made by the observation of lice or nits among the pubic hairs. Treatment is with permethrin cream applied to the area.

CONDOMS

Condoms aren't perfect, but after abstinence they are the best protection against STDs. However, the condom failure rate for adolescents is higher than for adults. The key to condom effectiveness is correct and consistent usage. Inexperienced, impulsive adolescents don't always use condoms right—or at all.

Parents who know their child is or will soon become sexually active might consider buying some condoms and talking with their teen about how to use them correctly. Sound too embarrassing? Admit your embarrassment, but don't let it stop you from providing life-saving information.

And what if you do not approve of your teen's having sex? Talk about abstinence as the best choice. But if you are concerned that your child will have sex anyway, say that your child's health and safety are of paramount importance to you, and you want to make sure he or she knows how to correctly use a condom.

Here's what to include in a condom show-and-tell.

Correct Condom Use

- Practice makes perfect. Get used to opening up a condom package and putting on a condom so you are comfortable with it. Then you'll be more at ease with your partner, and safer.
- Always use latex condoms; polyurethane are next best. "Skin" condoms are too porous to protect against STDs.
- Check the expiration date.

- Be careful not to tear the package with teeth, fingernails, or jewelry.
- Don't use a dried-out condom. Do not keep condoms in locations where they can become dried out, such as a wallet or the glove compartment of a car.
- Breathe. Don't be in such a hurry that you put the condom on wrong.
- Check to see which way the condom unrolls. Place it on the erect penis (put the condom on two fingers or a small banana to demonstrate), squeeze air out of the tip to create a reservoir for semen, and unroll the condom all the way down the shaft of the penis, smoothing out any air bubbles.
- If your partner is wearing the condom, feel with your fingers to make sure it's on before as well as once or twice during intercourse. If you can't feel the condom, stop and make sure it hasn't slipped off inside your body. If it has, pull the condom out of your body with your fingers and insert spermicide into the vagina. Better still . . . have spermicide already inside the vagina before intercourse (see page 212).
- If a condom slips off or breaks, call your doctor or a Planned Parenthood clinic as soon as possible to ask about the morning-after pill (see page 216) or STD risks.
- Never reuse a condom. Use a new condom every time you have sex.
- Use a condom for vaginal and anal sex and for oral sex on a man's penis.
- To use a condom for oral sex on a woman, create a flat barrier by using scissors to trim off the rim of the condom and make a vertical cut through the condom so it is no longer a tube but forms a flat sheet of latex. Place this against the vulva so that there is no direct contact between the mouth and vaginal fluids. This barrier can also be used to prevent contact between the mouth and the partner's anus. Other oral sex barriers include latex squares called dental dams, or sheets of plastic wrap, but these have not been FDA-approved as barriers against sexually transmitted disease.
- After intercourse, withdraw the penis, holding on to the base of the condom to make sure it doesn't slip off and stay inside.
- Wrap the condom in a tissue and dispose of it in a trash can. Do not flush it down the toilet; it will come back to haunt you or will mess up the plumbing. Do not dispose of the condom where it can be found and played with by curious small children.
- Feel proud of yourself and your partner that you practiced responsible sex.

"Negotiating" condom use is a phrase often used in sex education. But the negotiation should be as basic as thumbs-up or thumbs-down: *No condom, no sex*. Don't assume it's only males who object to condoms. Girls, too, may urge a partner to leave off the condom. They may dislike the sensation of a condom, want to offer greater intimacy, or want to make a baby. Advise your daughter or son to be prepared with rebuttals.

Words That Keep You Safer

- If a partner says, "Condoms don't feel natural" . . . say, "But I'm not willing to have the 'natural' thing happen, which could be pregnancy or an STD."
- "I don't have a condom with me" . . . say, "Let's not have sex now. We'll be prepared next time."
- "I'm not comfortable wearing a condom" . . . say, "I'm not comfortable having sex without one."
- "I don't have any diseases; we don't need a condom" . . . say, "I'm not saying either of us has an STD; I'm saying the condom will make me feel safer and sexier."
- "I'm allergic to latex condoms" . . . say, "That's okay, we can try polyurethane condoms or you can wear a skin condom with a latex one over it."
- "Don't you want to feel me without a rubber between us?" . . . say, "The rubber makes me feel like you love and protect me."

CONTRACEPTION

Can I get pregnant (or cause pregnancy) at this age?

How can we prevent pregnancy if we don't have any condoms or birth control with us?

Should I tell my parents that I need birth control?

A Parent's Perspective

Abstinence is the only sure method of contraception—and teens not only should be encouraged to abstain, but also should be assured that it is the healthiest, most appropriate choice, and will free them of worry about diseases and pregnancy.

But for teens who have decided to have intercourse, condoms should be mentioned in the same breath as contraception. Using a folksy image, the American Academy of Pediatrics (AAP) calls the use of condoms and birth control "the belt and suspenders approach." Since condoms can protect against STDs as well as pregnancy, use of a second method may seem excessive. But when it comes to preventing teen pregnancy, there's no such thing as being too careful. The AAP says that the "optimal" approach is condoms used together with hormonal contraception such as birth control pills.[18]

According to a contraception update in the journal *Pediatrics*, the "comparative failure rates of contraceptives are as follows: 'Depo-Provera and Norplant, 0.4 percent; IUD, 0.5 to 0.7 percent; oral contraceptive pills, 3 percent; condom, 12 percent; diaphragm, 18 percent; and vaginal foam, 21 percent.' "[19] Note that failure rates are usually quoted as actual or theoretical; actual takes into account human error and theoretical is assuming perfect usage. The 3 percent failure rate of the Pill is nearly all due to human error; when taken properly, the Pill is nearly 100 percent effective. An adolescent must consider a number of factors when deciding about birth control.

- Does she want a systemic hormonal method, such as the Pill, that offers round-the-clock protection? Or a local method, such as the diaphragm, that she uses only when having intercourse? A young woman who has sex infrequently may be less inclined to take the Pill than one who has a steady boyfriend and an active sex life.
- Medically, is she a candidate for hormonal methods? A physician must evaluate her medical history to determine this.
- How focused, responsible, and motivated is she? Will she remember to take the Pill every day? Will she have the discipline to insert her diaphragm before sex?
- Is her partner supportive? If he will object to her use of a device and she still wants to be with him, maybe she'd be better off with Depo-Provera or the Pill.
- Is she comfortable touching herself? If so, she may be fine with the diaphragm or female condom. If not, she needs to increase her comfort level or choose a "hands-off" method like the Pill or an IUD.

Perhaps the most important indicator of whether an adolescent girl will use contraception correctly is that she genuinely believes she is at risk of pregnancy and doesn't want to get pregnant. She is well informed and does not buy into myths, such as that pregnancy can be avoided by having sex while standing or that suppressing orgasm prevents fertilization of an egg.

Girls should be taught that even before they have their first period they might be fertile. They should always mark the first day of their periods on a calendar, but never rely on "safe periods" (the rhythm method) as okay for abandoning precautions.

The Most Common Contraceptive Choices for Adolescents

Most adolescents and young adults choose one of the following methods of contraception.

Condom Plus Intravaginal Spermicide

The condom is not only a method of disease prevention, it is also a method of birth control. But because condoms are not always used correctly, may break, or can slip off, it is far better to use a spermicide along with them. While the male puts on the condom (see Correct Condom Use, page 208), the female partner inserts spermicide into her vagina, giving the couple a second barrier to sperm in case there is a problem with the condom. (Spermicide on the surface of the condom is not sufficient since it will have no benefit if the condom breaks or falls off.)

Spermicides come in several forms. Foam (Delfen, Emko) is immediately effective upon insertion and comes with an applicator. Suppositories (Encare, Semicid) take about ten minutes to dissolve and become effective. There are also various jellies and creams that come with applicators. Condoms and spermicides are available in drugstores without a prescription and are therefore the best initial methods of contraception if intercourse occurs before the teen has had a chance to see her doctor.

Hormonal Methods of Contraception

These are generally the most effective, and include several old faithfuls, as well as some newcomers.

THE PILL was introduced in the 1960s and perhaps single-handedly brought on the sexual revolution. An oral contraceptive pill contains synthetic forms of the female hormones estrogen and progestin. These "combined" pills are packaged with four weeks (a cycle) of pills per pack. The "real" pills are taken for three consecutive weeks (twenty-one days), followed by one week of "blank" pills (containing no hormone). It is during the week of blank pills that a girl gets her period. After completing a four-week pack of pills, the teen starts the next four-week pack the next day.

The Pill acts primarily by preventing ovulation each month. A girl must take a pill every day (at approximately the same time each day), whether or not she is having intercourse. Some girls and women experience generally mild side effects, such as nausea, headaches, and moodiness, when they first start the pill. These symptoms usually go away after a few days or one or two cycles.

There are approximately thirty different formulations of the Pill, each with slightly different dosages of estrogen and types of progestin hormone. If side effects do not resolve, a different pill may be tried to see if it causes fewer or no side effects.

Serious medical complications related to the Pill are very rare, especially in healthy adolescents and young adults. However, a doctor will screen patients to make sure there are no risk factors that would rule out the Pill for a particular female. If risk factors are found, the doctor should not prescribe the Pill except after a thorough medical history, physical, and gynecologic examination. Teens who smoke are strongly advised to stop smoking if taking the Pill. (Of course, *all* teens are advised to stop smoking!)

Several positive side effects associated with the Pill include shorter, lighter, and less-painful periods; improvement of acne; and a lower incidence of ovarian and endometrial cancer. The Pill can be obtained only with a doctor's prescription. Because the Pill does not protect against sexually transmitted infections, it should always be used along with a latex or polyurethane condom.

THE PROGESTIN-ONLY PILL (POP, "MINI-PILL") is unlike the standard "combined" oral contraceptive Pill. The progestin-only Pill contains no estrogen, only progestin. With a slightly higher failure rate than the combined Pill, it is prescribed for teens who cannot tolerate estrogen or who for medical reasons (such as migraines, high blood pressure, or sickle cell disease) should not use the combination Pill. POPs suppress ovulation in only half of the women who take them but are effective contraceptives because they decrease cervical mucus and produce other local changes in the uterus and fallopian tubes that interfere with establishing a pregnancy.

These Pills are best taken in the late afternoon. Their effectiveness is more vulnerable to misses (pills forgotten or taken late) than the combined Pill. They come in packs of forty-two pills (six weeks) and are taken continuously from one pack to the next. The most common reason for discontinuing the "mini-Pill" is irregular menstrual bleeding.

DEPO-PROVERA, an injectable contraceptive, contains medroxyprogesterone, a synthetic progestin. Administered by injection into the muscle on the upper arm every three months, the shot prevents ovulation, thickens cervical mucus, and produces other local changes in the uterus and fallopian tubes (similar to the changes induced by POPs) that interfere with successful implantation.

Depo-Provera appeals to teens who have a hard time remembering to take a birth control pill every day. It is highly effective, but may cause weight gain, depression, breast tenderness, and other problems. If side effects occur, the teen must wait at least three months before the progestin is eliminated from her body.

214 *Healthy Teens, Body and Soul*

Most users stop menstruating after three shots, which some girls like but others don't. In girls who stop menstruating and have low estrogen levels, Depo-Provera may be the cause of lowering bone density at a time in life when bones should be strengthening. Despite these disadvantages, some teens find Depo-Provera to be the best choice for them.

NORPLANT, a subdermal implant, consists of six rods that are inserted under the skin through an incision on the upper arm. The rods release levonorgestrel, a synthetic progestin that prevents pregnancy. Norplant rods prevent pregnancy for five years after they are inserted and then need to be removed and replaced. They work in much the same way as Depo-Provera and the POPs.

Because there can be scarring or infection problems upon insertion or removal, it is essential that the implants be inserted by an experienced and careful practitioner. Other side effects are similar to those of POPs and Depo-Provera, but irregular bleeding and spotting are the most troublesome problems that may lead to discontinuation of this method. Teens more than adult women may object to the bumpy appearance of the rods under the skin.

Hormonal Newcomers

Four new hormonal methods of contraception are of great interest. Of these Lunelle and Ortho Evra are already in use, and the two others are soon to be released.

LUNELLE is a "combined" contraceptive injection containing both estrogen and progestin. It is administered monthly and has similar effectiveness and side effects as the combined birth control Pill. It is an excellent alternative to the Pill for those teens who have a hard time remembering to take a daily pill but are willing to go monthly to their doctor or clinic for the injection.

ORTHO EVRA is a combined contraceptive patch that contains and releases estrogen and progestin. It is about the size of a matchbook and is applied to the buttock or lower abdomen. The patch is changed weekly for three consecutive weeks and then no patch is used for a week, during which time menstruation occurs. The patch is similar to the Pill in effectiveness and side effects.

NUVA RING is a soft, flexible ring containing estrogen and progestin. It is inserted deep into the vagina near the cervix. It is left in place for three consecutive weeks and then removed for a week before being reinserted. The Ring is similar to the Pill in effectiveness and side effects.

MIRENA is a new intrauterine device (IUD) that releases a progestin and may be left in place for five years. Like other IUDs that are currently on the market, it is unlikely to be the most appropriate method for most adolescents (see "Intrauterine Devices," page 215).

The Diaphragm

The diaphragm is a barrier method of contraception, which means it blocks the movement of sperm into the uterus. Although it has been around for many years, and was likely used by the grandmothers (and mothers) of many of today's adolescents, it is still a good method for those teens motivated to insert it into the vagina each time they have intercourse. The diaphragm is a dome of soft rubber. It is surrounded by a firm rubber rim that contains a spring that allows it to pop into place after insertion, in order to cover the cervical os (opening to the uterus).

The diaphragm is used along with spermicidal cream or jelly, which a girl spreads along the rim and inside surface of the diaphragm before inserting it into her vagina, preferably within a half hour before having intercourse. The diaphragm is then left in place for six to eight hours. If a girl has intercourse again within that time, the diaphragm should be left in place and additional spermicide should be inserted into the vagina with an applicator.

The diaphragm is very reliable if used consistently and correctly, and has no serious side effects. In some users, it may increase the likelihood of a bladder infection, but this is very easily treated. The diaphragm is especially suitable for a teenager who is having infrequent intercourse, because it is used only when needed. Diaphragms come in several sizes and they must be fitted to the individual user by a health professional. They are available only by prescription. Diaphragms do not protect against sexually transmitted diseases, so they should be used along with a condom.

Intrauterine Devices (IUDs)

The intrauterine device (IUD) is a small object that is inserted inside the uterus by an experienced practitioner. A string attached to the IUD hangs into the vagina so that a woman can check to make sure that the IUD is in place, and so it can be extracted in the future.

Exactly how IUDs work is not known for sure, but it is thought that they prevent pregnancy mainly by interfering with fertilization of an egg by sperm. Two IUDs are currently licensed for use in the United States (also see "Hormonal Newcomers" on page 214), the Progesterone-T and the Copper-T, which must be replaced annually and every ten years, respectively.

IUDs have had a difficult history, with some IUDs, such as the Dalkon Shield, being pulled from the market because they caused pelvic inflammatory disease (PID) or miscarriages in a number of users. Today's IUDs appear to be safer, but there is still a risk of PID. Therefore teenagers are generally not considered the best candidates for this method due to their higher risk of acquiring infection, which could reduce fertility.

THE MORNING-AFTER PILL/EMERGENCY CONTRACEPTION

The morning-after pill, also referred to as "emergency contraception" (EC) should *not* be considered a method of contraception. However, adolescent girls should know that if they skip Pills and neglect to use another method when having sex, or are relying only on a condom for contraception and it breaks or falls off during intercourse, emergency contraception can be obtained in a doctor's office, clinic, or emergency room.

Approved by the Food and Drug Administration in 1997, EC, or the "morning-after pill," when taken within seventy-two hours of intercourse, is highly effective in preventing a pregnancy from taking place, either by impeding ovulation or by preventing implantation.

Several forms of EC are available. Teens may be prescribed a pack of combined birth control pills and be instructed to take several pills at once in two doses twelve hours apart; the same method has recently been packaged as Preven. Because the dose of estrogen and progestin is fairly high (several times greater than that in a daily birth control pill), nausea and vomiting are common side effects. They can be lessened or prevented by taking an antinausea pill, which the doctor should prescribe, prior to each dose. Another technique of EC is called Plan B; it contains only progestin and is less likely to cause nausea and vomiting.

IF PREGNANCY OCCURS

To encourage both daughters and sons to use contraception, parents can initiate a conversation about the wrenching decisions teens must make when faced with unintended pregnancy. Each of the three options—abortion, adoption, or keeping the baby—has the potential of offering both relief *and* regret. Each affects the girl's health; there are health risks associated with pregnancy and with abortion, especially later abortion. (Abortion in the first trimester carries fewer health risks than pregnancy does.)

Moreover, in making the decision, a young woman, preferably in coordination with her partner and both families, must take into consideration a myriad of factors. These include her values, personal goals, and religion; her ability to support and raise a child at this time; the support and mores of her community; and her ability to continue her education.

The decision about what to do when an unplanned pregnancy occurs is so monumental that only after thorough counseling, such as at a Planned Parenthood clinic, should a young woman make her decision. Counseling explores

each option, and the counselor remains impartial. Reputable counselors encourage young women to inform and involve their parents as well as their partners.

While the male partner may want and deserve to have a say in the matter,
the final decision is the woman's. Even if a young man wants the baby and she
does not, he cannot compel her to carry the pregnancy to term. Because it is her
body that must go through the pregnancy, she gets to decide whether that's
what she wants and is prepared to do.

- *Abortion* is legal in the United States, and especially in the first trimester
  carries fewer medical risks than does carrying the pregnancy to term. A
  young woman may feel relieved after an abortion, but she may also grieve
  or feel guilty. Counseling afterward can help her work through this emotionally charged and difficult experience, and reinforce her efforts to take
  measures to help assure that she will not get pregnant again until she is
  ready.
- *Adoption* used to mean that surrendering the baby meant having no knowledge of that child again. Today there are more "open" adoptions, in which
  there is some level of communication between the birth mother and the
  adoptive parents, and perhaps eventually the child. Thus a decision to place
  a child for adoption means not only proceeding with the pregnancy but also
  determining what type of adoption to seek. Again, counseling should be
  part of both the decision-making process and the adjustment period after
  the baby is born.
- *Keeping the baby* will affect the young parents' day-to-day lives forever.
  Will they marry or stay single? How will they cope with the disruption of
  their education, job prospects, family, relationship, and life goals? How can
  they afford to raise the child? What financial and other help will they need
  and can they count on? Young men should be made aware that they are
  responsible for paying child support until the baby grows up, which can
  affect their future earnings for decades.

The longer adolescents can delay pregnancy, the greater their chances of
someday being able to make the kind of home they want for the children they
can have the pleasure of planning.

HEALTH-PARTNERING TIPS FOR PARENTS

- *Affirm that sexuality is an intrinsic part of the life force.* Never let your
  warnings about the risks of sex eclipse the message that sexuality is a wonderful, joyful, and fundamental part of life.
- *Talk to your opposite-sex child.* Dads should talk to daughters as well as to
  sons; moms should talk to their sons as well as their daughters. Give your

teen the wisdom of your experience and the gift of your perspective. Let your teen know you're available to talk, whatever the topic.

- *Talk about sex before it happens.* Have regular conversations with your child about your values and beliefs, and about health issues associated with sex.

- *Prepare your teen to cope with peer pressure.* Role-play what to say and brainstorm what to do in a situation that feels coercive. Make it clear that no one has the right to pressure, guilt-trip, or manipulate another person into having sex.

- *Discuss abstinence as a self-empowering choice.* Saying no (right now) to sex frees teens from worry about disease, pregnancy, and relationships they are not ready for. Help your teen focus on his or her life goals, friendships, and schooling.

- *Help your child identify and avoid situations that may lead to sex he or she does not want.* Being alone in a home or attending a party where parents are not present, and going out with an older teen who expects sex, are two examples of risk situations you should discuss with your teen.

- *Make sure your sexually active teen has protection from diseases and unwanted pregnancy.* Thank your teen for trusting you with the information that he or she is sexually active. Whether or not you approve of the decision, discuss how to stay healthy. Provide condoms or give your teen money to buy them. Offer to accompany your teen to a doctor's appointment to discuss contraception. (See chapters 2 and 5.)

- *Talk with your teen about the connection between sex and alcohol and drugs.* Adolescents' experimentation with alcohol and other drugs often goes hand in hand with sexual experimentation. (See chapter 9.)

- *Remember that teens with chronic illnesses or disabilities have sexual desires, too.* Talk with your teen about protection. (See chapter 7.)

- *Focus on the "relationship" part of "sexual relationship."* Ask your teen how the partner treats him or her, if your teen is happy, if this relationship feels good and caring and fun and kind. If not . . . why is your teen continuing it?

NINE: No Teen Is Immune: Substance Use and Abuse

Adolescents have assets they don't always appreciate. Their fine pink lungs, for example, tirelessly drawing life out of thin air. Their thousands of busy brain cells, inventing interesting theories and witty remarks. Their miraculous child-becoming-adult bodies, revealing destinies tapped out by unique genetic codes.

Yet every day many adolescents choose to use substances that can stain their lungs, shorten their breath, destroy their brain cells, and damage their body and soul. They underestimate the addictive power of nicotine. They don't realize the havoc drinking can cause. They want to believe that "recreational" drugs really are just harmless chemical toys, and that warnings of dangerous consequences are just hype. They may not be aware that alcohol and other drugs are implicated in the three leading causes of death of adolescents ages 15 to 24: accidents, homicides, and suicides.[1]

It seems that some adolescents who use tobacco, alcohol, and other drugs escape unharmed. When they grow up they may look back at their substance use as coming-of-age escapades. But no one can tell which adolescents will be the lucky ones and which will find themselves ensnared in the worst that these substances have to offer: a lifelong smoking habit; derailment of academic and social functioning; physical or psychological drug or alcohol dependency; arrests for use or selling of illegal substances; damage to their lungs, liver, nervous system, or other organs; and death.

Adolescents who use substances may also suffer psychological harm. Those who get into the habit of turning to drugs or alcohol at times of stress may find themselves less equipped to deal with the inevitable stresses of school, dating, family life, and employment. Drugs are simple nonanswers to complicated questions. They may seem to offer respite, but real life waits on the other side of the high.

It is important for parents to understand the degree and context of any substance abuse their child may participate in. Not all teens use substances the same way, at the same frequency, and for the same reasons. Not all substances are the same, although none is innocuous. There is a spectrum of use and abuse that runs the gamut from occasional experimentation, to regular use on weekends, to daily use, to addiction. The age of the child, the number and specificity of the substances, the effect on the child's overall functioning, and the role substances play in his or her life are all factors that contribute to the potential seriousness of a problem.

WHY ADOLESCENTS USE

There is an alarmingly neat fit between certain innate characteristics of adolescence and the appeal of substance use. Teens' perceptions of risk and the future, their search for individuation and connection at the same time, and the stresses they inevitably encounter may lead to substance use by those who are vulnerable.

- *Adolescents are natural experimenters*—and in the right context, their curiosity and risk taking lead to expansion of their creative abilities and their understanding of how the world works and what their place in it can be. To naive adolescents, substances can be just one more thing to experiment with—as a one-time indulgence or as an ongoing adventure with friends.

- *Adolescents are impulsive, short-term thinkers*—so they are not inclined to focus much on the long-term implications of their experimentation. Impulsiveness can be an endearing and joyful quality, but when it comes to substance use, it can result in their failure to connect today's impulse to tomorrow's consequence.

- *Adolescents think they will live forever*—and they exude an infectious optimism. Addiction? Overdoses? Accidents? Those things happen to *other* people.

- *Adolescents want to fit in with their peers*—and in the right context, they can learn the soul-strengthening power of mutual support on a team, working on the yearbook, or hanging out. But when peers are offering alcohol and other drugs, adolescents may focus more on "going along to get along."

- *Adolescents often feel awkward and intimidated in social situations.* It can be intimidating to walk into a party, unsure of how to act or whether people like you. Grabbing a cigarette or a beer can seem like a shortcut to relaxing and feeling part of things. Teens hope that using a drug may help them feel more daring, have more fun, give them better sex, or connect more deeply with others.

• *Adolescents are eager to explore adult lifestyles and privileges*—and to emulate the adults in their lives. Indeed, a family history of substance abuse makes it more likely that an adolescent will try substances, too.[2] And trying these substances is easier when there is ready access to a well-stocked bar or stash at home.

• *Adolescents are often overwhelmed and confused by the pressures of growing up.* Substance use does not occur in a vacuum. Conflicts at home, educational challenges, disappointments with friends, and political strife and violence within communities and in our world may make adolescents wonder whether they have much of a future at all.

• *Adolescents are ambitious.* But sometimes, like everyone, they fail— and may seek the so-called solace of drugs or alcohol. Young people need to know that conflict, failure, and confusion are not *exceptional* aspects of life but *expectable* ones. Substances may offer escape, but ultimately they can deprive adolescents of their forward-moving momentum.

• *Adolescents are stressed, trying to do it all.* These teens are so overextended, they feel taut as rubber bands stretched to the limit. Come the weekend, that rubber band snaps free—time to cut loose with drugs and partying. Drugs may also provide the means of staying up late to study or of "coming down" after a particularly frenetic day.

Whatever comfort substances offer is temporary and double-edged; the time lost and the impaired development are very real. Many adolescents manage to stop or limit their substance use before it sabotages them. But others never manage to regain the ground they lost. The less they feel capable of navigating in the "real world," the more they become invested in substance use. Some will remain dependent on substances all their lives, or delay indefinitely the time when they can become emotionally, socially, and financially independent.

TALKING WITH TEENS ABOUT ABSTAINING
Connected Adolescents Abstain or Wait
As harmful as tobacco, alcohol, and other drugs (referred to as TAOD) can be at any age, there is good news. The longer adolescents delay trying them, the

likelier they are to avoid lifelong substance abuse problems. Adolescents entering their twenties who have not tried tobacco, alcohol, or drugs in their teens are less likely to start as adults. The presence of supportive, caring parents, educators, health care providers, and other adults in preteens' and teens' lives is one of the most pivotal factors in influencing adolescents to avoid or delay substance use.

Informed parents are empowered parents. It is important to know what substances your adolescent may be invited or tempted to try. As with so many other adolescent health issues, communicating with your adolescent about substance use is critical. You may be surprised to find that your child is both receptive and relieved when you initiate this discussion.

Perhaps the best way to prevent substance use is to promote family and community involvement, and participation in constructive activities. Substances often rush in to fill a void. When adolescents' lives are filled with positive people and enjoyable, meaningful activities, they are less likely to use substances that can derail their own sense of purpose.

Not Everyone Is Using

The pull to be similar to peers is very powerful for adolescents. If they believe that most of their peers are smoking, drinking, or using drugs, they will be more likely to experiment themselves. But a reality check is in order. The fact is, most teens are not habitual smokers, drinkers, or drug users. Adolescents who insist that "everybody is using" are likely to be mistaken. They may have friends who glorify substance use because they think it sounds cool or grown-up to complain about a hangover or boast about how stoned they got at a party.

On the other hand, if your adolescent is habituating "raves" (all-night dance parties, often featuring electronically synthesized music and drug use) and hanging out with teens or young adults who use, then your adolescent indeed will have a skewed perception that "everyone" is using.

Abstinence versus "Harm Reduction"

When talking with adolescents about substance use, parents often find themselves coming up against the dilemma of what to do and say if they know or have reason to expect that their teens are using substances anyway. The dilemma is: Do you just urge teens to abstain? Or do you also talk with them about harm reduction—namely, strategies that help ensure that teens who do use substances will be safe?

Proponents of discussing only abstinence believe that it gives a clear, unambiguous message, while harm reduction messages are "mixed" and confusing for a teen to interpret.

Parents who opt for harm reduction messages, on the other hand, believe that they are being realistic in their advice and rules and are ultimately enhancing their child's safety and comfort level about coming to them for help.

For example, parents may prefer that their adolescent not drink. But they are aware that in their community drinking is commonplace at teen parties, and they do not want to deprive their teen of being able to attend. So they may ask their child to limit drinking to one beer. They may tell their child to call them for a ride at *any time* instead of driving with friends who have been drinking or using drugs. They will pick up their child "no questions asked." They may even serve alcohol at home, giving their teen a glass of wine at dinner to teach how to drink responsibly and appreciatively, rather than with the more puerile goal of getting drunk. The theory is that it's better to keep the child safe than to be so punitive that an adolescent may be afraid to call home for help.

A key element in this "debate" must be consideration of the age, maturity, and reliability of the teen. You may feel it is more appropriate to take a more flexible approach with a senior in high school who has earned your trust than with a middle school child who appropriately should be abstaining from all substances. Yet discussing harm reduction with your teen, while better than saying nothing, is clearly a distant second choice from urging adolescents of any age to use nothing.

TOBACCO

In *Thank You for Smoking*, a satirical novel, Christopher Buckley captures the clash between health and profits. Antismoking advocates say smokers are "victims, their lives stubbed out upon the ashtray of corporate greed," while a tobacco industry spokesman defends "the cigarette industry's right to slaughter half a million Americans a year."[3]

Indeed, those half a million tobacco-related deaths each year in the United States make tobacco use the number-one preventable killer in this country.[4]

Tobacco companies know that most people who start smoking do so as adolescents or even preteens. The vast majority of adult smokers began smoking as teenagers, 90 percent before the age of 19.[5] Adult nonsmokers are unlikely to start smoking—and are no longer prospective customers. Tobacco companies view adolescents as prime targets, and market their toxic goods accordingly. Cigarette ads portray happy, sexy, slim, confident people, smoking as if they hadn't a care in the world about their health or anything else.

Adolescents continue adding to the tobacco industry's profits. Findings from the National Youth Tobacco Surveillance 2000 survey conducted by the

Centers for Disease Control and Prevention (CDC) are startling. Nationally, over 8 percent of students had first smoked a cigarette before age 11. Among middle school students (grades six to eight), 36 percent had ever smoked cigarettes, and 15 percent were current users (at least once in the past thirty days) of a tobacco product (most commonly cigarettes, then cigars and smokeless tobacco). Among high school students, 64 percent had ever smoked cigarettes and 35 percent were current users of a tobacco product.[6]

Cigarettes as Social Accessory

To many adolescents, a cigarette is just a cool social accessory. The many celebrities puffing away in films and on some TV shows help foster the perception that smoking is a stylish thing to do.

Teens have many motivations to smoke. A cigarette gives you something to do with your hands and lets you gaze flirtatiously through lowered lashes as you light it. It gives you a moment of connection with someone else: "Got a light?" It even gives you an excuse to do nothing: "I'm going out for a smoke." It allows you to carve out a space of time to think, to take a break: When you sit on a step to smoke, you're doing something; when you sit there not smoking, you're doing nothing and you think you look strange.

When you're waiting on a street corner to meet a friend, a cigarette helps pass the time. You think you look relaxed and casual. Holding the cigarette just so, you learn to shape your lips like an *O* and blow out perfect smoke rings.

A cigarette is punctuation; it's the pause as you think of what to say, it's the dessert after a meal, it's the B-movie way to conclude a sexual encounter. A cigarette keeps you company as you walk to school, brood in your room, watch TV, or read the paper. A cigarette helps you keep your weight down, manage your fidgeting, join your friends, proclaim your independence, and show that you're tough enough to defy health warnings.

After a while, a cigarette is your steady companion, even when you wish you could make it go away. The cigarette calls to you when you wake up in the morning, after you eat, before you go to bed, when you're anxious, when you're stressed, when you're studying, when you're with friends. Activities seem incomplete without a cigarette in your hand. You want to quit, but you really want a cigarette. You *need* a cigarette. And that's addiction, getting stuck with a habit when all you really wanted was something to do once in a while.

Effects of Smoking, Now and Later

Because tobacco is legal and commonly available, many adolescents do not view it as a drug. Adulthood seems far away, so the threat of side effects like lung cancer, respiratory trouble, and heart disease likewise seems remote.

However, tobacco is harmful in the short-term, too. Adolescents who smoke cough more, get more colds, have less stamina, and get short of breath more quickly. If they have asthma, smoking will make it worse. Smokers have bad breath (the dreaded "ashtray mouth"). Their hair, skin, and clothes stink. Their teeth and fingers get dark stains. Getting turned down for a date by someone who thinks smoking is disgusting may be one of the most compelling catalysts for quitting.

If those aren't enough reasons to avoid smoking, here's another one: Cigarettes are expensive. Adolescents who are given plenty of spending money may not care, but those who have after-school or summer jobs may think twice about seeing their hard-earned dollars go up in smoke.

Bidis, Cigars, and Smokeless Tobacco Are Risky, Too

Bidis are small, hand-rolled, "herbal" cigarettes that are imported from Asian countries. The tobacco is wrapped in various types of leaves, and bidis are available in many flavors, including chocolate and cherry. Bidis have become popular "cigarette alternatives" in some areas. In one survey of urban youth in Massachusetts, for example, 40 percent of teens said they had tried bidis, and 16 percent said they were bidi smokers now.[7]

Many adolescents believe that bidis are a more "natural" choice and are less hazardous than cigarettes. But bidis can be just as dangerous as cigarettes, have a higher nicotine content, and, unlike cigarettes, are not regulated by the Food and Drug Administration.

Cigars were once viewed as the province of corporate men and rakish entertainers. In recent years cigars have been promoted for stylish iconoclasts, as if wielding a chubby wad of tobacco were proof of independent thinking. Women have gotten in on the act, too.

Over the last decade, cigar smoking has increased by 50 percent,[8] and more than 17 percent of high school students have tried smoking cigars. Some adolescents think cigars and smokeless tobacco are less hazardous than cigarettes, but such is not the case. Cigars increase the risk of cancer of the lungs, mouth, tongue, lips, throat, esophagus, and possibly pancreas and bladder, and of respiratory and heart disease.[9]

Chewing tobacco, tucked between cheek and gum, and snuff, which is sniffed, can cause cancer of the mouth and pharynx, mouth sores, gum and dental problems, and halitosis. More than 7 percent of high school students, mostly male, use smokeless tobacco.[10]

Quitting the Tobacco Habit

A majority of middle school and high school cigarette smokers surveyed tried to quit (unsuccessfully) within the past year,[11] and about half of current smokers reported they want to quit. The youngest smokers, and those smoking the least quantity, would have the easiest time, but may lack the motivation and any strategies to go about it. They could certainly benefit from working out a plan with a supportive parent, doctor, teacher, or even a friend.

Setting a quit date is the first order of business. The quit date should not be far off, preferably within a few weeks of making the decision to quit, or chosen to coincide with a special date such as a birthday, graduation, or right after (or before) the prom.

Going "cold turkey" is one option. This strategy is more likely to be successful if it is thought through ahead of time. The teen (with help from another person) should identify and write down the situations or stressors that lead him or her to grab for a cigarette, then make a plan for how to address each stressor. For example, if a teen smokes while doing homework, substitute carrot sticks. If a teen smokes after a stressful event like an argument with a parent, then call a friend, go for a walk, or take a bubble bath. A simple act like drinking a glass of water instead of reaching for a cigarette substitutes a healthy habit for a harmful one.

Experiencing withdrawal symptoms, such as irritability, insomnia, headaches, gastrointestinal symptoms, fatigue, and increased appetite, should be expected for a few weeks if the smoking habit was daily and more than just a few cigarettes.

Chewing Nicorette gum may ease the urge for a cigarette. Each piece contains 2 milligrams of nicotine and should be chewed for fifteen to thirty minutes, up to ten to fifteen pieces per day.

Using a nicotine patch can also help. The patch is available over-the-counter under several brand names. It is recommended only for people who smoke at least ten cigarettes per day. Patches come in several strengths, depending on the severity of the habit. It is important to refrain from smoking while using the patch so that you do not take in even more nicotine than you are accustomed to and become ill. Read package inserts about possible side effects.

Gradually reducing cigarette use is another method, such as smoking one or two cigarettes fewer each day (or for several days or a week) until the number is zero. The concept of evaluating vulnerable times of the day and tricks to get through them may prove worthwhile for this tapering approach.

Joining a smoking cessation group at a school or a local organization such as the Y may prove the difference between success and failure. The best motivation to staying a nonsmoker will be how much better the teen feels: easier breathing, fresher breath, no cough, colds easy to break, and a lot more energy . . . not to mention a lot more spending money.

How Parents Can Help

Certainly it is easier for adolescents to stop smoking if they live in a smoke-free home. Parents who smoke can increase their child's likelihood of success if they join their teen in quitting. They can also spare other members of the household the substantial health hazards of secondhand smoke.

Toss the ashtrays and banish smoking in the home by family and guests alike. Stock up on raw veggies like celery sticks to munch on when the oral urge hits. Beginning an exercise program at the same time helps control weight, reduce stress and irritability, and provide constructive distractions. Every non-smoking day should produce increasing degrees of stamina and lung power—a wonderful, tangible reinforcement of what a great thing parents and adolescents are doing for their individual and family futures.

Tobacco as a Gateway Drug

If your child smokes, it is important to assess that decision in a broader context. Not only is tobacco use dangerous in and of itself, but it can also serve as a gateway to other drugs. An adolescent who uses tobacco is demonstrating a willingness to introduce a toxic substance into his or her body. That willingness may extend to other drugs, too.

Look at the adolescent's life overall to determine what might have contributed to the decision to smoke. Is the adolescent excessively stressed? Associating with reckless friends? Socially ill at ease? Vulnerable to peer pressure? In addition to encouraging and helping your child to quit using tobacco, find other ways to strengthen your child's self-esteem, increase health awareness, and participate in healthy activities, including physical activities.

Dr. C. Everett Koop, the former surgeon general, wrote in his autobiography, "I have been with ex–drug addicts who say something like this: 'You know, I kicked heroin, I kicked pot, I kicked cocaine, I kicked morphine; why can't I kick cigarettes?' "[12] He pointed out that although tobacco use by a teen is often considered to be less serious or worrisome than alcohol or drug use, for most teens it is the *most deleterious* to their current and future health. Most teens who use alcohol or a drug do so sporadically and usually don't continue to abuse them into adulthood; this is said not to condone such use but to point out that most teens do not become alcoholics or drug-addicted adults. By contrast, high percentages of teens are regular and addicted smokers, and are likely to continue the habit into adulthood and thus suffer considerable consequence, including premature death. For this reason, rather than thinking of tobacco use as simply a gateway to harder substances, it should be considered dangerous in its own right.

ALCOHOL

Alcohol is the inspiration for "happy hour." It is a rationale for a rendezvous: "Let's meet for a drink." It flows through parties, toasts, rituals, religious rites, dinners. People drink to celebrate, to savor, to be sociable.

But there is little subtlety in adolescent drinking. Adolescents tend to drink to get drunk. Their drinking is furtive, hidden from parents' eyes, done with friends or alone. Alcohol, along with tobacco, is the easiest drug for adolescents to get hold of, and often the first they'll try. Adolescents whose parents drink, especially those with alcoholic parents, are more likely to drink themselves, and alcoholism is a disease that runs in families.

According to the Youth Risk Behavior Surveillance survey, 50 percent of high school students in grades nine to twelve were current users of alcohol (had at least one drink of alcohol during the preceding thirty days); use increased with grade, and higher percentages of males than females were current users (67 percent of male twelfth graders compared to 57 percent of female twelfth graders). Approximately one third of students reported drinking more than a few sips of alcohol before age thirteen, one third of ninth to twelfth graders had had at least five drinks or more on at least one occasion within the preceding thirty days, and nearly one third of twelfth grade boys had driven a vehicle after drinking alcohol within the last thirty days.[13]

Alcohol and Health

Alcohol presents health risks at the time of drinking, the day after, and years later:

• *Health Risks While Drinking:* Adolescents may say things they shouldn't say and do things they didn't intend to do—like vomit in front of their friends, or worse. Because drinking impairs judgment, adolescents who drink are more likely to engage in high-risk behaviors such as unsafe sex, taking on dangerous dares (for example, diving off a rock into a too-shallow river), and getting into fights. Adolescents' perilous lack of control is even worse if they pass out or black out, unable to remember what happened while they were drinking. Binge drinking, infamous in fraternity hazing and drinking games on college campuses, can cause coma or death from alcohol poisoning. Alcohol also impairs coordination, making falls and other accidents more likely. (See the discussion of drinking and driving on page 229.)

- *Health Risks the Morning After:* Hangovers are the unwelcome souvenirs of a night of drinking. Headaches, gastrointestinal distress, wooziness, and nausea can ruin a next day. The morning after can also bring a feeling of panic: *Did we have sex? Did we use a condom? Who was there? Did someone put something in my drink?*

- *Health Risks Years Later.* Ongoing heavy drinking can damage the liver, causing alcoholic cirrhosis, a disease in which inflamed liver cells die and scar tissue forms. The liver becomes less capable of carrying out its various important metabolic functions, which eventually will lead to death (or the need for a liver transplant). Nutrient intake is less likely to be adequate. Alcohol also damages the heart and brain cells, and increases the likelihood of certain cancers (liver, throat, and esophagus).

Legal and Lethal: Drinking and Driving

Many potentially dangerous things are legal. Cars, for instance, when crashed, can kill. Heavy machinery, mismanaged, can maim. Alcohol can kill, too. Minimum-age laws were passed to reduce the problem of teen drinking and driving, and although they have helped, there are still too many adolescents who die or are injured through drunk driving (see chapter 12).

Adolescents need to understand that what they consider a modest amount of alcohol can increase their blood alcohol level enough to impair reflexes and judgment. How quickly alcohol causes intoxication is related to gender, weight, how much food the person has eaten, and how quickly the alcohol was consumed.

An adolescent girl who protests "All I had was a beer" is failing to consider that a 12-ounce beer ingested by a petite 100-pound girl within an hour of driving can make her too intoxicated to drive safely.

Adolescents also often have the impression that beer and wine are less likely to cause inebriation than hard liquor. But a 12-ounce bottle of beer, a 1.5-ounce shot of whiskey, and an 8-ounce glass of wine have the same alcohol content. Teens sometimes drink wine coolers to get a buzz without getting drunk, but these beverages, too, may have as much alcohol content as regular wine. Furthermore, teens who drink a lot of wine coolers, justifying them as being "light," may take in enough alcohol to cause impairment.

You Don't Have to Stumble

Teens sometimes say "He [or she] didn't *seem* drunk" when explaining why they got into a car driven by someone who had been drinking. The fact is, people hold their liquor differently. After a single drink one person may giggle, stumble, and have slurred speech. After five drinks another person may seem stable and controlled—but will not be able to react quickly enough behind the wheel of a car to avoid an accident.

Teens are not trained to assess reflexes and impairment levels; they do not carry devices to measure someone's blood alcohol level. So their best bet for safety is to avoid driving with someone who has had anything to drink. Appointing a designated driver or arranging in advance for parents to pick them up are lifesaving strategies to which teens should agree.

Help for the Adolescent Problem Drinker

If you suspect that your adolescent has a drinking problem, enlist the help of your child's health care provider, who can screen your adolescent and determine the extent of the problem. For example, the practitioner may ask about the quantity, frequency, timing, and circumstances of alcohol use, as well as the adolescent's own assessment. Does the adolescent feel compelled or pressured by others to drink? Drink secretly or alone? Experience blackouts or hangovers? Feel guilty or worried about drinking? Participate in risky behaviors while drinking? Have friends or family members expressed concern about the adolescent's alcohol use?

Depending on the extent of the problem, treatment may range from substance abuse counseling, enrollment in a peer support group, participation in Alcoholics Anonymous or Alateen programs, or referral to a residential treatment facility that is experienced in working with adolescents. In some instances, the medication Disulfiram (Antabuse) may be used; if an adolescent drinks, the medication interacts with the alcohol to make the adolescent vomit or feel nauseated or dizzy, or cause headache.

ILLICIT DRUGS

Like products in the mainstream consumer culture, illicit drugs are ever-changing. Drugs fall in and out of fashion, new ones appear on the scene, and both sellers and users are always looking for the newest sensation. Dealers tinker with recipes to cut costs or to make a drug more intense or addictive. Prescription medications assume unsavory new identities as experimenters find ways to use them to get high. Household products lose their innocent utility as users discover ways to sniff or otherwise redeploy them for intoxication.

Even old familiar drugs can't be depended upon to be what they used to be, as growers and processors boost their level of psychoactivity. A "natural" drug like marijuana is not the mellow weed of yesteryear; it now has a higher level of THC, its psychoactive ingredient. Even marijuana initially sold as "pure" can be laced with other drugs, with or without the user's knowledge.

Unlike the legitimate marketplace, there are no product liability laws to protect users, no Better Business Bureau to censure unscrupulous entrepreneurs, no Food and Drug Administration to test new drugs for safety before they go on the market. Adolescents who sample illicit drugs often do not realize how vulnerable they are.

They trust that the pill they're given is really what it's supposed to be.

They trust that an administered dose is the "right" amount—enough to get high, not enough to make them unconscious, brain-damaged, or dead.

They trust that a high will be fun, not dangerous.

And they trust that they can get out of whatever situation they've gotten into.

MARIJUANA

Marijuana poses a particularly delicate dilemma for some parents. Having smoked marijuana themselves, whether during their own youth or to this day, can they honestly counsel their child to avoid it? Indeed, if asked whether they ever tried it, what should they say?

Parents are under no obligation to part the curtains of their lives and let their child see all. The decision to disclose is deeply personal. Some parents disclose their pasts as cautionary tales. Others chuckle as they shake their heads, remembering their wild days, then quickly add, "But you shouldn't smoke." There are also parents who take the Fifth or simply lie, fearful that admitting their own drug use will subvert their abstinence message for their kids.

Marijuana (also referred to as "grass," "pot," "weed," and "dope") is derived from the plant cannabis. It is the most widely used illegal drug in the United States (overall, about 50 percent of students in grades nine to twelve reported ever using it, and one fourth used it at least once in the preceding thirty days).[14] It can be smoked in a joint (rolled cigarette) or from a pipe, or be ingested orally when baked into cookies or brownies. Its active ingredient, delta-9-tetrahydrocannabinol (THC), is present in much higher percentages these days than in the 1960s, thus increasing its potency to produce a euphoric high—but also adverse toxic reactions such as panic, disorientation, paranoia, seizures, or psychosis. For regular users, the more potent marijuana available today is much more likely to result in addiction and withdrawal symptoms similar to those seen with opiates (agitation, insomnia, sweating, drug craving).

Indeed, parents' ambivalence about marijuana may dissipate as they learn more about it. Smoking marijuana not only causes immediate adverse effects;

chronic use can also impair physical health—lung damage with respiratory ailments, possible effects on female and male fertility, and diminished cognitive brain function (memory and comprehension). Combined with alcohol or other drugs, marijuana can contribute to dangerous toxic effects. Most notably, marijuana inhibits nausea and vomiting. But vomiting, in fact, protects against alcohol poisoning and death.

Marijuana use can also divert an adolescent from studies and friends. One effect of chronic marijuana use is "amotivational syndrome," a pattern of apathy that causes an adolescent to turn away from constructive activities.[15]

Help for the Adolescent Marijuana Smoker

Adolescents often are uninformed about the health risks associated with marijuana. Explain to your child that marijuana can become habitual (or addictive) and interferes with learning, the ability to develop close relationships with others, and constructive engagement with life. Ask your child's health care provider to assess your child's extent of use.

INHALANTS

Inhalants are the vapors from common household products such as glue, aerosol spray cans, gasoline, and paint thinner. Unlike other "drugs," inhalants are most popular as methods of intoxication among younger adolescents and preteens. They are sniffed from inside paper or plastic bags or rags soaked with the substance, to initially produce a stimulant state. Oftentimes, the setting is an enclosed space with poor ventilation, which enhances the hazard of the teen's eventually drifting into sleepiness, dangerous central nervous system depression, and even death. Inhalants can be toxic to the liver, heart, lungs, kidneys, and other organs. Because they are so easy to obtain and are popular among the very youngest users—those with the least ability to judge the seriousness of their behavior—they are particularly dangerous and scary.

There are about a million new inhalant users each year. Twice as many eighth graders are likely to have used inhalants in the past month as twelfth graders. A recent National Household Survey on Drug Abuse, however, revealed that first-time use among 18- to 25-year olds has risen from 4.8 to 11.2 per 1,000 potential new users.[16]

The range of consumer goods used as inhalants is mind-boggling. They include:

- *Industrial, household, art, or office supply solvents* (such as paint thinners, dry cleaning fluids, gasoline, glues, correction fluids, felt-tip marker fluid).

- *Household, aerosol, or medical anesthetic gases* (aerosol propellants such as those in hair sprays, deodorants, and spray paints; butane lighters, propane tanks, refrigerant gases, and medical gases such as ether, chloroform, and nitrous oxide).
- *Nitrites* (such as amyl nitrite, available by prescription, also known as "poppers" and often used in clubs).

Help for the Adolescent Inhalant User

Chronic inhalant users may suffer psychological problems and social maladjustment, and are known to be harder to treat than many other substance abusers. Depending on the extent of the problem, family counseling and treatment in a residential or community facility may be recommended. Evaluation of blood lead level should be done for adolescents who have sniffed gasoline.

STIMULANTS

Amphetamines

Adolescents may use amphetamines to overcome sleepiness (for example, so they can stay up late to study) or to suppress appetite. They are highly sought-after drugs by the many adolescents who feel it is very important to be thin. As street drugs they are often referred to as "speed," "mollies," "bennies," and "uppers."

Crystal methamphetamine ("ice") is a smokeable and especially potent and dangerous form of amphetamine. Its acute toxic effects can be profound, including seizures, coma, cardiovascular collapse, and death. Adolescents may also use amphetamine "look-alikes" (such as ephedrine and pseudoephedrine, and the herbal drug called ma huang), caffeine, and Ritalin (sometimes "borrowed" from a friend for whom it was prescribed for attention deficit disorder).

Whether they are obtained as illicit drugs or as over-the-counter "diet aids," amphetamines can be addictive, and a heavy user who wants to stop may experience withdrawal symptoms such as depression (perhaps with suicidal or other violent thinking), profound fatigue, and intense appetite. Amphetamine psychosis primarily affects habitual users but may also occur when a person takes one large dose.

Cocaine

Cocaine, a stimulant, is a highly addictive drug. It can be inhaled (snorted), injected, or smoked. When processed with baking soda or ammonia, it is known as crack cocaine. Crack produces a particularly intense and addictive high, but a briefer one—which makes users crave repeating the experience again and again. With all forms of the drug, repeated use increases tolerance to the drug, which means that increased quantities must be used to achieve the desired high. While high on cocaine a person may feel euphoric, clear-thinking, and spared of the need to sleep.

When people who have become frequent users try to stop, they may experience a depression so intolerable that they return to using. Repeated cocaine use can make a person feel paranoid, anxious, and restless. Over time, snorting cocaine can cause ulcers in the membrane of the nose and weaken the septum, causing it to collapse. Many people have died from respiratory and cardiac arrest caused by cocaine. In some instances deaths have occurred after using the drug for the first time. It is impossible to predict which users will be susceptible to this sudden death.

When adolescents combine cocaine and alcohol, the synergy of the two substances in their body creates a third substance, cocaethylene. The resulting intoxication is especially intense. It can also cause sudden death.

Nearly 10 percent of high school seniors say they have tried cocaine at least once.[17]

Help for the Adolescent User of Stimulants

Adolescents addicted to amphetamines or cocaine should enter a chemical dependency program that contains the following components: immediate cessation of the substance, individual and group therapy, family counseling, supervised urine testing at least twice a week, and careful monitoring to prevent or respond effectively in case of relapse.

HALLUCINOGENS AND CLUB DRUGS

At clubs frequented by older adolescents, Ecstasy and other drugs are often an integral part of the scene, and are known as "club drugs." Of course, they are not only used in clubs but also at parties, by couples, or by a person alone.

Adolescents often buy into the idea that these drugs are harmless fun and give them the energy and verve to party for hours and hours. Yet used alone or (frequently) in combination with other drugs or alcohol, they can lead to medical emergencies, long-lasting damage, or even death.

Ecstasy

One of the most popular club drugs among adolescents is Ecstasy (MDMA, or methylenedioxymethamphetamine), a stimulant and a hallucinogen. Young people often continue to use Ecstasy as a way to elevate their mood, feel closer to others, energize themselves so they can dance all night ("raves"), and alter their sense of reality. Ecstasy is illegal, and young people cannot be sure what is in the pill they are taking or how they will react. They are playing Russian roulette with their bodies. Is the pill really MDMA, or is it adulterated, or is it something else altogether?

Ecstasy appears to work by increasing the release of neurotransmitters in the brain. These include serotonin, a chemical that affects mood, emotions, appetite, sleep, and other behaviors.[18] When MDMA causes the release of a large quantity of serotonin, the user feels an increased sense of well-being. However, the release depletes the brain's supply of this important chemical, and the effect of this depletion, especially when Ecstasy is used frequently, appears to be varying degrees of damage to brain cells. While the degree of damage is likely associated with such factors as an individual's reaction and the quantity and frequency of use, it is not known whether any particular level of use is "safe." Some people have suffered ill effects after a single use. Ecstasy can lead to impaired thinking, memory, and sleep.[19]

Ecstasy has also been associated with a number of deaths. Hyperthermia is one cause. MDMA impairs the body's ability to regulate its own temperature, while also giving a person the energy to dance all night. The combination of increased body temperature (hyperthermia), severe dehydration, and substantial expenditure of energy through hours of dancing in hot and poorly ventilated dance halls has proven fatal in a number of instances. Fatalities have also been caused by MDMA-associated heart attacks and stroke.[20]

Rohypnol

Known as a "date rape drug," Rohypnol (flunitrazepam) is a colorless, odorless, and tasteless substance that can be added to someone's drink without that person's knowing it. The drug (also referred to as "rophies," "RZs," and "RIP") can make a person feel drowsy and confused—therefore more susceptible to sexual assault—and it induces amnesia, so a person has no memory later of what happened to her or him. Rohypnol can also lower blood pressure and cause dizziness and an upset stomach.[21]

Teens—especially older adolescents who are more likely to go to a bar—need to protect themselves against Rohypnol. When ordering a drink, they should watch it being made. They should never leave a drink unattended at a bar or party. When they go to the bathroom or turn away for a conversation, they should take their drink with them.

GHB

GHB (gamma-hydroxybutyrate, also known as "G," "Georgia Home Boy," and "Liquid Ecstasy") depresses the central nervous system, relaxing users and making them feel less anxious. Excessively high doses increase the sedative effect and may make the user fall asleep, or even lapse into a coma or death, especially if the user has also drunk alcohol. Indeed, GHB is usually sold as clear liquid and is used to spike alcoholic beverages. According to the National Institute on Drug Abuse, GHB is responsible for more overdoses than other club drugs, and GHB-related emergencies in the United States have soared from 56 in 1994 to nearly 5,000 in 2000.[22] It is not hard to imagine that a young person could become unconscious in a hot, crowded club, without anyone's noticing or obtaining help for quite a while.

Ketamine

Also known as "Special K" or "K" or "Vitamin K," ketamine is used as a general anesthetic in veterinary medicine. It is used as an illicit drug in liquid or powder form for its sedative, hallucinogenic, and hypnotic qualities. It takes effect rapidly and lasts about an hour, but for up to two days afterward the user may have impaired judgment, coordination, and memory, and possibly psychotic symptoms.[23]

LSD

LSD (lysergic acid diethylamide), or "acid," had its dubious heyday in the 1960s, when the Beatles and other luminaries claimed that taking a tab of acid let them break through into new realms of higher consciousness. This liquid hallucinogen may not have the high-profile devotees of several decades ago, but it has certainly not gone away. According to the Drug Enforcement Administration, doses today are somewhat less than those in the sixties.[24] But LSD can still cause severe disorientation, fearfulness, psychosis, sleeplessness, loss of appetite, and other immediate or long-lasting effects. Flashbacks to acid "trips" can occur among both healthy users and those who have been impaired by chronic use.

Help for the Adolescent User of Hallucinogens

Adolescents must be informed of the potential toxicity of Ecstasy and other hallucinogens. They must be alerted to the fact that not only do these drugs present their own risks, but that combining drugs (especially stimulants with hallucinogens) compounds the danger, and so does combining drugs and alcohol. The club scene is fraught with dangers that teens are best advised to avoid.

OPIATES

Heroin, perhaps the best-known opiate, has been associated with hard-core addicts and jazz greats, addicting and harming people of despair and people of talent equally. While in the same family as such painkillers as morphine and codeine, heroin, derived from the opium poppy, is one of the most addictive drugs known. As users build tolerance to the drug they must use more and more to achieve the sought-after euphoria it produces. Heroin can be injected, snorted (preferred by adolescents), or smoked. Users who share needles risk HIV infection, viral hepatitis, and tetanus. Acute opiate overdose produces coma, respiratory and cardiac depression, and eventual death if not medically treated.

"Designer drugs" are synthetic chemical formulations of opiates that mirror or exceed the effects of heroin and morphine, and can be just as dangerous and potentially lethal. These drugs include 3-methylfentanyl, known as "China white," which has been linked to multiple deaths.

Help for the Adolescent User of Opiates

People who try to end heroin or other opiate use suffer a physically and psychologically agonizing withdrawal, an experience so wrenching that in some instances it has caused death. Detoxification to manage withdrawal should always be done under medical supervision, followed by enrollment in a dependency treatment program. Some users find it impossible to quit and enter a methadone maintenance treatment program through which they receive daily doses of methadone, a long-acting synthetic narcotic, to manage opiate craving. For many addicts, methadone maintenance is a lifelong commitment that allows them to stabilize their lives.

ANABOLIC-ANDROGENIC STEROIDS

Young people who want to become more muscular, usually with the goal of improving their athletic performance or appearing more "bulked up," may turn to injectable or oral anabolic-androgenic steroids. These synthetic derivatives of the male sex hormone, testosterone, can cause an ironic swapping of sexual characteristics, impairing a male's reproductive system and "masculinizing" a female. Steroids may be injected or taken orally.

Males may lose hair prematurely, become impotent, have difficulty or pain when urinating, and develop shrunken testicles, a lowered sperm count, an enlarged prostate gland, and increased breast size (gynecomastia).

Females may grow facial hair, develop shrunken breasts, have irregular menstrual periods or none at all, and acquire a deeper voice and an enlarged clitoris.

Both genders may experience severe acne, jaundice, trembling, swollen ankles and feet, high blood pressure, and reduced HDL (the good cholesterol).

" 'Roid rage" refers to the sudden, inexplicable rages to which users of steroids are prone.

Help for the Adolescent User of Steroids

Parents should make sure that steroid use is not encouraged, condoned, or ignored by athletic coaches and other adults in their child's world. The health care provider must do a comprehensive assessment of the steroid's effects and make recommendations accordingly.

SIGNS OF DRUG AND ALCOHOL USE

Long before parents "know" their child is using drugs, there are usually indications. But parents have to know what to look for and be willing to consider the possibility—it is easy for adolescents to explain away signs when parents are eager to believe that there is no problem.

On the other hand, there can indeed be innocent explanations of seemingly suspicious signs. Maybe your child stinks of cigarette smoke because everybody else was smoking. Maybe that pipe did roll under the bed when a friend's backpack spilled. Maybe that wine bottle truly was scavenged for a candlemaking class. Maybe your child is drug-free even though several of his best friends were just arrested for drug possession. Every one of these explanations is possible.

Or maybe not.

Know your child. Here are some questions to ask of yourself:

- Have your adolescent's friends, activities, and/or overall state of mind been changing recently?
- Does your adolescent seem newly defiant, breaking curfews and other rules?
- How is your adolescent doing in school? Are grades dropping, either suddenly or consistently over a period of time? Does your child seem distracted, forgetful, less motivated to do well?
- Have you found liquor bottles, cigarettes, rolling papers, drugs or drug paraphernalia in his or her room? Are there posters on your child's walls that glorify drug or alcohol use?
- Is your adolescent increasingly secretive? Does your child seem to have something to hide?
- Are you missing money or valuable items? Could your adolescent be "borrowing" from you to pay for cigarettes, alcohol, or drugs?
- Does your adolescent stay out all night? Do you believe what your adolescent is telling you about her or his evening activities?

- Does your adolescent go to clubs that are known for drugs? If you have no idea which clubs those are, do you think it is time to find out?
- Does your adolescent have sudden rages? Seem paranoid, depressed, or anxious? Seem to have lost motivation and interest in old friends and favorite activities?
- Are new buddies suddenly calling or visiting, people you've never heard of before? Could your child be dealing drugs? Could these individuals be customers?

If the answer to any of these questions produces some concern, then trust your gut feeling—do not push the worry aside. Your observations may be related to your child's use of tobacco, alcohol, or drugs, or perhaps may be due to something else. But if you feel concerned about changes in friendships, school performance, mood, activities, attitude, or behaviors, then certainly it is a good time to contact your adolescent's health care provider for a consultation.

HEALTH-PARTNERING TIPS FOR PARENTS

- *Be a responsible role model.* There is no question that by abstaining from substance use yourself, you are sending a powerful antiuse message. But what if you are a smoker? Having an adolescent to set an example for can be just the motivation you need to quit. If you choose not to quit, perhaps use yourself as an example of someone who got hooked as a teen and now regrets it. You can still speak up about not wanting your child to become addicted, too.
- *Do not drink and drive.* If you drink in moderation and never drive while drinking, you are setting a responsible example. But a child who sees a parent drunk or driving while intoxicated is less likely to take seriously that parent's admonitions not to follow suit.
- *Talk frequently with your child about tobacco, alcohol, and drugs.* Initiate discussions when your child is at an early age (preteen or even younger) and continue them periodically throughout the adolescent years so that your child knows that substance use is something you are concerned about. Use various opportunities to initiate a discussion, such as a TV show, news item, incident in the community or at school, or observations of teens on the street. Just as a single conversation about the birds and the bees does not suffice, neither does a single conversation about substance use.
- *Encourage your child to participate in after-school activities.* Much substance use occurs in the after-school hours, when adolescents are unsupervised and have time on their hands. Adolescents involved in sports, music

lessons, clubs, volunteer work, or enrichment classes are less likely to have the opportunity or inclination to use.

- *Set clear limits.* Specify where your child may go and set a time for returning home. Require your child to keep you informed. *Where are you going? With whom? Will the parents be home? What are the phone number and address? How do you know this person?* Be clear about whether your child is allowed to have friends over when you are not home, or visit friends whose parents are absent. Your child may protest your limits—but they are a sign of love and will help protect your child.
- *Work cooperatively with other parents.* Network with other parents to discuss substance use and support one another's efforts to promote substance-free parties and events. Especially during early adolescence, call parents in advance of a party to ask if they'll be home and if they will be banning alcohol and drugs at the party. Make the call even if your adolescent claims that this will cause her or him lifetime embarrassment.
- *Make the same phone call before sleepovers.* These get-togethers are sometimes pretexts for drinking. When kids "sleep over" you really don't know when they are getting in or if there is tobacco or alcohol on their breath. Encourage sleepovers regularly at your own house.
- *Urge the school and community to support a peer culture of abstinence.* What are the consequences if a child is caught with drugs or alcohol at school? Does the school tolerate smoking in the schoolyard? Does the school actively ban drinking at proms and take steps to enforce it? If your child's school does not have clear, well-thought-out, publicized, and *consistently enforced* policies, join with other parents to create and advocate for them. Similarly, speak with youth organizations that your child goes to about their policies.
- *Stay informed.* Drug trends and fads, chemical formulations, and usage patterns are constantly evolving. Both parents and adolescents should stay informed about what's going on for the sake of their own family and the health of their friends. Go to a website such as www.theantidrug.com, which is set up as a support and information source for parents and educators.
- *Present accurate information about the consequences of substance use.* Be clear about the risks of tobacco, alcohol, and other drug use, and urge your child to take those risks personally. If appropriate, use examples from your family or neighborhood: "Aunt Katie started smoking when she was fourteen. She has tried to quit many times but can't. Now she has emphysema."
- *Describe but do not exaggerate the risks.* For example, don't say that a child will become addicted after smoking one cigarette. Tobacco is highly addic-

tive, but there are some people who are able to smoke occasionally and resist addiction. It is more constructive to say that it is impossible to know which people can avoid addiction and which will become addicted—and that therefore it is better not to take the risk.

- *Role-play* with your adolescent possible responses if peers offer tobacco, alcohol, and drugs. Practice excuses ("It would make me nauseous") or calm, assertive statements ("No, thanks, none for me" or "I don't drink beer. I'll have a soda.").
- *Review with your child how to avoid or leave a problematic situation.* It's the teenage version of the game "What would you do if . . . ?" For example: What would you do if you were at a party and somebody brought out some marijuana joints? Possible answers: Decline to smoke. Go into another room. Go outside with a friend. Call home and ask to be picked up.
- *Emphasize the danger of drinking/drugging and driving.* Offer to pick up your child anywhere, any time, providing an alternative to riding in a car with someone who has been drinking or using drugs, or to driving after doing so himself or herself.
- *Link privileges to abstinence.* Be explicit: "If you drink and drive, you lose driving privileges."
- *Express your concerns to the police.* If you know of a club that illegally admits underage adolescents, notify the authorities.
- *Do not permit your child's room to be a hiding place for drugs.* It is understandable to want to give your adolescent a certain degree of privacy, but if you suspect drug use, you owe it to your child to check. This is your home, after all, and your child, and you are responsible for protecting both.
- *Seek help*—for your child, for yourself, for your family. If your adolescent is using tobacco, alcohol, or other drugs, don't feel like you should— or even can—handle the problem alone. Ask your health care provider for assistance or referrals. Join organizations such as Toughlove (see "Resources," page 342) for help in coping with a resistant adolescent. If your gut feeling is that something is wrong, there is a good chance you are right. Do what you need to do for your child's health and future, and for your own peace of mind.

TEN

Panic at the Mirror:
Teens and Eating Disorders

Given that countless adolescent girls are tormented by society's idea of the perfect body, it seems especially apt that it was Eve, not Adam, who reached for the apple in the Garden of Eden, setting a disastrous precedent. For so many of today's young Eves, eating is not a simple pleasure but an act fraught with peril. To those who see calories as enemies, even an apple can seem like forbidden fruit, and eating it can lead to a dire fate.

A report from the U.S. Surgeon General in 1999 stated that about 3 percent of female adolescents suffer from eating disorders. Such disorders include anorexia nervosa, bulimia nervosa, binge-eating disorder, and eating disorders "not otherwise specified" that resemble but do not fully meet the diagnostic criteria of the first three.[1]

And although the great majority of adolescents with anorexia nervosa or bulimia nervosa are female, Adam is not exempt. Boys also develop eating disorders, often in association with dieting to improve their appearance or to meet the weight restrictions of such sports as wrestling or track. (Due to the fact that 90 percent of individuals with diagnosed eating disorders are female, in this chapter we mainly use female pronouns to refer to those so afflicted.)

In addition to the eating disorders listed above, eating behaviors resulting in obesity are even more prevalent among adolescents, although such behaviors and obesity are not classified per se as eating disorders. Obesity is a major health concern among adolescents, putting stress on various organ systems of the body and causing considerable mental anguish. Indeed, adolescents' various and profound struggles with food can be wrenching for the whole family.

EATING DISORDERS AND THE HAZARDS OF THINNESS
The Runaway Body

In striking ways, eating disorders are generated from the inevitable and dramatic physical, psychological, and social changes that preadolescents and adolescents begin to face even as young as age eight or nine. Their bodies begin to grow uncontrollably, and they are expected to become more mature and independent, social and sexual, goal-oriented and mindful of their futures. Ready or not, adolescents are carried along by great waves of hormones and social expectations, swept into new shapes and feelings they don't feel ready for. The body they once knew is morphing daily. It's a runaway body, speeding toward sexual maturity. Peer, parental, and academic demands to function in new ways are potentially overwhelming.

Many adolescents welcome these changes; they are exciting, though sometimes disorienting. But other adolescents mightily resist the idea that they must cooperate with the direction in which their bodies are heading. There is a powerful disconnect between the lengthening and rounding of their bodies and the "Hey, wait a minute!" response of their brains. These adolescents can feel trapped inside bodies that no longer feel like "them." They want to turn back the clock, return to the prepubescent bodies that were so much less threatening—and so much leaner.

Compounding the problem is the fact that what is causing their bodies to become so much curvier is not just hormones but *fat*. It's fat as well as muscle that gives breasts their bounce and hips their contour. But in our can't-be-too-rich-or-too-thin society, *fat* is a dirty word.

Rich Fashion Models, Poor Role Models

A healthy body is a fit, well-nourished body, and may or may not be thin. Most normal people can achieve the extreme thinness of top fashion models only when they undertake a punishingly stringent regimen of self-control that involves taking in fewer calories than they probably need and want, and perhaps doing more exercise than their reduced-calorie diet can support.

Normal bodies have a layer of fat. Fat is necessary for estrogen production, for reproduction, for life itself. But if fat is the enemy, then normalcy is the enemy. Adolescents who are at once rebelling against their "new bodies" and trying to meet unrealistic aesthetic standards are caught in a terrible bind. Fasting, vomiting, and obsessively exercising are ways out of the bind. They see these as "control mechanisms," strategies that enable them to impose their will on their runaway bodies and at the same time feel more in control of their fast-moving lives. By putting their bodies through these torturous rites, adolescents keep their weight down and gain access to the fat-free status so prized by our society.

What adolescents don't realize is that they may be heading their runaway bodies down a hazardous hill. They can lose control of their "control mechanisms."

Eating less and less in order to continue to lose weight can lead to eating nothing at all; the dieter is now an anorexic, zooming toward possible death.

Vomiting regularly can lead to vomiting unwillingly; the bulimic has lost control of her own peristaltic reflexes.

Overexercising without taking in enough calories can lead to perilous exhaustion; the exerciser has barely enough energy to walk down the hall.

The Lost Aesthetic of Body Diversity

Genes spell out a dazzling array of noses, necks, and knees. Basic parts turn out not to be so basic after all. Each part, in each person, is honed in a unique way. How much happier people would be if there were more appreciation of body differences. A round-bellied woman can be as lovely as a flat-bellied one; a very thin man can be as pleasing as a muscular one. Sculptors know this. From the elegantly attenuated forms of Alberto Giacometti to the magisterial, voluptuous nudes of Gaston Lachaise, all human silhouettes can be celebrated in art.

Unfortunately, such aesthetic breadth is beyond the narrow scope of most of today's image makers. From magazines to movies, the media almost purposefully sow discontent. They rub our collective noses in the message that most people can't possibly attain the perfection of the rarefied creatures who grace the glossy page and the big screen. And they lie. Their computer technicians are "technosculptors." They airbrush and alter the images of models and celebrities to make them look even thinner and smoother-skinned than they really are. This digital prestidigitation is so widespread that we can no longer trust the commercial images we see.

And because adolescents tend to worry anyway about whether their changing bodies are normal and acceptable, they are especially vulnerable to the media's trickery. Perfect, toned bodies with long limbs, flat tummies, and trim thighs become the physiological holy grails that adolescents (and many adults) avidly desire. Eating disorders are just a short step from the diet merry-go-round that millions of people live on as they seek a perfection that is rarely humanly possible.

Family and Peer Pressures

The exhortations of family and peers and coaches ratchet up the pressure. Several studies have shown that girls are more likely to diet and worry about their bodies if their mothers are doing the same.[2] Parents who make weight-related comments to their adolescents may unwittingly trigger a plunge in self-esteem and the resolve to resort to unhealthy weight-control practices. It is not unusual for adolescents with eating disorders to recall verbatim some of these pivotal, inadvertently hurtful comments:

You're looking a bit pudgy today.

You shouldn't wear that sweater; it makes your stomach look big.

I don't think you should buy that bikini. Try this one-piece instead.

You're so cute; you never lost your baby fat.

Such comments can be so devastating that they lead to what's called "pinpoint onset" of anorexia nervosa in a vulnerable teen. An adolescent's decision to embark on a drastic weight-loss campaign can be pinpointed to the moment when that comment was made, or to when some incident or piece of clothing made the adolescent feel fat.[3]

Interestingly, one study noted that while a mother's concerns about weight often spurred her adolescent to adopt poor weight-control behaviors, a father's concerns held even more weight, so to speak.[4]

Parents' own views and efforts regarding weight control have a tremendous effect on their children. Adolescents are more likely to eat healthy meals and exercise if their parents do, and are more likely to obsess about weight if that's the attitude that permeates their home.

Parents are most helpful when they model healthy eating and fitness behaviors, love and value their child regardless of appearance, and support their their child's growth into a healthy, secure, and responsible young adult by respecting the child's preferences, interests, views, and opinions starting at an early age.

Peers and Community Play a Role

Peers' comments, of course, are also very meaningful to adolescents. Peer pressure or the urge to feel like one "fits in" is an inescapable fact of adolescent life. It takes an emotionally sturdy adolescent with a strong support system to withstand the constant weight-control comments and behaviors of her peers. Competition to see who can fit into Gap clothes in size zero can be devastating to an adolescent girl who wears size eight or ten. If shrinking body size can lead to magnified standing among peers, it can be hard to resist taking the steps to achieve it—even though they may be harmful to health.

Schools and community groups should endeavor to expose the thin-is-better mentality as superficial and unhealthy. Through class discussions and establishing an overall good-health environment (for example, by asking neighborhood businesses to reject billboards and advertisements that glorify emaciated bodies), they can help counteract society's weight obsessions and redirect peers' efforts to more constructive pursuits.

ANOREXIA NERVOSA

After getting badly bruised in a car accident, Angie, fourteen, is taken to a hospital and hooked up to an IV.

"What's in that IV?" she screams. "How many calories are you giving me?"

The doctors, nurses, and family around her are just trying to make sure that she stays alive. But Angie has virtually starved herself for months. She does not want the IV to steal the "progress" she has made in achieving a near-skeletal body.

Angie has anorexia nervosa. The word *anorexia*, from the Greek words *an* ("without") and *orexis* ("appetite"), is actually a misnomer, since loss of appetite is usually not the case. Rather, there is a marked refusal by these individuals to fulfill one of the most essential human urges: to eat, to take in nourishment. In fact, individuals with anorexia nervosa eat little but think *a lot* about food, often to the point of an obsessive preoccupation about their food choices, meal planning, calorie counting, or elaborate cooking for others.

Anorexia Nervosa: Both Defining and Threatening Life

An adolescent who develops anorexia nervosa often starts dieting and exercising simply to lose some weight. But the more she loses, the more she wants to lose. The goal is no longer to be slender but to be the thinnest among her peers. Weight loss is her mission, and it's something she has turned out to be very good at. Losing weight makes her feel effective and better about herself, and therein lies the incentive to keep it going. The single-minded focus on losing weight obliterates painful thoughts and feelings and provides her with a newfound identity. The intense fear she develops of gaining any weight back, even when emaciated, is linked to the intense fear of losing control, self-esteem, and this new identity around which she organizes her life.

She is not stupid. She would not perpetuate the starvation if she didn't "have to." Anorexia nervosa is a disease that actually distorts her perception of herself. When she looks in a mirror, she "sees" fat. Others may see only a skeleton veiled by ever-drying, increasingly translucent skin. But in her eyes there is no such thing as thin enough. Ergo, she is fat, and must continue to starve.

Her quest to get even thinner requires ever stricter routines in order to perpetuate the weight-loss trend. She increasingly restricts her food intake, obsessively aware of the calorie count of each bite. There are fewer foods she is willing to eat, and none have fat. No matter how much she loses, she still feels fat, or deeply fears becoming fat again if she eats even an extra morsel. Occasionally, she may slip and eat just a little more than she feels she should, and may follow her lapse by vomiting or exercising even harder. Her pursuit of thinness takes on a life of its own—until eventually the act of starving becomes her life.

But something is threatening her extraordinary achievement. People around her are getting worried while her weight continues to drop. They implore her to eat. They tell her over and over that she is not fat. If fat is the enemy, now these family members and friends are also part of her defiant fight. If she gives in to them and starts eating again, the fat will win and she will lose.

Indeed, this is the first time in her life she feels truly assertive, having been a compliant "good girl" while growing up. Her family always stressed the importance of her being obedient and meeting their expectations. She rarely expressed disagreement or discontent. In fact, she never felt the need to act or speak or dress differently from other members of her family and hated more than anything to displease them. Now she has an arena for her fight for independence. It may be a lonely fight, but it's all her own. Without realizing it, she is turning herself against her own body and its most basic needs.

Diagnosing Anorexia Nervosa

When does a simple diet become a dangerous disease? The diagnosis of anorexia nervosa is based on the following criteria [5]:

- Refusal to maintain body weight at or above a minimally adequate level for age and height (usually 90 percent of normal weight). However, diagnosis may be apparent even above this level, especially in someone who starts off overweight. In a growing early adolescent, *a failure to gain* the expected amount of weight may also be diagnostic, even if no weight loss has occurred.
- Intense fear of gaining any weight or becoming fat, even when emaciated.
- Preoccupation with thoughts and behaviors pertaining to food.
- Distorted perception of weight and body shape, denial of the seriousness of current low weight, and overreliance on body weight and shape for self-esteem.
- Amenorrhea (cessation of menstrual periods in females) or cessation of pubertal development in younger adolescents (males and females).

Health Risks of Anorexia Nervosa

Anorexia nervosa is a hazardous hunger strike. One by one, body systems deteriorate. The progression of the disease demonstrates the body's biological triage, as less vital body functions cease or slow down (for example, menstruation) to reserve ever-diminishing supplies of energy for those body functions that are essential to survival (for example, heart, liver, and brain).

Loss of menstruation (amenorrhea) and cessation of pubertal development are among the first casualties of inadequate caloric intake (the body's source of energy). Most females with anorexia nervosa become amenorrheic as a result of weight loss (and lack of estrogen and other hormonal secretions); however, some cease to menstruate even before significant weight loss has occurred, and others may continue to menstruate even after becoming substantially emaciated.[6] Inadequate estrogen secretion combined with low weight and poor nutrition contribute to the development of diminished bone mass, which increases the risk of bone fractures. This condition is called *osteopenia* if relatively mild and *osteoporosis* if more severe. (For a discussion of the related female athlete triad, see chapter 5.)

Gastrointestinal problems also afflict people with anorexia nervosa. Because the body goes into a general slowdown to conserve energy, including a slowing down of the motility of the entire gastrointestinal tract, adolescents with anorexia nervosa often complain of symptoms of stomach fullness, bloating, and constipation. Quick feelings of fullness will make it more difficult for them to feel comfortable increasing their intake of food when treatment of their disorder begins, and so this process must proceed gradually.[7] In a way, the body has gotten used to starving and must relearn the processing as well as the pleasures of food.

Similarly, elimination becomes a problem. Constipation, bloating, and abdominal cramps are common. These symptoms may discourage an adolescent from "refeeding" if she fears that everything she eats will stay inside her. Indeed, it can take weeks or months to restore normal bowel function.

Anorexia nervosa can also have devastating effects on the cardiovascular system, initially showing up as diminished energy or such marked fatigue that performing even routine daily activities becomes exhausting. On physical examination, patients typically have very slow pulses and low blood pressure. Cardiac failure is the most common cause of death associated with this disease.

Malnutrition also causes dysfunction of the endocrine and immune systems, and temperature regulation. These adolescents usually feel cold all the time, and circulation of blood to their hands and feet is usually low, resulting in cool, bluish, and clammy extremities. Severe malnutrition may cause the body to sprout a growth of fine hair similar to the lanugo hair of premature newborns; this hair growth may be the body's attempt to help keep itself warm in the face of lost subcutaneous fat. The skin may acquire an orangeish tinge from the ingestion of vegetables rich in beta-carotene, as well as become dry and scaly. The hair and nails may become brittle and fall out or break easily.

Significant psychiatric and neurological symptoms are associated with anorexia nervosa, and most are attributable to the starvation and malnutrition.

Like any individual who is deprived of adequate food for whatever reason, adolescents with anorexia nervosa often display impaired concentration and ability to complete tasks, irritability and apathy that contribute to isolation from their peers, various psychiatric symptoms including depression, obsessive-compulsive behavior, decreased libido, and sleep difficulties. In fact, suicide is one of the more common causes of death. However, it is often gratifying to see all these very disturbing symptoms improve once better nutrition is instituted as part of a treatment plan. Most people can relate to what it feels like to be sleep-deprived or jet-lagged and then finally get a good night's sleep. Likewise, finally eating a better meal can reap an immediate improvement in mood and sense of well-being.

Laboratory Tests

When a doctor evaluates the medical condition of an adolescent with anorexia nervosa, several laboratory tests will be performed. Blood tests may turn out to be pretty normal (even in a very sick patient) and should not be interpreted in an overly reassuring way. But many patients will have abnormalities in their blood count (low red, white, or platelet cell counts), liver function tests, electrolytes, other blood chemistries, levels of zinc or vitamin B_{12}, and various hormone levels (thyroid, adrenal, sex hormones). An electrocardiogram will likely show a slow heart rate and possibly rhythm abnormalities.

Treatment of Anorexia Nervosa

Anorexia nervosa is a complex disease with profound medical, nutritional, and psychological manifestations. Therefore, its treatment requires a team of professionals and the full involvement of the adolescent's family.[8]

The health care team should consist of, *at a minimum*, two professionals.

1. A medical specialist (adolescent medicine, pediatrician, internist, family physician) with expertise in evaluating and treating the medical and nutritional complications of eating disorders.
2. A mental health professional (psychiatrist, psychologist, social worker, psychotherapist) with expertise in treating the individual patient with an eating disorder and the patient's family.

These two professionals are the overall providers and coordinators of the medical/nutritional and psychological care of the adolescent with an eating disorder. It is crucial that they communicate with each other regularly to be certain they are both on the same page with the patient and that their work is truly complementary and not in any way contradictory. Members of the treatment team share information and strategize treatment together in order to optimize the outcome. Sometimes the medical specialist may arrange for the patient to work as well with a nutritionist, and sometimes the mental health professional will recruit a colleague to do the family therapy and/or group therapy. As more members are added to the team, it remains crucial that team members maintain regular communication with each other. Of course, as the team enlarges, the time commitment and financial costs of treatment increase, but often this is necessary.

If outpatient treatment, even with several team members, is unsuccessful in stabilizing and moving the patient toward health, then various types of more intensive care should be considered, including full- or half-day programs, residential treatment centers, and inpatient programs in medical or psychiatric hospital settings.

Through Treatment, a New Direction

The goals of treatment are, first and foremost, to stabilize any medical complications, facilitate weight gain, and ease anxiety about weight gain. But in order to achieve lasting change, the adolescent must come to understand that anorexia nervosa is a disease that is not really about weight and starvation at all, but rather stems from a need to feel better about herself and to be in control of various facets of her life.

Family involvement is key to finding improved means of communication and examining family dynamics that may have contributed to the adolescent's problems. There should be no assigning of blame, but rather a cooperative examination of how the adolescent, the family, and the therapeutic team can work together to help the adolescent regain good health and feel confident that she can move forward in her development and be successful in life. The road to recovery can be rocky and slow, with detours along the way.

At first the adolescent may be secretive and sneaky, and even dishonest with the doctor, therapist, and parents . . . anything to avoid having to gain any weight. Many anorexic adolescents wear bulky sweatshirts or sweaters and baggy pants to conceal their boniness. Some girls pad their bras to maintain a feminine silhouette, even as their bodies look increasingly boyish.

Anorexic adolescents also may go to elaborate lengths to hide or throw away food or to exercise in secret. To get people to back off, these adolescents will use such ruses as hiding coins or magnets in their underwear or body cavities, or loading up on food or water so that when they step on the scale in the doctor's office it will seem as if they have gained weight. Those experienced in treating adolescents with anorexia may need to resort to such unpleasant measures as not permitting them to go to the bathroom alone, not permitting them to eat alone, and searching their rooms to make sure they are not hoarding food that they were supposed to eat.

But eventually, with persistence and hard work, the adolescent begins to feel comfortable in a larger body, gradually allows herself to derive true pleasure from food, and no longer needs the eating disorder as an identity or means to feel safe.

BULIMIA NERVOSA

Sherise binges, shoveling food into her mouth as if it is all going to disappear tomorrow and this is her last night to eat. She eats fast, going for quantity, and she mixes it up: a chicken leg, a chunk of cake, leftover potato salad, bread and butter, a pickle—whatever's around.

When her binge ends Sherise feels sickened and ashamed by her lack of control. She is terrified that the calories she just consumed will throw off her carefully maintained weight. So she heads to the bathroom, sticks her fingers down her throat, and forces herself to throw up the food she just ate. By minimizing the amount of time she allows the food to stay in her body, she hopes to keep it from turning into fat. Food is only safe when stuffed in and purged as soon as possible.

Her binge-and-purge pattern is a secret, a bizarre weight-loss practice, and a way to release stress. To Sherise, bulimia is a way to have her cake and vomit it, too. But it also makes her feel uneasy and worried. Although she can have her treat without gaining weight, she begins to realize that she is compromising her physical and psychological health in many ways.

Bulimia nervosa is binge eating (consuming large quantities of food within a relatively brief time period) combined with "compensatory activities" that are intended to reverse the potential resulting weight gain. The cycle of bulimia is accompanied by feelings of self-loathing, guilt, and depression. The bulimic adolescent also often feels burdened by and ashamed of this "secret life."

The compensatory activities taken to forestall weight gain after a binge include vomiting, using laxatives or diuretics, or exercising obsessively after eating.

Hidden Rituals

Like anorexia nervosa, bulimia nervosa often involves a series of clandestine practices and rituals. In fact, it is often easier to hide the binge-and-purge pattern of bulimia nervosa than the steady starvation of anorexia nervosa. After all, the bulimic adolescent is eating and may appear to maintain normal—or at least not excessively low—weight. That she steals away to the bathroom to vomit after meals is something she views as her private affair. But it can also be a clue for alert parents. By the same token, in order to continue their purging, bulimic adolescents rely on their parents' failure to notice this pattern or to suspect what it might mean.

Food is the fuel that propels one forward; rejection of nourishment is rejection of life. The "tools" of bulimia—diuretics, laxatives, and vomiting—further abrade life. When used in excess and for long periods of time, they can harm the body in a number of ways, as discussed below. Malnutrition is paired with various forms of toxicity. And the loneliness of bulimia can tear at an adolescent's self-esteem. She condemns herself for her frenzied bingeing and her humiliating purging, but on her own feels unable to get the cycle under control.

Diagnosing Bulimia Nervosa

This secretive illness may exist for years without anyone except the affected individual knowing about it. However, when the illness becomes known, an adolescent will describe the following:

- Recurrent episodes of bingeing and purging (vomiting, laxative or diuretic use, or other compensatory behavior such as excessive exercise or restrictive eating) occurring at least twice a week for three months, during which the individual feels unable to control what or how much is eaten.
- Body weight and shape unduly influence and affect the individual's self-evaluation of her appearance and worth.

Health Risks

The health risks of bulimia nervosa are related to the method(s) used to compensate for binges, the frequency and severity of the recurrent episodes of bingeing and purging, and the individual's weight. If the bulimic individual's weight is too low, she will suffer similar consequences to those experienced by someone with anorexia nervosa. These may include irregular or no menstrual periods, fatigue, dizziness, cold intolerance, and osteopenia/osteoporosis. Some individuals with anorexia nervosa may also purge or exercise excessively, but typically these behaviors do not follow recurrent episodes of bingeing. Most adolescents with bulimia nervosa maintain a fairly normal weight, although they may experience considerable yo-yo-ing of their weight as the result of fluctuations in their eating and purging behaviors.

Specific to bulimia nervosa are problems associated with the purging behaviors.

The vomiting can cause erosion of tooth enamel and dental decay as well as erosion of the esophageal lining (esophagitis) from repeated exposure to regurgitated stomach acids. Bulimic patients may develop gastroesophageal reflux (or spontaneous vomiting without even trying) and, rarely, esophageal tears. Loss of stomach acid results in electrolyte deficiencies of potassium, chloride, and sodium, which can cause fatal heart arrhythmias. Some patients develop swelling of their parotid (salivary) glands. Adolescents who use ipecac syrup, a substance sold in pharmacies to keep on hand to induce vomiting in case of an accidental poisoning, risk toxicity to their muscles, including the heart muscle, and this complication can result in death.

Bulimic adolescents who rely on laxatives usually find that they must continue to increase their dose over time in order to produce the desired effect of massive watery diarrhea and the resultant feeling of emptiness they seek. Sometimes dozens of laxative tablets are taken each night. In addition to the dehydration that results from massive losses of fluid from the lower intestine, dangerous electrolyte losses may also ensue. Laxatives, in fact, act on the large intestine (the colon) after all calories have already been absorbed in the small intestine. Therefore, the weight loss experienced is "water weight" and not fat at all. The laxative abuser then feels very thirsty, drinks back the weight lost, and feels compelled to repeat the cycle of laxative abuse over and over again.

Treatment

The treatment of bulimia nervosa, as with anorexia nervosa, is best provided by a team of professionals including at a minimum a physician and a mental health professional experienced in treating eating disorders. The physician cares for and monitors any medical complications of the bulimia nervosa, and the mental health professional performs psychotherapy. Together they coordinate and provide the various components of care.

- Cognitive-behavioral therapy (CBT) aims to help the bulimic adolescent resume eating regular meals and snacks, avoid restrictive eating that can lead to bingeing, and examine the function of the bingeing and purging in her daily life. An important component of CBT is for the patient to keep detailed daily logs of everything she eats and drinks, any bingeing and purging episodes that occur, and a running written analysis of thoughts and feelings associated with eating and purging. In this way, the patient learns to identify triggers of the dysfunctional behavior (certain foods, moods, feelings, thoughts, locations, companions, or other stressors) and is taught strategies to deal more effectively with such difficult situations. CBT may be done with an experienced physician or a mental health professional.

- Interpersonal therapy aims to engender self-examination, enhance understanding of self, and bring about personal change within a trusting and safe relationship with the mental health professional. Family or group therapy may also be recommended in addition to individual work.
- Medications, especially certain antidepressants such as the SSRIs (selective serotonin reuptake inhibitors)—for example, Prozac and Zoloft—are often helpful in relieving the depressive and anxiety symptoms and urges to binge of patients with bulimia nervosa. Such medication would be prescribed by the medical physician or a psychiatrist added to the team if the mental health professional is not a psychiatrist. (See chapter 11.)

BINGE-EATING DISORDER

Colette eats carefully, watching calories, selecting nutritious meals. But every week or two, she is seized by an uncontrollable desire to binge. Suddenly she feels transformed from human to vacuum cleaner, cramming whole cakes, entire pints of ice cream, a bucket of fried chicken into her mouth. On and on she eats. Her hands can't stop grabbing food, her mouth gobbles bite after bite. When the binge is over she is consumed by self-loathing.

Binge-eating disorder (BED) is characterized by recurring episodes of out-of-control eating that are similar to those experienced by people with bulimia nervosa. However, these episodes are generally not followed by the compensatory activities of vomiting, laxative or diuretic abuse, starvation, or excessive exercise. BED often results in obesity, with its concomitant health risks, described later in this chapter. Individuals with BED also experience shame, disgust and guilt, and sadness associated with their behavior.

The treatment of BED is less well researched than that of bulimia nervosa, but the same methods and medications that are listed above seem to apply. Attending meetings of Overeaters Anonymous or other groups that address compulsive overeating may also prove helpful to these adolescents, as well as to those with bulimia nervosa.

EATING DISORDERS "NOT OTHERWISE SPECIFIED"

Many adolescents suffer from obsessive eating concerns and distressing eating behaviors that do not completely meet the diagnostic criteria of anorexia nervosa, bulimia nervosa, or binge-eating disorder. Such individuals are designated as having eating disorders "not otherwise specified," and they require a similar kind of care and attention to restore health and relieve anguish.

Some of these individuals resemble patients with anorexia nervosa, are too thin, but have normal menstrual periods. Others may have all the intrusive thoughts and anxieties about eating and their body's size and shape, eat rigidly and restrictively, but maintain a weight near or within the normal range. Others may vomit or abuse laxatives at times, not necessarily following a binge, but after eating something they wish they hadn't had, such as a piece of cake or a large muffin. Others may binge and purge but less frequently than a person with bulimia nervosa. And others may chew up food and then spit it out.

Sometimes people with these disorders eventually develop anorexia nervosa or bulimia nervosa, and sometimes these disorders follow a full-blown case of anorexia nervosa or bulimia nervosa. Not infrequently, the same individual may move from a classic case of anorexia nervosa to bulimia nervosa, or vice versa, and this pattern can repeat itself. And so, although these various eating disorders seem to fit into nice distinct cubbyholes, in real life a person may suffer sequentially or repeatedly with more than one pattern of disordered eating.

OVEREATING TO OBESITY

Overweight and obese adolescents need help as surely as their anorexic or bulimic peers. Obesity is a serious health problem, and assisting or "coaching" an adolescent to overcome it can be pivotal for lifelong health. Obese adolescents are at risk for developing precocious (early) puberty, menstrual irregularities, hypertension, diabetes mellitus, respiratory difficulties, and orthopedic conditions, and for becoming obese adults who are at increased risk for cardiovascular disease and cancer as well. Unfortunately, an increasing number of adolescents are overweight—14 percent of adolescents ages 12 to 19, compared with 11 percent only a few years ago, according to the National Health and Nutrition Examination Survey.[9]

As an adolescent becomes increasingly ungainly, parents sometimes watch helplessly, unaware of how they may be enabling their child's weight gain. At one home, guests at a dinner party were treated to an up-close view. The hosts' overweight twelve-year-old son preferred to dine at his computer. The guests watched as his parents took turns carrying food to him: first one plate piled high with fried chicken, whipped potatoes, peas, buttered corn, and rolls; then another, followed by chocolate cake with ice cream. Later on, as the guests prepared to leave, the boy wandered in to say good-bye. The last thing the guests heard as they headed out the door was this exchange:

"Mom, I need pizza!"

"Okay, honey, I'll go get some for you."

"Oh, and some of those cinnamon buns, too!"

What made this situation especially disquieting was that the parents had reported to their guests that the pediatrician had advised them: "Don't do anything about the child's obesity; surely, you don't want to precipitate an eating disorder!"

Clearly, this doctor—like many others—had no idea how to help an obese child, or much interest in doing so. Unfortunately, many doctors feel that treating obese adolescents is fraught with frustration and likely to fail. So they don't even attempt it and simply hope that the adolescent will grow out of the fat.

Obesity as a Social Hardship

One Fat Summer, Robert Lipsyte's novel for adolescents, relates the tale of Bobby, a 200-pound, 14-year-old boy who worried that "somebody was going to make fun of my fatness in front of people I cared about."[10] Bobby hated the arrival of summer, because winter coats that concealed his fat had to be abandoned for shorts and T-shirts that revealed it.

The obese adolescent experiences a wide range of emotional and social disadvantages that may contribute to perpetuating the problem. Being obese is socially hard on a kid. The self-consciousness, embarrassment, and shame that many obese adolescents feel can be debilitating. They often don't feel part of things, are at a disadvantage in sports and other physical activities, feel unattractive to potential friends and dates, find it hard to find stylish clothing that fits, and may be subjected to teasing, bullying, or discrimination.

Having a poor self-image may lead obese adolescents to isolate themselves, become depressed or withdrawn, or conversely, to feel compelled to compensate in various ways. These compensations can be somewhat positive, such as entertaining others (the stereotype of the fat, jolly teen) or focusing on schoolwork or hobbies. But compensation may also be expressed in deleterious ways. For example, some overweight adolescents court attention by making themselves sexually available.

It takes an exceptionally strong adolescent to withstand the humiliation that often attaches to obese young people. Of course, no one deserves to be rejected for being overweight, and people of all body types and conditions should be treated with respect. Nevertheless, it must be recognized that obese adolescents are burdened by more than their excess pounds. By helping them to lose weight, parents and health care providers are improving their long-term outlook for both good health and social comfort.

Is It "Baby Fat" or Obesity?

The pudgy contours of childhood sometimes persist into early adolescence, then diminish nicely as increased height and changes in body composition result in the appearance of more evenly distributed weight. Especially boys, who naturally become more muscular and less fat as adolescence advances, seem to simply "outgrow" chubbiness, and any weight problem simply becomes a thing of the past. Nature is less kind to girls, who become "fatter" as they mature, and the trend may be an ever-increasing degree of overweight. However, the more pleasing scenario is more likely to occur for any adolescent, girl or boy, who is physically active and eats a variety of nutritious foods containing a moderate amount of calories.

Obesity is defined as a state of excessive storage of body fat. The determination of whether an individual is overweight or obese is made in several ways, each with its limitations and inaccuracies. One technique relies on the concept of an "ideal weight" for age and height as listed in various published tables—which, in fact, differ somewhat from each other. A child is "overweight" if between 10 and 20 percent above the "ideal weight" for the child's age and height, and is "obese" if 20 percent or above.

The "body mass index" (BMI) concept also relies on weight and height measurements (weight in kilograms divided by height in meters squared). An individual with a BMI greater than 30 or above the 95th percentile is considered "overweight"; and if at 30 or above the 85th percentile, is "at risk."

Neither tables nor the body mass index directly measures fatness, nor takes into account variations in body habitus (body build and constitution), leg length, or body composition. Therefore, some doctors prefer a direct fatness assessment, easily done in an office setting using an instrument called skinfold calipers. They measure the thickness of subcutaneous fat by grasping a thickness of flesh with the calipers at various sites on the body, most commonly the triceps and subscapular (under the shoulder blades) areas, and compare the measurements to published standards for age and sex.

Diets Are a Detour

For Lana, every day is a battle with food. At 5 feet, 4 inches, she tips the scale at 210 pounds and continues to gain. Every so often she plunges into a new diet: grapefruit and cottage cheese, the cabbage soup plan, the protein-intensive diet. Each diet brings her fresh resolve, fresh hope. But the diets don't make her feel well. They are hard to stick to. She feels deprived and always hungry. To add insult to injury, whatever pounds she takes off leap right back on. The bathroom scale taunts her with failure.

Many people think that the response to a weight problem should be "going on a diet." But a diet is a detour that misses the main point: Weight loss should result from healthful eating practices that a person can learn to maintain and enjoy for life.

Adolescents should not go on the restrictive diets that are all too familiar to many adults. These diets do not supply the nutrients and calories that growing adolescents need. They may even backfire, contributing to even greater obsessiveness about food and, in a vulnerable adolescent, slippage into an eating disorder. Diets by design are also intended to be temporary. While one is "on" a diet, life is different, and the duration of the diet is set aside as a time of great sacrifice. Then, once the weight-loss goals are achieved and the diet is set aside, the pounds tend to quickly pile back on because the diet never taught how to eat properly in the first place.

Reveal Remedies by Identifying the Causes

Eating too much, exercising too little is a shorthand description of many people's weight problems. But in fact every adolescent with a weight problem has a unique set of particular factors that led to and perpetuate the excess weight. Some of these factors are environmental in nature—that is, the adolescent is subject to broad categories of "risk factors" such as family history of obesity or belonging to groups or living in conditions that increase their risk of obesity.

Other factors are very personal in nature: the individual's particular practices, habits, knowledge, and feelings. It is gaining an understanding of the specific and personal eating behaviors of an overweight individual that sheds light on how to begin to tackle the problem.

Eating is among the most emotionally laden of activities. Food is associated with love ("Aunt Sophie always has an apple pie waiting") and comfort ("Stop crying, honey, have a cookie"). An adolescent, therefore, may overeat when feeling lonely, unloved, or stressed. Eating produces a full feeling that may seem to fill an emotional void. During anxious times, crunching on chips may take the place of biting fingernails or nervously tapping a foot.

Eating can be a response to feelings, a setting, or a situation rather than to just hunger. People often eat because it's time to eat, or a meal is served, or a bowl of candy is on the table, or they're at a party. Many adolescents habitually eat while watching TV, doing homework, reading a magazine, or talking on the phone. This is "automatic eating," the gustatory equivalent of background noise. Food "goes with" the activity; it is part of the package. And the pounds pile on.

Some people (including many adolescents) who are trying to lose weight postpone eating each day as long as possible, but then are so famished that they binge, consuming great quantities of high-calorie foods in one sitting.

A Weight-Loss Coach

To manage their weight problems, teens must analyze their particular eating patterns and identify the feelings, foods, and situations that trigger their overeating. Doing this alone can be near impossible, and doing it with a parent often spells disaster (but not always). Most teens trying to tackle a weight problem should find a "coach" who can help them see more clearly what the problem moves are and help them design strategies to be better players. Their coach may be a doctor, a nurse, a nutritionist, a teacher, or anyone else qualified to help, but not someone who is emotionally tied to the teenager's problem. Too often well-meaning relatives or friends only make the situation worse because of their close relationship to the teen and the difficult nature of this problem.

Reshaping Habits

Habits can be the greatest assets or the worst impediments to good health. Habits harden fast and cling tenaciously. Once set, they're tricky—though not impossible—to change.

Good habits are marvelous allies. For example, you are probably in the habit of brushing your teeth before going to bed. Just try to resist doing so one night. Unless you are extremely tired, you're liable to discover that the feel of unbrushed teeth is so distracting you can't fall asleep until you get up, brush your teeth, and go back to bed.

Weight loss is more likely to be lasting if adolescents learn to harness habits to their advantage and create new habits to replace the old, counterproductive ones. Then not only will the weight stay off, but the process of maintaining a happier weight will be easier and pleasurable.

Here are some common habits of overweight teens and some new ways parents can encourage them to approach food.

Old habit: Speed eating.
New habit: Savor eating. Learn how to install brakes on your fork. Rest the fork on the plate between bites. Breathe. Chew longer. Chat with someone at the table. Don't read or watch TV while eating. Take time to concentrate on the pleasurable texture and taste of the food. Enjoy every bite.

Old habit: Skip meals; snack on chips or candy.
New habit: Eat every meal, and then some; eat healthy snacks. Always eat breakfast, lunch, and dinner. Have something for breakfast and lunch even if it is only an egg or a cup of soup. Breakfast provides energy after the nighttime fast. Lunch keeps energy up (and raises the metabolic rate to burn more calories) and prevents late-afternoon bingeing. Between meals and after dinner,

have small snacks with built-in portion control—such as a banana, a granola bar, or a container of yogurt. Plan ahead and tuck snacks in your backpack if you won't have ready access to food.

Old habit: Eat on the run.

New habit: Eat seated. Avoid frenzied eating in your fast-paced life. Don't grab quick, high-calorie snacks and fast foods. Plan ahead and build in time to sit down to eat, which in turn will allow you to think about food selections and to taste and derive more pleasure from your food.

Old habit: Eat your heart out.

New habit: Find other ways to feed your heart. Reach for the phone, not for a doughnut, when the going gets tough. Food is no substitute for friends—and in excess, food is no friend at all. Keep a food diary to help you become more aware of what you eat and also your state of mind when you eat it: *Tuesday, 4:15: Home from school. Snack: Apple and two graham crackers. 5:15: Feeling lonely and bored. Snack: Frozen Girl Scout cookies.* Better choices: Call a friend and talk, take your little sister to the park, write about your feelings in your journal, play your flute.

Old habit: Quench thirst with sodas, juices, and milk.

New habit: Learn to love water. Aim for eight cups of water per day. Eight cups of juice or milk add up to 800 calories, a sizable amount indeed if you are trying for about 1,500 to 2,000 calories total. The water habit is no-calorie and highly beneficial in many ways. (See chapter 3.) You can also try seltzer mixed with a little juice.

Old habit: Eat rich desserts.

New habit: Eat low-fat, lower-calorie alternatives such as fruit salad, sorbet, and low-fat or no-fat frozen yogurt.

Old habit: Ride.

New habit: Walk. Exercise makes weight loss so much easier. Burn calories, boost your metabolism, feel energized, reduce stress, and feel really good about yourself.

Old habit: Suffer in silence.

New habit: Seek support. Talk to someone about your food habits. Take advantage of the opportunity to reflect on your food choices and eating triggers. Learn from—and support—others who are going through the same thing.

Weight Watchers, Overeaters Anonymous, and other groups are open to teens and may even have special teen groups.

A Parent's Words

It is important that adolescents "own" their weight-control efforts and don't feel as though their parents are constantly monitoring them. There can be nothing more insufferable for a teen than having a parent constantly say, "Are you sure you should eat that muffin?" or "Do you really *need* a second helping?" or "Did you take a walk today?" The pressure can drive a kid "underground," resentfully eating in secret.

Express your confidence that your adolescent can take charge of his or her health. Ask what you can do to help. Find your adolescent a weight-management coach. Offer support through actions. Stop buying high-fat, high-sugar foods (ice cream, cheese, and cookies) your adolescent can't resist. Serve delicious, low-fat meals (lots of vegetables and salads, lean meats, poultry and fish, fruit for dessert). Learn food preparations that use little or no fat (steam, microwave, grill, broil, bake; avoid fry, sauté). Stock the house with appetizing, healthful snacks (fruit, nonfat or low-fat yogurt and frozen yogurt, whole-grain crackers). Engage in fitness activities as a family. Take walks with your adolescent. Buy your child a good pair of walking shoes that he or she will enjoy wearing. Model good eating and fitness behaviors yourself. (See other suggestions in chapter 3.)

Setting Realistic Goals

Not every obese adolescent will become thin or even average. But it is also a worthy goal to at least slow down weight gain. Learning about healthy foods, gaining insight into eating patterns, and choosing to walk up the stairs instead of taking an elevator may lead to small but ultimately cumulative changes that may at the very least forestall overwhelming weight gain and help adolescents achieve a sense of control.

It is so easy to get discouraged. If goals are modest, they will feel more achievable. Rather than trying to make a fat adolescent into a thin one, go for achievable goals the young person will feel more inclined to pursue. The first goal: Gain a sense of control. Make it through one day without sweets. Then make it through another day. Lose a pound. Make it to the next lowest clothing size. Go for progress little by little, remembering that nothing succeeds and motivates . . . like success.

HEALTH-PARTNERING TIPS FOR PARENTS

It is a difficult but essential challenge for parents to help their adolescents (especially preteens and young teens) to feel comfortable and take pride in their maturing bodies, in order to avoid eating disorders and resist behaviors that can lead to obesity.

- Model and help your child take pride in his or her body and appearance *via avenues other than weight and shape*. Encourage your adolescent to participate in dance, sports, and other forms of exercise. Compliment your child's gracefulness, sense of balance, flair in clothing, hairdos, jewelry, and other expressions of creativity, individuality, and skillfulness.
- Try hard to avoid preoccupation and *comments about your own weight and shape*. Try to model healthy eating and an enjoyment of food.
- Avoid *overinvolvement with your child's weight,* body shape, and food choices. Overvaluing and complimenting a very thin child may put undue pressure on her to stay thin as her body begins to change. Excessive emphasis on your concern about a child's overweight may make that child feel that his or her weight is all that matters to you.
- Model by your comments, actions, and activities how much you value aspects of yourself, your children, and your friends for *qualities having nothing to do with weight and shape,* such as kindness, humor, creativity, and intelligence.
- Within the family, *acknowledge negative as well as positive feelings*. Talk about anger, fear, and sadness as normal human emotions. Such openness will help your child feel less ashamed of his own difficulties growing up and achieve "emotional literacy," an ability to identify and express feelings in words rather than in harmful actions (over- or undereating).
- Above all, don't forget to tell your child that she is beautiful and he is handsome—for truly they are.

ELEVEN Your Teen's Mental Health

In life, as in a self-defense class, it is essential to learn how to fall safely, then get back up. Adolescence is a destabilizing time of life, presenting young people with plenty of opportunities to fall and recover. Their hormones and moods and bodies and schools and friends and family relationships and feelings change; some of the changes are thrilling and others are scary.

Having no choice but to cope with change, teens usually learn that they can. Most emerge from adolescence as more resilient, self-confident, and mature individuals.

But along the way, being (and living with) a teen can be rough. Stress, anxiety, and insecurity come with the territory. Previously well-adjusted children may lose their equilibrium. Some adolescents adopt prickly attitudes that keep parents at a distance. Others develop serious problems that threaten their ability to function.

From their respective sides of the generational divide, parents and adolescents ask the same question: *How do you know when a problem is part of the normal travails of growing up and when it is a mental health problem that needs outside help?*

Every chapter in this book addresses emotional issues that may cause or exacerbate medical problems. However, some of these issues demand separate attention. This chapter will describe the mental health continuum—from common adolescent stresses to mental illnesses, and provide guidance on how to recognize when your adolescent needs help.

THE FIRST STEP: SEEING MENTAL HEALTH IN CONTEXT

If you are concerned about your adolescent's mental health, the following questions offer a good way to begin exploring what the problem may be. Along with your adolescent, a doctor, or a therapist, see if you can identify any of these connections between your adolescent's state of mind and other health issues or life events.

1. How is your adolescent doing with "the basics"—nutrition, exercise, and sleep?

The three basics discussed in chapter 3 affect mental as well as physical health. Poor diet, a sedentary lifestyle, or sleep deprivation may affect how an adolescent feels emotionally as well as how he or she performs at school or in activities. A snappish and irritable adolescent may be sleep-deprived. Insufficient food or erratic eating habits (just like insufficient or erratic sleep) can cause irritability, depression, and inability to concentrate (and, linked with low self-esteem and body image anxiety, may be the result of an eating disorder). A sedentary lifestyle devoid of exercise and fresh air may contribute to a depressed mood, whereas a brisk walk home after school would clear the head and lift the spirits.

2. How is your adolescent's physical health?

Whether it is caused by an acute illness like mononucleosis or a chronic health condition (see chapter 7), poor health may affect an adolescent's mental outlook. An undiagnosed illness (such as anemia, a kidney disorder, or thyroid disease) may sometimes be the explanation for depression or anxiety. Various medications—such as steroids, bronchodilators, or birth control pills—may contribute to an altered mental state, which clears after the medication is stopped. Check out the "body-mind connection" to see if your adolescent's case of the blues is related to his or her physical health.

3. Did your adolescent's changed state of mind coincide with certain events?

When did you begin to notice your adolescent's sadness, irritability, or withdrawal? Consider whether the change is linked to an event such as a divorce, death, breakup, argument with a best friend, or moving to a new community or school. Antonia stopped seeing her friends and became increasingly moody as she began spending more time with a possessive and controlling new boyfriend who was several years older. When Jack's friend was killed in a car accident, he developed insomnia and did not want to go to school. Lydia's despondence and eventual eating disorder could be traced to her dad's ill-considered teasing about her "cute" baby fat.

An adolescent may also have a delayed reaction to a traumatic event. Michael, age eighteen, plunged into a depression during his first semester of college. His father had died during his junior year of high school, but leaving home brought forth renewed feelings of loss and separation from his family.

4. Could your adolescent's changes be drug-related?

Secretiveness, mood swings, depression, and other problems may be associated with drug use (see chapter 9). For example, Robert's schoolwork began to suffer when he started hanging out with a new group of friends. It was his parents' first clue that he had starting using drugs.

5. *What is happening within your adolescent's family, school, and friendships?*

Family, school, and peer relationships are the three interlocking spheres that form the heart of most adolescents' worlds. Try to get a sense of whether your adolescent is having problems in one, some, or all of these areas. For example, an adolescent who withdraws from family, friends, and school may be depressed. But an adolescent whose school performance drops but whose family relationships and friendships are solid is likely to have a more limited problem, such as a learning disability. Difficulty that originates in one sphere (such as school) can cause mental anguish that spills over and affects other areas or activities in the adolescent's life. Following are examples of some of the common stresses that occur in each of these three spheres.

COMMON FAMILY STRESSES

Much as adolescents may seem to want to pull away from their families, they still need to depend on their family's "being there," being a solid home base. Problems at home can affect adolescents deeply and affect every part of their lives.

Illness or Death of a Family Member

A teen whose mother is ill with AIDS may fear that she will die. He may react in various ways. For example, he may pull away from other activities to devote energy to caring for his mother, or use drugs to numb his sorrow, or withdraw from friends if the disease is being kept a secret. A death in the family—even if the person was not a close relative—may devastate an adolescent, rocking her sense of safety. Some schools and community-based organizations have excellent bereavement support groups for teens.

Parents' Unemployment or Financial Problems

When one or both parents are laid off, the adolescent may feel anxious, not only about money but also about the family's ability to remain in their home, stay together, or pay for medical bills. Having friends whose families are financially secure or affluent may make the adolescent feel isolated or ashamed. An adolescent who works an after-school or evening job to supplement family income may feel proud of her contribution but stressed by the pressure to balance school and job responsibilities.

Abusive or Substance-Using Parents

An adolescent with physically, sexually, or verbally abusive parents may feel overwhelmed by fear, shame, and/or the need to hide the secret. Such situations are usually complex. An adolescent may have mixed feelings about informing a teacher, social worker, or the police. Abused teens may love, fear, pity, and depend on their parents—all at the same time. If parents have a drinking or drug problem, a teen may assume responsibility for younger siblings, even to the point of skipping school in order to stay home and baby-sit, cook, and clean.

Parental Conflict, Separation, or Divorce

How parents handle their conflicts can spell the difference between whether their children manage to cope or spin into a traumatic reaction. Assure your child that he or she is not to blame for your relationship problems, and avoid using your child as a sounding board for your troubles. As painful as it is to have these problems with your partner, do not permit your considerable distress to distract you from your adolescent's needs.

In the event of separation or divorce, keep to a minimum the effect on your child's daily life. Try to let your child stay in the same school and neighborhood, participate in normal activities, and see friends. As much as possible, stay in touch and available. Family counseling can help everyone in the family adjust to the new situation and figure out ways to solve logistical and other problems. For seventh grade Samantha, for example, just learning how to manage shuttling clothes and books from one parent's home to the other's on her alternate half weeks there was a demanding process that required both parents' involvement and cooperation.

Keep in mind this vision: Years from now, when you and your partner have long been apart, it would be wonderful for you both to be able to attend your child or children's important events. Whatever cooperation you can muster now, during your breakup, will build goodwill that will pay off in years to come. So whether through weekly phone calls, letters, messages left on one another's answering machines, E-mails, or communicating through intermediaries (not the children), do what it takes to address the child's needs and maintain each parent's involvement.

COMMON SCHOOL STRESSES

There are many reasons adolescents may start doing poorly in school, want to stay home, or be truant. Family problems can distract or diminish an adolescent's motivation, or—if an adolescent is acting out because of family discord—even make an adolescent actively seek to do poorly in order to "get back" at parents. Or an adolescent may be cutting classes to use drugs and be less able to concentrate as a result of drug use (see chapter 9). Following are additional common problems with school.

CREATING A LOW-STRESS HOME

It's a stressful world out there. To help your family reduce and manage stress, try these suggestions for making your home a pleasant and supportive place:

- *Have family dinners.* Ask everyone to talk about what happened during the day—including *one good thing.* This can be small ("I didn't have to wait for the bus; it came right away") or major ("I got a B on my chemistry test").
- *Encourage the whole family to take care of the three basics*—described in chapter 3—eating well, sleeping enough, and exercising.
- *Make laughter a priority.* Watch funny TV shows and movies together. When you hear a joke that you like, repeat it at home.
- *When conflicts or bad moods seem to get out of hand, call for a time-out.* Any argument can benefit from a walk around the block to cool off.
- *Create quiet times.* No TV, no music, no computer—just an environment conducive to meditation, reflection, reading, or rest. You may need to negotiate this with a teen who is used to practically round-the-clock sound.
- *Practice yoga.* Buy yoga videos to help family members do yoga exercises alone or together.
- *Touch.* Hug, kiss good-night, or at least "high-five" your adolescent.
- *Pitch in.* As a family, help one another. For example, if a teen is struggling to complete a school project, other family members can collate resources, staple exhibits on a display board, or bring in a snack.
- *Celebrate.* Not just birthdays, but accomplishments like an adolescent's improved report card. No gifts required. Saying "Congratulations," initiating a round of applause, or writing a note will get the point across.
- *Welcome friends.* Encourage your adolescent to invite friends over, have them stay for dinner, or sleep over.
- *Inspire.* Talk with your adolescent about goals, making plans, thinking ahead. Show that you take your adolescent's goals seriously and will do what you can to help.
- *Affirm that some stress can be healthy and yield rewards.* It is stressful to host a party, run for school office, or apply for a job when you're a high school kid with little experience. Reassure your adolescent that in order to grow it is necessary to venture beyond the usual, safe boundaries.

Overwhelming Academic Demands

The work may be too difficult, and an adolescent may feel increasingly hopeless about being able to keep up. Parents may need to contact teachers, identify after-school tutoring or remedial programs, or talk with their adolescent about selecting courses that are more in keeping with his or her interests and abilities. (See "Learning Disabilities and Attentional Disorders," later in this chapter.)

Problems with Peers

Poor school attendance or performance may have little or nothing to do with academics. Perhaps the adolescent is being bullied or teased by other students, sexually harassed, or pressured to join a gang. Discuss the situation with your child, but also with the school. Schools are legally obligated to provide a safe environment for learning and must take appropriate steps to protect your child from harassment.

School Phobia

A fear of attending school, common in young children, is in fact a very serious problem in an adolescent. Adolescents with school phobia often complain of physical symptoms that they claim make it impossible for them to go to school. Determined efforts must be directed at understanding the phobia's source. The longer this pattern continues, the harder it is to break. Family or peer problems are often involved.

COMMON STRESSES WITH PEERS

During adolescence, peer approval and relationships are more important than ever. Adolescents may feel devastated when friendships go awry, romances burn out, or they find themselves the scapegoat of classroom bullies.

Loneliness

Some lucky adolescents attract friends as easily as a dancer picks up new steps. After a tentative moment or two, their self-confidence kicks in. They flow from one step to the next and know how to smile, recover, and move on if they trip along the way.

To adolescents on the social fringe, watching such a performance is an exercise in envy and awe. Just about all adolescents long to feel a sense of belonging. But some teens can't figure out how to crack the code of making friends. Some are spared acute pain because they have been with the same group of peers since elementary school. By virtue of their "seniority" they are often automatically included, even if they do not feel close to anyone. This was true for Jeffrey until eighth grade, when at age thirteen he already looked and spoke like a six-teen-year-old and his friends started to withdraw.

Adolescents who enter a new school, relocate from another town or coun-try, feel isolated by a disability, or just don't fit in can feel unbearably lonely. They feel at an utter loss about what to do. Their morale can sink lower and lower, sometimes into depression. When they lament "Nobody talks to me" or "I feel like I'm invisible," it doesn't dawn on them that others feel the same way. (See "Making Friends," on the following page.) Cliques especially make adolescents feel excluded—at least until they figure out how to create one of their own.

Peer Pressure

Countless adolescents have done things they didn't really want to do because they were dared, pressured, or coerced into doing so, or simply didn't want to draw attention to themselves by turning away. Joining in is a way of belonging and avoiding loneliness, even when joining peers means doing bad things. Chugging liquor, having unwilling or unsafe sex, shoplifting, joining a gang, taunting a peer, playing a cruel practical joke, vandalizing a rival team's school . . . the list goes on and on. Adolescents who alone are fairly decent peo-ple can get swept up in group mentality and find themselves doing dangerous, stupid, illegal, or unethical things that can get themselves or others into trou-ble. Later, regretful or ashamed, they just can't explain what they did: *Well, everybody was doing it. I didn't really think about what could happen.*

Very often alcohol and other drugs are the catalysts, loosening adolescents' inhibitions and impairing their judgment. Catherine was an honor roll student and president of her class, yet got arrested twice in her junior year in high school. Once she was caught dumping empty beer cans at the town dump at midnight and another time shoplifting a roll of film while rushing off to a rock concert with friends.

To reduce the chances that your adolescent will become involved in such activities:

- *Emphasize the role that alcohol and other drugs play in leading people to do things they'll regret later.* (See chapter 9.)
- *Be aware of where your teen is and agree on a time to come home.* Adoles-cents may protest such limits, but they also want and need them.
- *Talk about such events that have happened in your community.* Initiate discussions and ask "What would you do if . . ."
- *Encourage your adolescent to get involved in constructive activities.* Play-ing sports, tutoring, volunteering, baby-sitting, becoming involved in a

MAKING FRIENDS

Loneliness is passive; action is an antidote. Instead of waiting for others to reach out and rescue them, adolescents have to take the responsibility themselves for making friends.

- *Improve social skills.* Let's call them "popular mechanics"—the basic skills of making friends. A crucial concept: *Instead of being wrapped up in yourself, focus more on others.* Suggest that your adolescent practice a few icebreaking, friend-making skills:
  - » Smile. Say hi.
  - » Be a listener. Ask people about themselves.
  - » Remember what people say, even if you have to take notes, then follow up later.
  - » Don't gossip; people will think you'll talk behind their backs, too.
  - » Be trustworthy. Keep people's secrets.
  - » Offer to help.
  - » Relax.
- *Get involved in school, volunteer, or community activities.* Build a set for a school play, serve meals at a homeless shelter, or answer phones for a charity. Such activities at the very least distract adolescents from their loneliness. But they also have the potential to help them develop new skills, have interesting things to talk about, and meet new people with whom they have something in common.
- *Look ahead.* Some adolescents have such different values, backgrounds, interests, or philosophies than other teens in their community that they really cannot bridge the gap. This especially may be true for those in rural communities or small towns who have limited access to a variety of people. But that doesn't mean that the future won't be better. Adolescents who go away to college or take a job in a larger city often meet people with like values and for the first time in their life feel that they are not alone. *What a relief, to find that within this world are many worlds.* Poets find other poets. Odd ones out find people who appreciate their unique points of view.

community or church/synagogue/mosque youth group, or getting an after-school job can improve your teen's skills and self-esteem and reduce the idle hours in which trouble is more likely to occur.

Teasing and Bullying

From sexual harassment to scapegoating, many young people suffer from the insensitivity or cruelty of others. Being the target can lead to school phobia, low self-esteem, isolation, debilitating anxiety, substance abuse, depression, suicide, or violence against others, including homicide. Some school shootings have been committed by teens who were taunted by fellow students.

It is not just the victims who suffer. Teens who bully have often been abused themselves, at home or by peers, and turn their rage on others.

The indifference or inaction of adults makes adolescents feel abandoned and deprives them of the protection to which they are entitled, especially in school. We have all read too many accounts of this kind of occurrence in recent years.

If you know or suspect that your child is bullying or being victimized:

- *Seek counseling for your child.* Do not simply hope that the problem will go away. That may happen, but it could get worse—not a risk worth taking.
- *Enlist the school's support.* Advocate for conflict resolution and antibullying programs, as well as antiharassment school policies that are consistently enforced. Your child is entitled by law to a safe school environment.
- *Contact the police* if you feel your child may be in danger.

Heartache

John Donne captured the all-or-nothing passion of adolescent love when he wrote, "Ah, what a trifle is a heart/If once into love's hands it come! . . . I brought a heart into the room/But from the room, I carried none with me . . . My rags of heart can like, wish, and adore/But after one such love, can love no more."[1]

Even if you think of your adolescent's relationship as infatuation or puppy love, don't say so aloud. To adolescents, a breakup can feel as devastating as a divorce, even if the relationship lasted only weeks or months, and they may be convinced that they will never love again. Your adolescent may find some comfort in the book *How to Survive the Loss of a Love.*[2] If nothing else, it may help your adolescent feel less alone in experiencing this pain.

You might also point out that breakups happen for all kinds of complex reasons, often having nothing to do with the person being left. For example, sometimes a teen feels too much in love and just can't handle such strong feelings now. And yet the rejected partner may not be able to shake off a feeling of self-hate or an intense sense of vulnerability. Depression, eating disorders, drug use, sexual acting out, or school failure may follow.

If your adolescent does not seem to recuperate from a breakup after a reasonable amount of time (within a month), consider the possibility that he or she may be depressed, even suicidal, and take the steps discussed later in this chapter.

Although no person is replaceable, your adolescent may be comforted by the idea that it is not only possible but indeed likely to find joy and love with someone else. Talk about all the people your adolescent loves—parents, siblings, grandparents and other relatives and friends, perhaps neighbors or teachers. All lovable, but all different, and the difference doesn't make the love any less meaningful. So can it be with romantic love. There may be only one first love. But there can be a next love.

Dating Abuse

High school teachers are often appalled to see some of their most appealing students submitting to boyfriends' abusive demands. Such boys demand that their girlfriends abandon favorite activities and friends, avoid speaking to other boys, or dress or act a certain way so as not to "provoke" jealousy. Abuse may consist solely of such mind games and verbal abusiveness, or progress to physical abuse. In some cases, it has even led to murder.

Abusiveness is not limited to boys. There are some girls, too, who make their boyfriends feel strangled, who verbally or physically abuse them.

It is agonizing to see your adolescent in an abusive relationship. You feel infuriated by this person who dares treat your child this way. Yet your adolescent may feel so invested in the relationship as to be unable to envision living without it. When one mother, who happened to be divorced, talked with her daughter about her concerns, the daughter curtly deflected them this way: "Mom, you're just jealous that I have someone and you don't." The relationship got even worse before the daughter was finally able to acknowledge how damaging it was and end it.

Your adolescent may or may not want to talk with you. But do not stay silent. That could give your adolescent the impression that you do not see or object to the abusiveness. Tell your adolescent that genuine love does not make a person feel threatened, scared, defensive, or confined. An abusive relationship constricts one's world; a genuinely loving one expands it. You may want to suggest that your adolescent see a therapist or call a domestic abuse hot line for help. Or you can call to obtain guidance yourself.

There are other ways to intervene, but you must consider the risk of alienating your child. With an early adolescent, it may be appropriate for you to enlist the support of a school counselor, other family members, or friends, or perhaps contact the boyfriend's or girlfriend's parents to discuss the situation. However, mid or late adolescents would most likely insist on handling the situation themselves, and you should let them.

However, if you feel that your adolescent is in danger—for example, if a boyfriend or girlfriend is threatening or stalking your child—insist that your adolescent take it seriously. Talk with the police about what can be done and, with your adolescent, ask their advice about whether to obtain a restraining order or take other actions.

THERAPIES AND THERAPISTS

For some teens, talking with parents or other trusted adults, older siblings or good friends, or a school counselor is all they need in order to feel better when times are rough. Other adolescents benefit from seeing a therapist, whether for help in dealing with stress or for treatment related to a mental illness (discussed later in this chapter). Some schools have mental health clinics or provide referrals for mental health services, and of course your child's doctor can also provide referrals.

The terms *psychotherapy* and *psychotherapist* are often confusing for parents and teens because there are so many different types of therapies and therapists. Psychotherapy is a treatment process designed to bring about helpful change in a person's behavior, feelings, and thoughts. First a specific diagnosis must be made by a psychiatrist, psychologist, or licensed clinical social worker. Then treatments, consisting of various combinations and types of psychotherapy (individual, family, and/or group therapy; or psychodynamic, behavioral, or cognitive therapy) and medications, are used to help bring the mental health problem or mental illness under control and allow the adolescent to return to normal life activities. This process can be a smooth path or a rocky road and usually requires the full support and involvement of the adolescent's family.

- *Individual therapy* involves the teenager meeting alone with the therapist.
- *Family therapy* usually includes the teenager's entire nuclear family (but this could vary to include fewer or more family members).
- *Group therapy* includes several teenagers struggling with similar problems who meet together with a therapist (or sometimes with more than one therapist).
- *Psychodynamic/psychoanalytic/interpersonal psychotherapies* are similar forms of "talk" therapy in which the teenager, with the therapist's inter-

pretive help and feedback, explores new insights and understanding of self and relationships in an attempt to change behavior and feel better.

- *Behavioral therapy* aims to modify a teen's actions, reactions, or thoughts using various direct interventions. The teen learns through experiencing more positive results and fewer frustrations and failures.
- *Cognitive therapy* helps an adolescent think and feel more positively and optimistically about himself or herself and the world by the therapist's challenging irrationally negative and pessimistic thoughts and beliefs.
- *Cognitive-behavioral therapy* aims to change behavior by learning problem-solving skills, self-management, and by the therapist's challenging irrational thoughts and beliefs.

Psychotherapists include psychiatrists, psychologists, social workers, school guidance counselors, and others who have received training in mental health. It is usually best to find a psychotherapist who has received extensive education, training, and supervision in preparation for doing this work. Some individuals may call themselves "psychotherapists" after minimal amounts of training and supervision. Therefore, checking and understanding a psychotherapist's credentials is important.

Psychiatrists are medical doctors who have graduated from medical school and completed a minimum of three years of residency training in psychiatry afterward. Psychiatrists are the only psychotherapists who can prescribe medications. Most psychiatrists also do psychotherapy, but some only do psychopharmacology (prescribe medication).

Psychologists have advanced graduate school education and training. Many psychologists have a Ph.D. (and are called "Dr."), and others have a master's degree in psychology.

Social workers often become psychotherapists, although many social workers do other kinds of work. Social workers usually have a master's degree (M.S.W.) and take a certifying examination (C.S.W.).

Find someone with whom your adolescent is comfortable. If possible, ask your doctor to recommend several people. Your adolescent may need to meet two or three therapists before finding a "match." This screening process helps an adolescent feel more in control and invested in the therapy process.

When Adolescents Resist Therapy

What if your adolescent doesn't want to go to therapy? One issue may be age. Some younger adolescents are resistant because they are not ready or able to articulate their feelings. They may also feel insulted by the idea that something is "wrong" with them, or not want to feel "different" by going into therapy, and they are not mature enough to understand that therapy can help. When Mona's dad died, Mona's mother wanted her to see a therapist to work through the loss. But Mona wanted to be as normal as possible, and her mother had to back off. The mother's own therapist, however, helped her identify ways to reach out to Mona at home.

If a young adolescent's problems do not interfere with his or her functioning in school, at home, and with friends, it may be best to postpone therapy. However, consult a therapist if functioning is impaired—for example, if the adolescent seems depressed and unmotivated to do schoolwork or get together with friends.

By mid or late adolescence, teens may be more receptive to therapy, but also may be wary of it if they were forced to participate when younger. Sometimes a doctor who wants to refer an adolescent to a therapist will initiate a discussion so the teen can see that talking can be a pleasant experience.

A resistant adolescent may do well with short-term therapy, for which the therapist specifies a limited number of sessions and spells out the therapy goals. Adolescents like to know what to expect. Having a set number of sessions reassures them that therapy is not going to stretch on indefinitely—that there *is* a light at the end of the tunnel.

Whether or not an adolescent resists therapy, there is always something parents can do. They can go to therapy or support groups themselves. The counseling, advice, and opportunity to gain insight into their own behaviors will in turn help their child. Eventually their children (not only the "identified patient") may join them for family therapy. Going to therapy as a family can make an adolescent feel less singled out. By revealing family dynamics and providing an opportunity for everyone in the family to be heard, family therapy may lead to a happier home for all family members.

For some adolescents or other family members, however, family therapy may feel too threatening. And where there is mental illness, further professional help should be sought.

LEARNING DISABILITIES AND ATTENTIONAL DISORDERS

Learning disabilities and attentional disorders often go unrecognized. An adolescent who cannot follow directions or remember facts may be accused of not listening or being lazy. One who mixes up the placement of numbers or letters may be penalized for carelessness. One who is constantly losing books and homework is scolded for being disorganized. Of course, some adolescents *are* distracted, careless, or disorganized, and not learning disabled, and certain interventions can help them. But if a learning disability or attentional disorder is suspected, the adolescent must be tested and evaluated by an expert.

Learning disabilities and attentional disorders (such as attention deficit disorder, ADD; or attention deficit hyperactivity disorder, ADHD) may be diagnosed early in childhood or during elementary school. More subtle learning disabilities may not be suspected until middle or even high school, as school work becomes more demanding and complex.

Learning Disabilities

Learning disabilities pertain to an array of specific skills that students use to achieve proficiency in subject matters at school as well as in their daily life. Students with learning disabilities are usually of normal or superior intelligence. A student may have a learning disability limited to reading, mathematics, or written or verbal expression, or may have difficulty in more than one area. For example, an adolescent with dyslexia may have problems recognizing and understanding written words. Some students learn on their own to compensate for mild learning disabilities; indeed, most people recognize that they are stronger learners in some subjects than others or learn more easily in certain ways. For example, some are "visual learners" and others learn more naturally through listening. However, many students with learning disabilities really struggle to achieve on par with their intelligence.

Some individuals with Asperger's syndrome, a high-functioning form of autism, may have learning disabilities accompanied by social disabilities, such as an inability to pick up social cues, to show common sense in social relationships, and to demonstrate abstract thinking.

Educational testing to delineate the specific components of a student's learning disability, followed by an individualized educational plan (extra help at school, one-on-one tutoring after school, extended time on tests), lots of moral support from parents and teachers, and the passage of time (many learning-disabled students who have received help, in fact, do much better as they get older) can result in a very successful school career. Many extraordinarily successful adults working in a wide variety of fields have learned to overcome and live with (and thrive with) their learning disability.

Attention Deficit Disorder

Attention deficit disorder (ADD) refers to a constellation of behavioral symptoms that interfere with a student's learning. Such symptoms of inattention include an inability to stick with a task (such as homework), pay attention to details, organize work, listen when spoken to or during class, block out extraneous noises or distractions, and not lose or forget things. Some adolescents with ADD are identified by their teachers who see them staring off into space, not completing assignments, and acting fidgety in class. Other students, with more subtle difficulties, may "diagnose" themselves, realizing they have difficulty paying attention in class, tend to lose their focus while reading, and can't sustain the effort of trying to write a paper.

A true diagnosis of ADD should be made by a psychiatrist or psychologist based on a detailed history from the student, parents, and teachers—and often specific testing as well. Consideration may then be given to whether to treat the ADD with behavioral strategies alone or with the addition of medication.

The most frequently prescribed medication is Ritalin (methylphenidate). Regular Ritalin lasts for about four hours to alleviate symptoms of inattention and is often taken two or three times a day; newer preparations of methylphenidate (Concerta, Metadate) last for eight to twelve hours, which for many students provides a smoother effect and avoids the necessity of having to take a second dose during the school day.

The next most commonly prescribed medications for ADD are amphetamine derivatives such as Dexedrine and Adderall. These amphetamines generally act slightly longer than regular Ritalin (approximately six hours). Whether methylphenidate or an amphetamine derivative or other medication works best for your child must be determined by the physician prescribing the medication, who will review the effects over time and make changes as necessary.

Advocating for Your Child at School

Explore the resources at your adolescent's school. Talk with teachers, your child's guidance counselor or social worker, and the principal. Ask if there is a school psychologist or educational consultant you can talk to. Explore the availability of after-school tutoring or activities to improve social functioning, attendance improvement and dropout-prevention programs, substance abuse counseling, peer counseling, and the like.

Never hesitate to pursue the search if you seem to hit a dead end. If you expend the time and energy, you are more likely to get your child the needed attention and services. *Schools respect and respond to parents who advocate for their children.*

You can also enlist the support of community-based organizations that advocate for improved education and health services, or those that specialize in raising awareness about specific learning problems or disabilities. Ask the organization for advice on how you can get your child the services he or she needs. Check to see if your adolescent may be entitled to services through programs targeted to students with special needs.

MENTAL ILLNESS IN ADOLESCENTS

Mental illness is beyond the normal travails of growing up. It is not about a moody teen's hormones going awry, or dramatic outbursts seeking independence, or slamming doors asking for privacy, or testing the limits by coming home late or drinking some beer. Mental illness is very serious business that *always* requires professional help to diagnose, to understand, and to treat.

While not exactly "hormonal," mental illnesses are thought to result from aberrations in neurotransmitters—brain chemicals (such as serotonin, dopamine, and norepinephrine) that regulate mood and thought. Very often a specific mental illness runs in a family. A review of the family history of diagnosed or undiagnosed individuals (whose behaviors or moods were problematic), including parents, grandparents, aunts, uncles, and first cousins, can provide a clue to a teenager's disorder.

The mental illnesses discussed below often begin during the adolescent years,[3] or at least seem to become most troublesome then—even if in retrospect there had been signs earlier on in childhood. Sometimes a mental illness is triggered by a traumatic or stressful event from which the teenager does not recover within a reasonable amount of time. In this scenario the mental illness surfaces in a neurochemically vulnerable individual under stress.

Other times, a mental illness seems to come out of the blue during an otherwise uneventful phase of a teenager's life.

MOOD DISORDERS

Depression

I'm so sad and everything's hopeless.

I'm so ugly and stupid.

All I want to do is veg out on the couch.

I always have bad luck. Things never go right for me.

I want to kill myself.

These statements can mean such different things. They may be uttered in frustration, exasperation, disappointment, as manipulation, or even as punch lines for jokes. Or they may be deadly serious—cries for help or statements of intent.

Most people can think back on their lives and point to times when they felt discouraged, blue, or lonely. It is neither realistic nor desirable to aim to live on a plateau, with one flat view of the horizon unvarying through the years. Life derives its texture from losses as well as celebrations. Through the relationship of low notes and high notes, music touches our soul.

But depression is an unalleviated experience. Feelings of hopelessness extend and extend, and there seems to be no relief in sight. Beyond the inevitable disappointment, grief, or sadness that mark life's low points, depression reaches like a shadow into almost every moment, bleaching the color from life, leaving only the grays.

Signs of Depression

Depression is a disorder, and its symptoms distinguish it from more transient dejection. A major depressive episode is a period of at least two weeks during which the adolescent's mood is sad or irritable and there is a lack of interest and pleasure in most life activities. In addition, the adolescent may:

- Eat less and lose weight, or eat excessively.
- Experience insomnia, or sleep excessively.
- Complain of fatigue, lack energy, do not participate in usual activities, and withdraw from family and friends.
- Act restless and agitated—even sarcastic, angry, or rebellious.
- Express feeling worthless or guilty, and cry easily.
- Have difficulty thinking and concentrating and skip or do poorly in school.
- Express hopelessness and recurrent thoughts of death or suicide, or attempt suicide (see page 281).
- Stop taking pride in appearance, and have poor hygiene and grooming.
- Suffer frequent headaches, backaches, stomachaches, or other physical ailments that appear to have no apparent cause.
- Start to hang out with a new group of friends and increase use of alcohol and drugs.

An adolescent who has suffered more than one major depressive episode or a prolonged episode may have major depressive disorder.

Depression's Onset

An adolescent's depression may stem from losses, such as when a loved one dies, a romance ends, a best friend moves away, or a desperately needed scholarship that had been counted on falls through. But not all depression is tied to a specific event. Some people are simply "prone" to depression, perhaps because of their brain chemistry or other factors that are harder to define.

Whatever the cause, it is necessary—and fruitful—to seek treatment. Depression is not a disease one should have to live with. Indeed, it can be so

debilitating that an adolescent cannot bear to live with it, and attempts suicide.

Getting Help

The first step parents who suspect depression in their teen should take is to
find a mental health professional (psychotherapist) who can evaluate the symptoms, make a diagnosis, and recommend a treatment approach. Finding this
important resource is different in each community, but a good way to begin is to
talk with your teenager's doctor (or have the doctor meet with the teen first),
or to a counselor at your child's school, or to a member of your clergy.

Depression is a very treatable disease. Sometimes just talking with a psychotherapist in psychotherapy will help tremendously to lift some clouds. The
psychotherapist may meet with the adolescent alone, along with the family, or
in a group with other teens, or recommend some combination of these. Types of
psychotherapy that are used to treat depression include traditional psychody-
namic/psychoanalytic/interpersonal talk therapy, behavioral therapy, and cognitive therapy.

In recent years several new antidepressant medications have been developed that are often a very helpful component in the care of a depressed adolescent. The most often prescribed antidepressants are called selective serotonin
reuptake inhibitors (SSRIs). These include Prozac (fluoxetine), Zoloft (sertraline), Paxil (paroxetine), Luvox (fluvoxamine), and Celexa (citalopram). Well-
butrin (bupropion) and Effexor (venlafaxine) are other antidepressants that
may be prescribed for teens with depression. These newer antidepressants tend
to have far fewer side effects than those medications used in the past, and for
most adolescents they are acceptable and their benefits substantial.

How Teens and Parents Can Help Relieve Depression

Depression must be treated by a mental health professional (or mental
health team), but there are additional strategies that teens can use to try to
forestall or alleviate depressed feelings:

- *Get support.* Confide in family, friends, clergy, or a counselor. Make a short
  list of trusted people to call when times are tough.
- *Express the feelings.* Talk or write in a journal to help relieve some of the
  pain and pinpoint what may be causing it. Other ways of releasing pent-up
  feelings are drawing, dancing, singing, writing fiction or a play, or taking
  on physical labor such as clearing a yard of underbrush or cleaning and
  painting a room.
- *Exercise.* Take a walk every day or get other vigorous exercise.

- *Meditate.* Focused relaxation helps to unclench the mind and improve mood.
- *Stop drinking and taking drugs.* Enter a treatment program, if necessary.
- *Get out of a rut.* Shake things up a bit. Alter daily routines—walk or take the bus instead of driving. Use different routes. Eat different foods. Go somewhere new. Take a class in something you have always been curious about but never took time to explore.

Refocusing the mind in these and other ways helps the brain get the message: There are other possibilities, other people to meet, other ways to look at life. Change can recharge a spark and derail depression, perhaps only briefly, or perhaps in a more long-lasting way by opening a door in a wall that seemed to have no exit at all.

Bipolar Disorder

Also referred to as "manic depression," bipolar disorder may begin during adolescence and is characterized by at least one manic (or more mild "hypomanic") episode, often in an individual who has already experienced a major depressive episode (see above).

The manic episode, in sharp contrast to the depressive episode, is characterized by an elevated or expansive mood and is often accompanied by inflated self-esteem (grandiosity), boundless energy and a decreased need for sleep, pressured and fanciful speech, and increased involvement in activities that may either be productive or simply agitated and disorganized. If severe, a manic episode requires hospitalization to help contain the individual's behavior, generally with the aid of medication. The adolescent may feel unrealistically powerful or giddy, take great risks, spend money with abandon, talk nonstop or seem uncharacteristically aggressive, stay awake for days on end, and flit from one activity to the next, easily distracted and surreally energetic.

Manic and hypomanic episodes generally come on suddenly and must be distinguished from behavior resulting from substance abuse (such as cocaine) or medication (including certain antidepressants). Like major depression, bipolar disorder appears to be genetically linked; having a parent with the disease increases an adolescent's risk. Bipolar disorder must be diagnosed by a psychiatrist and can be treated with mood-stabilizing medications.

Suicide

Suicide is a real and growing risk for adolescents with depression or bipolar disorder, including those who have not been diagnosed. After accidents (and similar in incidence to homicides), suicide is a leading cause of death for youth ages 10 to 24. The incidence of suicide increases with age; it is relatively low but has increased dramatically in recent years among 10-to-14-year-olds, is higher among 15-to-19-year-olds,[4] and is highest in the 20-to-24-year-old group. Overall, about 5,000 youths in these age groups commit suicide each year (over 2,000 in the 10-to-19-year-old group).[5]

More girls attempt suicide, but most adolescents who "succeed" are male. Most adolescent suicides involve the use of firearms, with hanging and suffocation also used frequently. Although statistics are hard to firm down, several million adolescents attempt suicide each year, usually using less-lethal methods such as drug overdoses and self-inflicted wounds. Even if an adolescent happens to use a less-lethal means the suicide attempt must always be taken very seriously. In fact, the greatest risk factor for a completed suicide is a previous suicide attempt.

Signs of Suicidal Thoughts

Most adolescents who are contemplating suicide show the symptoms of depression described earlier, but in some instances they seem "fine" and the suicide comes as an even more profound shock. Adolescents may signal their suicidal thoughts in advance, and these signals must be taken seriously.

A suicidal adolescent may:

- Talk about suicide, even in a seemingly joking way, or say things like "It wouldn't matter if I died" or "People probably wouldn't care if I weren't around anymore."
- Have a history of suicide attempts; 20 to 50 percent of people who kill themselves have tried before.[6]
- Give away treasured items, such as a music collection or favorite clothes.
- Express not only sadness but also a profound hopelessness that things will never get better.

Contrary to what many people think, asking if an adolescent is contemplating suicide will not "put ideas in his or her head." The adolescent is more likely to be relieved to have someone express concern. If the adolescent admits having thought about suicide and (perhaps in response to your question) mentions having a plan, *seek help immediately.*

- Call a suicide hot line, your doctor, or a mental health professional, or take the adolescent to a hospital emergency room.
- Do not leave the adolescent alone.
- Remove things with which the adolescent could harm himself, especially firearms, heavy rope, knives, razor blades, and pills.

- Encourage the adolescent to talk with you about what is going on, and offer your support. But don't think you can talk the adolescent out of the idea. It is crucial to obtain help.

A Caring and Educated Community Can Help Prevent Suicide

Nothing can be more devastating to a family than a suicide. In its wake inevitably come feelings of profound sadness, guilt, regret, and even anger at the teen who has taken his or her own life—seemingly without much thought to the consequences for all involved. And "all involved" is the key. Parents aren't the only ones who should have noticed that something was very wrong.

The entire community can be helpful in preventing teen suicides by recognizing when an adolescent may be in deep trouble. School personnel—including teachers, coaches, and guidance counselors—see the teen many hours each day and know the school culture better than anyone. Friends may know some secrets and sense something serious brewing, and the parents or other adults in whom they confide should always heed their words of warning and worry. The adolescent's doctor is in a position to detect a problem if the teen comes into the office with a physical complaint such as fatigue or a bellyache for which no medical cause is found. The conversation should go further than a brief chat and physical examination.

Heightened awareness by family, friends, professionals, and others, and expressing concern and taking immediate action when a teen may be at risk for hurting herself or himself, can and will prevent suicides and lead to the restoration of sound mental health in our precious children. Mental health professionals who are invited to speak at schools, community groups, places of worship, and other family gathering places can spread the word about suicide prevention and make neighborhoods more sensitive to troubled adolescents' needs.

Self-Injury

Various forms of self-injury, sometimes practiced by troubled teens, should be distinguished from suicidal behavior, even though self-injuring teens may also be at risk for suicide. Self-injury, usually in the form of cutting, scratching, or burning one's own skin—such as on the arms, legs, or face—is rarely life-threatening and is done to provide some relief from overwhelming thoughts or feelings rather than to harm or kill oneself. Teens who self-injure themselves often describe the behavior as alleviating a sense of numbness or emotional pain or imparting expression to feelings of anger or despair that they can't put into words.

The behavior and resulting cuts, bruises, and ultimately scars are often shameful to and hidden by the teen, and are always very distressing to those who care about them. Adolescents who self-injure should receive professional help directed at assisting them to recognize and be able to verbalize feelings rather than act them out in this way.

OPPOSITIONAL DEFIANT DISORDER (ODD)

Adolescents are known for contrariness; they test parents' rules and patience, argue against limits, and demonstrate various annoying behaviors. Doing so occasionally is common, but a particular and persistent pattern of such behaviors over at least six months may indicate that the adolescent has oppositional defiant disorder (ODD).

An adolescent with ODD is argumentative with adults, quick to anger (and may throw tantrums), uncooperative with adults' rules, easily annoyed (but also purposefully annoys others), and blames others instead of taking responsibility for his or her own misbehavior. The adolescent may seem to seethe with resentment, want to get back at people for their perceived wrongdoing, and have an especially cutting way of talking back to adults. These traits interfere with the adolescent's ability to function, such as in social or academic settings.

While SSRI medications may be called for in some instances, both teens with ODD and their parents can benefit by working with a psychotherapist who is experienced with ODD. The therapist can help the teen learn more constructive ways of managing anger and communicating, and can coach parents in behavior-management techniques.

ANXIETY DISORDERS

Adolescents tend to live with a great deal of stress much of the time. This stress emanates from demanding academic programs, ambitious ventures into the arts or athletics, family problems, peer group upheavals, dilemmas around sexuality or substance use—all coming together for them in our fast-paced society.

Most teens manage to handle all this stress remarkably well. But some teens live with a pervasive sense of anxiety that incapacitates their ability to function or feel comfortable. They cannot escape a feeling of dread, just as a depressed adolescent cannot escape a feeling of sadness, and some adolescents feel both anxious and depressed.

Adolescents with any of the anxiety disorders described below should consult with a mental health professional. Psychotherapy and/or medication usually results in marked improvement of symptoms and a return to normal activities.

Generalized Anxiety Disorder

A teen with generalized anxiety disorder may have been an overanxious child as well, or has begun to experience excessive worry, nervousness, and fear only since entering adolescence. The anxiety often pertains to academic performance or achievement in sports or other activities. There may also be dread about things the teen cannot control, such as earthquakes, terrorist attacks, or riding in a car or airplane. The worries often interfere with everyday life by limiting the teen's ventures at school or play or travel, and are experienced as much more pervasive, prolonged, and distressing than simple stress or "normal" anxiety in reaction to a specific aspect of life.

Additionally, the teen may experience a myriad of physical and mental symptoms, including muscular tension and pain, fatigue, sleep difficulties, and trouble focusing and thinking straight. Sometimes teens with generalized anxiety disorder also develop phobias (including school phobia and social phobia), abuse alcohol and drugs, or feel depressed.

Suzanne vomited nearly every night during the fall semester of her senior year in high school, and didn't stop until her last college application was filed. As a young child, Lily was terrified when a balloon burst at a friend's sixth birthday party, and now in middle school she refuses to attend any parties for fear there may be balloons. She also suffers from chronic pain in her neck and shoulder muscles, especially on days when she has a test at school. Claude had great difficulty falling asleep in early elementary school; now, as the star forward on his high school basketball team, he has again developed insomnia, especially the night before big games, a problem that contributes to fatigue he can ill afford.

Anxiety disorders may be treated with various types of psychotherapy, including cognitive and behavioral therapy, and with medications, especially SSRIs (Prozac, Zoloft, Paxil, Luvox, or Celexa). In severe cases, and over short periods of time, a psychiatrist may prescribe a benzodiazepine such as Valium, Klonopin, or Ativan. These are addictive if taken on a regular basis and are usually used for a very brief period. Buspar is a nonaddicting antianxiety medication, and may prove to be a useful alternative.

Panic Attacks and Panic Disorder

Panic attacks sometimes begin in late adolescence. A panic attack is a sudden feeling of intense fear, danger, and doom that builds quickly (within ten minutes) and is accompanied by an intense urge to escape one's surroundings. By definition, a panic attack includes at least several physical symptoms that lead the individual to feel that he or she may die or suffer a stroke or heart attack. These symptoms include pounding heart, sweating, trembling, shortness of breath, choking, chest pain, nausea, dizziness, tingling or numbness, chills or hot flashes. Or the person may feel about to lose control or go insane or experience depersonalization (feeling detached from oneself).

Panic attacks may come "out of the blue," or be triggered by an actual situation, or occur in a situation that sometimes but not always triggers an attack, such as riding in the subway. Individuals with panic disorder experience recurrent panic attacks or persistent dread about having such attacks. SSRI medications are often prescribed for panic disorders.

Post-Traumatic Stress Disorder (PTSD)

Post-traumatic stress disorder (PTSD) is a constellation of symptoms that a person suffers (usually starting within three months) after experiencing, witnessing, or being confronted by a traumatic event that involved actual or potential death or serious injury to himself or others, and that at the time provoked intense fear, helplessness, or horror.

After September 11, 2001, survivors and witnesses of the terrorist attacks on the World Trade Center and the Pentagon, including many who witnessed these events solely on television, developed symptoms of PTSD. Victims of rape or other crimes or forms of abuse are also especially vulnerable to this disorder.

The symptoms may last only for a few months, or longer, or be delayed in their onset beyond six months after the traumatic occurrence. The symptoms of PTSD are varied and complex, and include recurrent distressing images and thoughts (including dreams) of the event; the avoidance of previously welcome thoughts, places, activities, relationships, and feelings that are now associated with the trauma; and symptoms of heightened arousal (and caution) including sleep difficulties, outbursts of anger, trouble concentrating, and hypervigilance. The symptoms of PTSD are often so severe that they interfere with work (or school), social life, and relationships.

Individual psychotherapy, group therapy, and medication specific to the individual's symptoms, such as antianxiety medications, can help a person find a way to co-exist with this trauma that will always be part of his or her life.

Obsessive-Compulsive Disorder (OCD)

Certain habits and rituals keep life humming along. But an adolescent with obsessive-compulsive disorder (OCD) feels an urgent need to maintain them in a particular way—or else. When eating peach yogurt for breakfast every day, for example, David felt he must stir the fruit up from the bottom with precisely four rotations of the spoon. Stirring three or five times could cause some sort of catastrophe. In the mind of a person with OCD, the well-practiced ritual wards off a dire fate.

Obsessions are intrusive thoughts, impulses, or images that cause distress and anxiety, and that a person with OCD tries to ignore or suppress, realizing they are the product of his own mind. One attempt to diminish the distress of the obsessions is through *compulsive* repetitive behaviors or rituals that the OCD sufferer feels rigidly compelled to perform, such as compulsive hand-washing and other extreme precautions against germs, repeatedly checking that doors are locked and coffeepots are turned off, and establishing patterns of touching objects, counting steps, mentally repeating certain phrases or numbers, and so on. Obsessive thought patterns may center on feared disasters or worry that one may cause harm to someone else.

Behavioral and other forms of psychotherapy, as well as antidepressant medications (SSRIs, such as Zoloft or Paxil), can help an adolescent with OCD overcome this emotional prison of intrusive thoughts and repetitive acts, and help to restore an ability to enjoy a more normal, spontaneous existence.

SCHIZOPHRENIA

Schizophrenia is a serious and chronic disorder of the brain that affects approximately 0.5 percent to 1 percent of the adult population and includes psychotic features (delusions and hallucinations). Most individuals with schizophrenia begin to show signs of the disease between their late teens and their early thirties; males tend to have an earlier age at onset (median onset, early twenties) and a worse prognosis than females (median onset, late twenties).

The onset may be abrupt or gradual. A teenager, for example, may begin to withdraw from peers, lose interest in school, appear disheveled, or display odd behavior including outbursts of anger. During such a time it may be difficult for family and teachers to understand what is going on. Eventually a fuller, more specific picture emerges that includes at least two of the following symptoms: delusions (false beliefs that often have a paranoid quality and that may be "bizarre"); hallucinations (most often hearing voices, but may also be visual, tactile, or of taste or smell); disorganized speech (ranging from jumping from topic to topic to completely incoherent); grossly disorganized or inappropriate behavior that may totally interfere with self-care; and a marked flattening of affect (lack of facial expression and body movement), minimal amount of speech, and lack of interest in performing any goal-directed activities.

This most profound mental illness of young people can be effectively treated with antipsychotic medications, especially the delusions and hallucinations. However, a full return to the pre-illness condition is unlikely.

Seeking Help

Parents, like their adolescent, are likely to feel caught unaware and at a loss to know what to do. Slowly at first, then with increasing urgency, they come to understand that their child needs help and must see a physician. However, symptoms may fluctuate somewhat, and the adolescent may resist reporting what he or she perceives—perhaps because the delusions are experienced as real. So there may be mental disconnects not only within the adolescent, but also between the adolescent and others. It is essential to consult with a psychiatrist who will delineate the illness and is experienced in its treatment and care.

Medications have greatly improved the outlook for people with schizophrenia, permitting many to work and attain more independent, well-functioning lives. But medication alone is not sufficient. An adolescent or young adult with this devastating disease must have ongoing support, care, and follow-up, including regular assessments by a psychiatrist of medication effects and side effects. As much as possible, the young person should be encouraged and helped to partake in activities that keep his or her mind active and engaged.

HEALTH-PARTNERING TIPS FOR PARENTS

- *Make mental health a topic of conversation in your home.* Talk about everyday problems and challenges that your adolescent and other family members are facing. Watch TV shows or films, and talk about the mental outlooks of the characters, and how they handle stress, frustration, loss, and disappointments.
- *Describe getting help for problems as a sign of strength.* Emphasize that people should not feel that they must face all of their problems alone. Seeking and giving support to family and friends are meaningful and comforting to everyone. Be open about your own needs for support, too. If you have seen a therapist, say so.
- *Seek professional help earlier than you think you need to.* If you sense that something is wrong, you are probably right. Better to have a doctor or psychotherapist help you determine if your child is just going through a normal adolescent phase than for you to look back later and regret not taking action sooner for what turned out to be a serious problem.

TWELVE: Preventing Accidents and Injuries

Looking back, it is often painfully easy to see how an accident or injury could have been prevented . . .

> *. . . if only someone had stopped her from driving after drinking.*

> *. . . if only there had been a No Diving sign.*

> *. . . if only he had been wearing a helmet.*

> *. . . if only her employer had made her use safety goggles.*

> *. . . if only that gun had been unloaded and locked away.*

> *. . . if only he had walked away instead of getting into a fight.*

Many public health experts claim that there is no such thing as an accident. Most accidents turn out to be almost inevitable outcomes to hazardous circumstances that could have been foreseen. It is a dizzying, agonizing experience, thinking back . . .

You want to snatch back that moment when everything went wrong, when a person now injured or dead could have been kept safe.

AN URGENT NEED FOR PREVENTION

About 15,000 adolescents die from injury each year, more than the number of adolescent fatalities from all diseases combined. About 60 percent of these deaths stem from unintentional injury, especially due to motor vehicle crashes. The rest are from homicide and suicide.[1]

Older adolescent males (15 to 19 years old) are especially vulnerable. According to the Centers for Disease Control and Prevention, they are more than twice as likely as females to die of unintentional injury, five times more likely to die from homicide or suicide, and ten times more likely to die from drowning.

CONVEYING THE SAFETY MESSAGE

Urging adolescents to be careful can feel like one of a parent's most frustrating tasks. Adolescents have a talent for denial. Even though they know intellectually that no one lives forever, this doesn't fit with the way they *feel*. To them life feels luxuriously long, with no abrupt punctuation mark waiting at the end. The concepts of caution and consequences seem out of sync with their conviction that nothing bad will happen to them.

Of course you can't let your adolescent's blithe faith in a safe future keep you from discussing precautions and risk taking. However, lecturing and dictating the rules are not always the most effective approach. Adolescents are more likely to learn and cooperate if you actively involve them in the process, as is shown in "Evading Emergencies," below.

EVADING EMERGENCIES
Six E's for Effective Communication with Your Teen

1. *Explore* safety facts together. Adolescents learn and retain information better when they are actively involved in discovering it. When your adolescent wants to learn to drive, play a sport, or take a job, suggest that he or she get safety information from the Internet, books, and pamphlets from related organizations. Together, comparison shop for safety gear, helmets, or auto insurance.

2. *Elicit* your adolescent's input on safety rules. Whether your 12-year-old is trying ever-more-challenging skateboard moves, or your 16-year-old will soon get a driver's license, collaborate on identifying the safety rules they will agree to follow and the consequences if they don't.

3. *Express your expectation* that your adolescent will adhere to these safety rules. Put them in writing, a contract for safety you will both sign. Post the contract on a bulletin board or refrigerator, or if being so public embarrasses your adolescent, make sure each of you has a copy.

4. *Enforce* consequences for breaching those rules. If your teen doesn't have the car home by the agreed-upon time, withdraw car privileges. *Be consistent.* Adolescents may forget or "forget," but either way a lapse should lead to a consequence. That doesn't mean you can't make exceptions or be flexible as warranted. But adolescents can be brilliant in exploiting loopholes. Don't let your teen poke so many holes in the contract that it ends up in shreds.

5. *Evaluate* the contract periodically. Tighten rules if necessary; expand privileges as your teen earns them. For example, you may require a beginning driver to call you after he or she has arrived at his or her destination, but might not need that reassurance from a responsible 20-year-old.

6. *Empower* your adolescent to avoid or get out of risky situations by posing scenarios that challenge your adolescent to think through strategies. For example, show your teen a newspaper article about teens who got injured during a fight over a girlfriend and ask how they might have avoided the fight by dealing with the conflict differently. Specific "what would you do if" discussions strengthen adolescents' decision-making skills and prepare them to be more clearheaded and self-confident when risky situations occur.

PREVENTING SPORTS INJURIES

Bravado and safety are not inconsistent, but they are likely to appear in that order. Adolescents swept up in the rush of action or the thrill of competition often put winning first, safety second. To them, the rewards of risk taking (such as "heroically" playing basketball on an injured ankle) are greater than the rewards of prudence and caution (teammates are less likely to urge a player to get an X ray than to do whatever it takes to defeat the opposing team).

Sports and other forms of exercise are valuable for many reasons—not only for fitness, but also for the development of leadership skills, coordination, self-esteem, camaraderie and teamwork with others; and the prevention of obesity and reduction of stress. Nearly half of all adolescents in the United States, girls as well as boys, participate in organized sports—a number that grows each year, which is great!

Yet injuries are part of the game. Most are minor, but others can be serious. Adolescents should be made aware of the potential for injury and the precautions they can take to prevent it.

First Step: Get Your Doctor's Go-Ahead

Sports teams generally require athletes to have a physical exam first—for good reason. In fact, the preparticipation examination (PPE) is now mandated in most states. However, the quality and thoroughness of the PPE vary dramatically depending on the form that is required to be completed (the items covered) and the skills and interests of the examiner. For many adolescents the PPE is the only reason they ever see their doctor, so this visit offers the potential for examination and counseling even beyond sports if time permits. Even though few athletes will actually be disqualified from participation in their sport as a result of this screening examination, it affords an outstanding opportunity, when done well, to uncover musculoskeletal problems requiring physical therapy, nutritional disorders requiring care, and previously unknown health problems such as high blood pressure that should be monitored.

A thorough PPE aims to identify:

- Any medical conditions in the adolescent that would make participation in the specific sport unsafe; a personal and family medical history and a physical examination are done.
- Any unknown musculoskeletal conditions and/or previous injury patterns (including concussions) that should be addressed prior to participation in the sport.

Ideally the PPE should be done one or two months prior to team participation to allow time for any recommended treatment (such as physical therapy) or additional screening (for example, by a cardiologist or neurologist).

The first part of the PPE is to take a thorough history from the adolescent and parent. Sudden death in a young relative of the adolescent can point to the possibility of an unknown heart problem. An adolescent with a history of wheezing during sports likely has exercise-induced asthma (which is easily treated).

Follow-up care would be warranted if there is a history of concussion, a recent bout of mononucleosis, loss of a paired organ (such as a kidney, testicle, or eye), lack of menstrual periods, use of certain prescribed medications or drugs of abuse (such as cocaine or amphetamines, also steroids or other performance enhancers), a seizure disorder, or injury to bones, ligaments, or joints.

In most instances, the adolescent can proceed to play, with the parents and coach reassured that he or she is healthy enough to do so. The PPE should not be feared as an obstacle to participation in sports; rather, it should be viewed as an opportunity to maximize safety and thus playing time and proficiency.

Check Out the Game, Gear, and Clothes

Karen, a dancer, signed up her son Gabe for gymnastics and tap classes when he was five, and he soon showed that he had inherited his mom's flair. But as an adolescent, his favorite performance platform turned out to be the skateboard. As his skills increased, he wanted to compete. Although concerned about injuries, Karen noted that her son's attitude and training provided some protection.

"Gabriel has always been a kid who *hates* to get hurt, more than I ever hated for him to get hurt. So that works in our favor. He is also incredibly agile and coordinated. Gymnastics taught him the art of falling."

Even so, there is no substitute for safety gear. Karen was pleased to see that skate parks mandated it.

"When we pay to go into a skate park, there is very little choice in the matter, and I like that. No option; all gear must be worn. That includes kneepads, elbow pads, wrist guards, and helmet."

Before participating in a sport, it is a good idea to get a basic understanding of how it is played. Watch games, read a summary of the rules, talk to players. Observe and ask about what the players wear. Find out whether there are required or recommended clothes, protective gear, and footwear. Some of this will be obvious, while other things will not (jockstrap, athletic cup).

The website of the American Academy of Orthopaedic Surgeons (http://orthoinfo.aaos.org) details gear and safety tips for various sports. Check your team's rules against the website's recommendations. Another good resource is *The Young Athlete: A Sports Doctor's Complete Guide for Parents,* by Jordan D. Metzl, M.D., with Carol Shookhoff (Little, Brown and Company, 2002).

Warm Up and Cool Down

Launching into vigorous exercise or stretching without warming up first is an invitation to muscle strain, pull, or tear, as well as to injuries to tendons (tissues that connect muscle to bone) and ligaments (which connect bone to bone).

Warming up sends blood flow to muscles, giving them oxygen and nutrients; increases body temperature; and stretches tendons and ligaments so they can be more resilient. It also provides a good transition into the activity, enabling the adolescent to focus and mentally prepare.

To warm up, get the blood moving by doing light aerobic exercise—such as walking, marching in place, or using a stationary bike—for five to fifteen minutes.

Follow this with moves that systematically warm up and stretch all parts of the body, holding each stretch for about thirty seconds. For example, some people like to warm up with "isolations," gentle moves that focus on individual body parts. You start with the head and work down to the toes. The routine may be something like this:

Look left and right, up and down . . .

Move shoulders up and down, forward and back . . .

Stretch triceps, biceps, shoulders, and back . . .

Gently twist from side to side to limber the spine . . .

Sway the hips . . .

Lift knees . . .

Stretch hamstrings, quadriceps, and calves . . .

Point and flex feet . . .

Which muscles, ligaments, and tendons to warm up and stretch will vary with the sport or activity. For example, ballet dancers regard a well-executed plié (knee bend) to be the heart of a warm-up, because the plié is so essential to fluid movement and to safe takeoffs and landings for leaps and jumps.

Cool-downs are just as important as warm-ups. It is not a good idea to stop exercising abruptly. A cool-down consists of progressively reducing the intensity of exercise. This restores normal body temperature and blood flow, and reduces the possibility of fainting or nausea after exercise.

As integral as warm-ups and cool-downs are to safety, many coaches and teachers do not insist on them. Parents should check to make sure their adolescent's coach or teacher has players do warm-ups and cool-downs. If not, they may be skimping on other safety measures, too. At the very least, insist that your child always does warm-ups and cool-downs.

Stay Cool

Competition is part of the game, and most people enjoy winning. But for parents and players alike, it is healthiest to focus on the joy of playing. Over-competitive parents and coaches can make the sporting environment tense and ruin the fun for everyone. Adolescents should be encouraged to play for enjoyment, and must be protected from the stress caused by rigid expectations and excessive disappointment when a team loses.

After a game, expand the focus beyond who won and who lost. Ask your adolescent:

Did you have fun?

How did you feel about the way you played today?

What were the highlights of the game?

What did you learn from today's game—anything you would do differently next time?

Avoid Steroids and Other Performance-Enhancing Drugs

Steroids are used to "bulk up." Creatine, androstenedione, and other "nutritional supplements" are used to improve performance. But any of these pose major dangers. An adolescent must know: *Do not take any drugs or supplements without checking with your doctor.* (See chapter 9.)

SAFETY ON THE JOB

Don't try to go too fast. Learn your job. Don't ever talk until you know
what you're talking about.

—Sam Rayburn[2]

Real-time, real-world job experience teaches teens more than the value of a
dollar. They gain skills, confidence, and insight into the workings of business.
(A restaurant never looks the same after you've been in the back, wearing a
hairnet and ladling lentil soup.) A job can inspire teens to pursue a certain
interest or make it very clear what they are *not* cut out to do.

Teens have a special niche in the economic landscape. They ring up sales,
put up drywall, flip burgers, swab floors, teach kids to swim, stack soup cans,
and urge customers to try the lime-green tank top with the turquoise skirt.

But then there's Angie, who handles vats of sizzling grease, scared that a
single slip will make the grease slosh over and burn her hands.

And Brian, who is only 15 but looks much older. He lies that he is 18 so he
can sneak into a job on a construction site that by law is off-limits to teens his
age. When asked to work on a high scaffold, he says sure, afraid he'll lose the
job if he says no. Once up there, he is terrified of falling.

Like all workers, teens should be aware that certain jobs have hazards—
and that some employers cannot be relied upon to look out for their young
employees' best interests. Workplace injuries kill about 70 teens each year and
send an additional 70,000 to hospital emergency rooms.[3] Teens get killed driving cars, trucks, and other vehicles on the job. They get hurt by equipment that
malfunctions or that they are too inexperienced or poorly supervised to operate
safely. They get burned in kitchens. They get hernias from lifting heavy boxes.
Alarmed by the health hazards many teens face, the National Consumers
League identified the five "worst jobs for teens" and urged teens to avoid them:

1. Delivery and other driving including: repairing, operating, or riding
   on forklifts and other motorized equipment.
2. Working alone in cash-based businesses and late-night work.
3. Traveling youth crews.
4. Cooking—exposure to hot oil and grease, hot water and steam, and
   hot cooking surfaces.
5. Construction and work at heights.[4]

Teens are often wronged by employers who fail in their legal obligation to
provide a safe and healthy workplace, and in their ethical obligation to avoid
asking inexperienced and poorly trained teens to perform dangerous tasks. But

teens have rights under the law. The National Institute for Occupational Safety and Health (NIOSH) website (www.cdc.gov/niosh/adolespg.html) addresses such issues as inappropriate responsibilities, unsafe settings, and excessive work hours. Some state laws exceed federal safety laws.

Talk with your teen about the safety and supervision on a job. Inexperienced teens may be so glad to get a job that they don't ask questions about the exact nature of the work and safety considerations. A teen may not think twice, for example, about being asked to tend a store alone late at night while the owner drives home to check on her kids. But that teen is a vulnerable target for thieves. Job-related homicide is second only to motor vehicle accidents as a cause of fatal injury for 16- and 17-year-olds.

Together with your teen, evaluate the possible safety risks of a job and investigate state labor laws pertaining to that work. Ask your teen about safety on the job and explore whether your teen should request additional training and supervision.

Pay close attention to your teen's uneasy feelings about a job. If your teen does not feel safe there, discuss what can be done to improve the situation. If an employer or coworkers do not support those changes, have your teen quit and find a job that will enhance, not threaten, her or his well-being.

LEADING CAUSES OF DEATH, Ages 15 to 20

Rank	Cause	Percent of Deaths	Number of Deaths
1	Motor vehicle crashes	35	6,209
2	Homicide	19	3,393
3	Suicide	13	2,254
4	Other Injury (falls, drowning, etc.)	9	1,562
5	Cancer	6	1,036
6	Heart disease	3	541
	Total	100	17,758

Source: National Center for Health Statistics (NCHS), Vital Statistics Morbidity Data 1997, Multiple Causes of Death (MCOD) File, NCHS, Centers for Disease Control and Prevention.

DRIVING SAFETY

Hell on Wheels

Your kid looks so grown-up behind the wheel, maneuvering the giant machine into a narrow parking space, or slaloming between the light poles when practicing in an empty parking lot. You want your adolescent to learn how to drive; it's such an essential skill—not to mention a relief for you when you don't have to chauffeur your child everywhere.

But then once your adolescent gets that license, how do you keep your heart from taking up permanent residence in your throat? That suspense . . . waiting until you hear the car pull up outside, the key in the front door, the footsteps heading right for the refrigerator . . .

There are good reasons for adolescents to drive and for parents to worry. Motor vehicle crashes are the leading cause of deaths for adolescents ages 15 to 20, accounting for 35 percent of fatalities.[5] (See chart, "Leading Causes of Death, Ages 15 to 20," on page 296.)

Adolescents are more likely to leave their seat belts unbuckled. If they have been drinking, they are more likely to get in a crash, even if they have had less alcohol than adults who drink and drive. More than half of all adolescent driving fatalities happen at night, even though adolescents do about 80 percent of their driving during the day.[6]

Learning to Drive

Many teens are so eager to drive, they beg for a chance to practice long before they are old enough to apply for a learner's permit, and on the very day of that long-awaited birthday, they rush to apply. But not all teens feel this way. Some show little or no interest, some procrastinate because they are scared, some suddenly decide they are ready to learn several years after their friends have gotten their licenses. In general it is best to let your teen decide when to learn, but it is an important skill and teens should be encouraged to learn—and reassured that if all the millions of people on the road could learn, they can, too.

Driver's education classes (some offered in schools) may be the best way for your teen to learn, although some parents take on the teaching themselves. This can be a great (though sometimes nerve-wracking) opportunity to pass on all the safety tips and driving techniques you have garnered over the years. But not all parents have the patience for this task, and not all teens are receptive to a parent's teaching. In either circumstance, it is a good idea to delegate the teaching to a professional or another reliable relative or friend.

The most dangerous time for many young drivers is after they have learned to drive, got the driver's license, and been on the road for a while. Greater self-confidence leads a teen to declare, "Now driving has become second nature to me. I no longer have to think about what I'm doing." Be careful. Often what comes next is a period of experimentation, testing of speeds, and saying "How close can I come to an obstacle without hitting it?"

Auto Attitude

Our nation's highways are the great democratic meeting ground. The fact that there aren't even more accidents is testimony not only to the skill but also to the decency of the majority of drivers. Safe driving is not just a matter of steering skill and staying sober. A calm attitude and sound judgment are also essential.

Mature drivers avoid the speeders who hog the left lane, the crawlers who hug the slow lane, and the volatile playboys who weave in and out of lanes as if the highway were an amusement park. Safe drivers refuse to get drawn into races, competitions, road wars, and dares. And they refuse to let feelings of frustration escalate into road rage.

The example parents set makes a difference. Teens observe how their parents handle the road and often emulate what their parents do. A parent who courteously waves another driver the permission to turn first at an intersection or has a "let it go" attitude when another driver shouts an obscenity is conveying powerful messages to his or her teen: *Treat other drivers as you want to be treated. Keep your cool.*

But a parent who screams at other drivers, calls them names (even if they can't hear), or pulls ahead so another driver can't ease onto the road is polluting the environment both within the car and on the road. A teen subjected to such behavior gets the message that—as in a video game—other drivers are antagonists who get in your way.

Is your teen emotionally equipped to cope with the challenges of the road? How would your teen respond to the following situations—and how would you?

- You overslept and you're running late. But the old guy in front of you is creeping along at twenty-five miles per hour. There are No Passing signs, but you know that just up ahead the road widens a bit. There is a truck in the opposite lane, but if you speed up and play your cards right, you'll just be able to make it . . .
- You're in the left lane of the highway and that truck driver has been tailgating you for miles. She has no right to be in this lane. Trucks are supposed to be in the middle lane. No way are you going to switch lanes and let this truck get ahead of you . . .

- For some reason a young guy you don't even know gave you the finger, then sped on as if daring you to catch up. Your car is just as fast as his. How dare he disrespect you and think he can get away with it . . .

Let it be. Let it go. Impulsive, in-a-hurry adolescents may find it difficult to tolerate poky drivers and cede to belligerent ones. But learning how to *let it go* may save their lives and the lives of others.

STEPS FOR KEEPING YOUR YOUNG DRIVER SAFE
How to Be a Healthy Driver

- *Don't drive sleepy.* Fatigue is responsible for numerous accidents (see chapter 3). A tired teen either should not drive or should pull off the road in a safe place and take a nap (after locking car doors), then perhaps also drink a cup of coffee. (Coffee without the nap will not suffice.)
- *Don't drive after drinking.* Require your teen to abstain from all alcohol and drugs before or while driving, to arrange with friends to appoint a designated driver if they will be drinking, and to call you for help *any time of the day or night* to avoid driving after drinking or accepting a ride from someone who has been drinking. (See Students Against Destructive Decisions, or SADD, in Resources, for a "Contract for Life.")
- *Do not allow passengers to drink or use drugs.* Not only are such activities illegal, they can increase the possibility of accidents or other problems. Furthermore, the car is an extension of the parents' home; behavior that is not allowed there should not occur in the car, either.
- *Always wear a seat belt.* Require all passengers to wear seat belts, too.
- *Check with your doctor or pharmacist about medications.* A teen may need to avoid driving while taking certain prescription or over-the-counter medications that cause sleepiness or impair coordination.
- *Check with your doctor about effects of illness on driving.* Adolescents with epilepsy and certain other conditions should be sure to get their doctor's approval and information about any limitations before taking to the road.
- *Calm down.* Teens should allow plenty of time to get places so they don't feel compelled to rush, keep their emotions in check when frustrations occur, and steer clear of drivers who drive erratically or dangerously.
- *Ban cell phones and headphones while driving.* They can distract your teen and prevent him or her from hearing sirens and other important sounds. Even if local law permits the use of cell phone headsets, they can still be distracting and should be used only when essential.

- *Avoid distractions.* Discourage your teen from eating, drinking coffee or other beverages, or other distractions while driving. The same applies when stopping at a light; your teen should not view this as an opportunity to apply lipstick or check notes for the upcoming history exam.

Car Care and Emergency Preparedness

- *Make sure the car is in safe condition.* Keep up with car maintenance and regular checks of brakes, tires, seat belts, etc.
- *Show your teen how to stay alert to car problems.* Make a point of asking your teen how the car is behaving. Follow up on any odd noises or quirks that your teen reports. If you do repairs yourself, have your teen assist you. If you take the car to a mechanic, have your teen go with you and learn how to describe a problem, assess the repair options, and read and check a repair bill.
- *Review basic on-the-go car-check skills.* Teach your teen how to use a tire gauge, check the oil and other fluids, and add fluids if necessary.
- *Equip your teen for emergencies.* Store a flashlight, flares, jumper cables, an extra quart of oil, a few rags, and an umbrella in the trunk. Tuck a notebook and a couple of pens in the glove compartment so your teen can write down insurance and contact information if there is an accident. A disposable camera lets your teen take pictures at the scene that may be helpful in insurance claims or in court.
- *Add emergency amenities.* To help your teen stay comfortable in case he or she needs to stay with the car until help arrives, use the trunk to store a blanket, bottles of water, and a few snacks that won't spoil (trail mix, dried fruit, crackers, juice boxes). Add reading material to help pass the time while waiting in the car or at a garage—perhaps a guide to car emergencies, a collection of short stories, and a magazine or two.
- *Join an auto club* that offers emergency road service. Some provide or offer discounts on driving lessons and safe driving refresher courses, and have pamphlets and other materials on safety for teens.
- *Encourage continuing education.* Many auto clubs publish helpful magazines. Encourage your teen to read articles on driving techniques, road safety, coping with various weather conditions, and auto maintenance. Such articles can make your teen more observant of road hazards and car problems, sharpen driving skills, and convey the message that even experienced drivers can always learn something new.

Family Driving Rules

- *Ease into driving alone.* Even after your teen has gotten a driver's license, he or she may still not be ready to drive independently. Indeed, some states limit driving alone for drivers under a certain age. You and your teen may be more comfortable, at least for an initial period of time, if a parent or another experienced driver accompanies him or her. This also gives a parent an opportunity to assess the teen's driving ability and maturity. Some parents do not permit their teens to drive with friends for the first twelve to eighteen months after getting their license.
- *Establish guidelines on where your teen may drive.* For example, driving might be limited to school and errands in the immediate community, eventually branching out to highway driving, and then to neighboring towns.
- *Set time frames.* Agreeing on what time your teen must be home adds greatly to a parent's peace of mind and encourages safe behavior and accountability. Be mindful of the increased danger of nighttime driving and your teen's skill level, and set limits accordingly.
- *Clarify your teen's responsibilities.* Driving is a privilege, a responsibility, and a way to help others. Do you want your teen to be responsible for putting gas in the car? Keeping it clean? Taking it in for repairs? Contributing toward car payments or insurance? Running errands for a grandparent or a disabled neighbor? Picking up younger siblings?

VIOLENCE AND ADOLESCENT LIFE

School killings do not happen often, but when they do they send shock tremors throughout the country. Metal detectors in some high schools testify to the need for constant vigilance to prevent further tragedies. Fighting has occurred in schools for generations, but the increasing availability of firearms has accentuated the need for young people to learn to avoid or de-escalate conflicts to minimize the chance of getting maimed or killed.

Gangs provide a sense of belonging for young people desperate for a sense of identity and protection, but are associated with violent behaviors and turf battles that endanger gang members and others.

Date rape has always been a hazard, especially when alcohol and drugs have been involved. Now "date rape drugs" such as Rohypnol (see chapter 9) have further increased the risks.

Seeds of Violence

According to the National Institute of Mental Health (NIMH), most violent behavior stems not from a single factor but from a convergence of environmental, family, intrapersonal, and peer factors.

Poverty can contribute to violence (most of the six or seven youths who are killed each day live in poor inner-city communities[7]), but violence is neither typical of poor people nor limited to them.

Violence in the media and in video games is increasingly believed to lead to violence in young people by portraying violence as sport or humorous and desensitizing youth.[8]

The NIMH states that risk factors for youth violence also include "ineffective parenting . . . poor monitoring; ineffective, excessively harsh, or inconsistent discipline; [and] inadequate supervision."[9]

Peer pressure, access to firearms, and inadequate education from parents and schools on how to manage anger, cope with conflict effectively and peacefully, and empathize with others are also compelling factors.

Protecting Teens

There are steps parents can take to discourage their children from committing or being the victim of violent behavior:

- *Keep your adolescent occupied with positive activities.* Busy teens are more likely to stay out of trouble, especially after school, when many fights or other youth crimes occur. Have your child enroll in an after-school program or get a job (twenty hours per week or less). Be aware of where your adolescent is; ask frequently and supervise.

- *Limit your adolescent's exposure to violence in films, TV shows, video games, and the like.* Encourage your adolescent to participate in positive family, community, and spiritual activities.

- *Advocate for conflict resolution and peer support programs at your adolescent's school.* Also explore whether students have adequate physical education classes, athletics, and arts programs that give them outlets for energy and creativity.

- *Consider enrolling your adolescent in a small school.* According to *Educational Leadership* magazine, schools with more than 1,000 students are more likely to be the sites of violent crimes, and teachers and teens in smaller schools (no more than 400 students) know each other better. This enables teachers to be "better able to anticipate potentially violent or disruptive behavior and deal with it before it erupts."[10]

- *Encourage your adolescent to avoid alcohol and drugs,* which greatly increase the possibility of date rape and other assaultive behavior and of the inability to cope with such behavior in others.

- *Get counseling for angry, bullied, or bullying teens.* Ask a doctor to help you and your teen assess and address medical, psychological, family, school, peer, or other problems that may be causing or worsening anger or depression. Angry and bullying adolescents may benefit from learning anger-management skills. Bullied youth may feel helpless and have low self-esteem, and should also have the opportunity to speak with a psychologist or learn assertiveness skills. Ask your doctor for a referral or consult your child's school social worker or psychologist.

• *Eliminate access to firearms.* If you have a gun, keep the weapon unloaded and the ammunition locked away separately. Do not allow your adolescent to know the location of the keys or to have access to the gun. Such measures could have averted numerous homicides, suicides, and injuries.

COPING WITH INJURY

An adolescent who suffers a physical disability stemming from a motor vehicle, sports, or violence-related injury suddenly tumbles into an alternate reality. In an instant, normal life is over. The adolescent faces the disorienting and urgent business of being rushed to treatment, and perhaps enduring a lengthy rehabilitation or adjusting to permanent disability.

Emotional, social, educational, and physical challenges abound. It is common for injured adolescents to withdraw and become depressed. They may go through a period of denial, mourning, and anger. They may feel ashamed or guilty for putting their parents and family through the grief, expense, and distress their injury has caused.

In *The Road Back: Living with a Physical Disability*, a book written for teens, Harriet Sirof describes the many facets of the newly disabled teen's experience, including hospitalization, physical or occupational therapy, support groups, altered relationships with family and friends, transportation difficulties, wheelchair sports and other kinds of exercise, and more. Through all the tumult, however, there is one thing the teen must remember and of which the family should reassure this new, reluctant, and distraught patient: The teen's intrinsic value and specialness is still intact. Ms. Sirof writes:

> *Your life could change in a minute. A truck might skid on a wet road and slam into your car. You might be thrown off your skateboard into a wall. Or you might wake up one morning unable to see out of one eye. You could suddenly be disabled.*
>
> *. . . Whether you had a broken hip that healed in a few months or a broken neck that left you paralyzed, you would still be you. You might face problems you never dreamed you would have. You might have to work hard at getting well. Or you might have to learn to live with your disabil-*

ity. But being sick or disabled wouldn't stop you from feeling or caring or hoping or dreaming. It wouldn't make you less of a person.[11]

HEALTH-PARTNERING TIPS FOR PARENTS

- Remember those health basics from chapter 3. Teens who are well-rested, well-nourished, and get adequate exercise may have an edge in preventing accidents and injuries because they are more alert, clearheaded, and generally healthy.
- Urge your teen to abstain from alcohol and other drugs; they significantly increase the risk of accidents and injuries.
- Know your own teenager's tendencies toward impulsivity, daredeviltry, bravado, lack of focus, impressionability, and other traits that may increase the risk of accident or injury. If your teen needs more help, supervision, or limit setting for these reasons. . . . *provide it!*
- Remember that some accidents may be related to carelessness with one's own life. If your teen seems to be uncharacteristically sad, withdrawn, lackadaisical, or reckless, seek professional advice. He or she may be depressed, even suicidal (see chapter 11).
- Always emphasize safety as a first and foremost consideration in any pursuit, be it driving, sports, a job, or any other activity. Discuss safety factors in advance, review them regularly, and respond promptly and consistently if your teen diverges from safe practices.

CONCLUSION

> The future starts today and tomorrow too.
> It starts and starts until it is through.
> In a way, all of life is an in-between,
> but never more in-between than age nineteen.
>
> —*excerpted from "Nineteen: A Poem
> for My Daughter," by Betty Rothbart*

Partnerships are fun and gratifying when both parties feel they have a vital role to play. For parents of teens, nothing can be more satisfying than continuing to connect and participate in a meaningful way in your child's life, even as he or she becomes more independent and self-sufficient. In fact, your involvement and ongoing dialogue are what help to assure your teen's steady growth and your eventual sense that the health partnership has reaped wonderful results.

The process of parenting teens and young adults remains challenging and at times frustrating and difficult, but emotional doors must remain open even as room doors may get slammed shut. When communication stops or feels blocked it is critical to try to figure out how to begin again.

Around age 18 many teens leave home. Your hope is that they are ready to manage their lives without your immediate words and supervision. This ability does not just suddenly happen because they have turned 18 or graduated from high school. It takes a lot of practice, some false starts, and falling on one's face from time to time to feel sturdy in one's independence. That is why from an early age parents need to let their teens practice decision making rather than deciding for them or telling them what to do. Share values and judgments and suggestions that make sense, then back off. Although parents can provide good tools, only the teen can build with them.

Most 18-year-olds living away from home, if they have come to value their parents' input and opinions, and feel respected and trusted by them, will continue to pick up the phone (or type out an E-mail) for advice or support. That dialogue, which started in earnest nearly ten years before, will continue—and continue to change—throughout your lives together.

Health challenges continue into late adolescence and young adulthood, the years after 18 or 21. Often the stakes go up. Many young adults are driving for the first time, or driving longer distances in unfamiliar territory. Will they drive sober and at a reasonable speed? Alcohol is now legal or more readily available. Will they drink in moderation? Sexual activity may begin or continue. At this older age, when sexual partners are likely to be more sexually experienced, a sexually transmitted disease is more likely to be lurking. Will they practice safe sex precautions and avoid casual sex and multiple partners?

Will these young adults be able to survive the breakup of a romantic relationship that was not just a fling but serious for five years? Will they manage to bounce back after being laid off from a job? Will they seek help for an eating disorder that has begun to plague them? Will they know what to do about an unplanned pregnancy? Will they go to bed at a reasonable hour? Will they eat healthy meals? Will they seek help for depression? Will they go regularly to a doctor and seek care if they feel sick or have an unexplained pain?

The time and effort invested in imparting health information and talking about health skills and decision making during adolescence will pay off during young adulthood.

Will young adults call their parents for advice? After so many years of a healthy partnership, you can now talk as friends or colleagues, connecting and collaborating.

And who knows? Next time, you may be calling *them* for advice!

Notes

CHAPTER 1: THE STAGES AND TASKS OF ADOLESCENT DEVELOPMENT

1. Philippe Aries, *Centuries of Childhood: A Social History of Family Life* (New York: Knopf, 1962), 25, 29, 30.

CHAPTER 2: A DOCTOR OF THEIR OWN

1. "Adele Hoffman, 74, Pediatrician Who Shaped Adolescent Care," *New York Times,* 21 June 2001.

2. Christopher J. Van Ness and Daryl A. Lynch, "Male Adolescents and Physician Sex Preference," *Pediatrics and Adolescent Medicine* 154, no. 1, (2000).

3. Jason Theodosakis and David T. Feinberg, *Don't Let Your HMO Kill You* (New York: Routledge, 2000).

4. *Guidelines for Adolescent Preventive Services,* American Medical Association, 1992.

5. Carol A. Ford, S. G. Millstein, B. Halpern-Felscher, et al., "Influence of Physician Confidentiality Assurances on Adolescents' Willingness to Disclose Information and Seek Future Health Care—A Randomized Control Trial," *Journal of the American Medical Association* 278 (September 24, 1997), 1029–1034.

6. Andrea Marks, J. Malizio, J. Hoch, et al., "Assessment of Health Needs and Willingness to Utilize Health Care Resources of Adolescents in a Suburban Population," *Journal of Pediatrics* 102 (March 1983), no. 3, 456–60.

CHAPTER 3: THE BASICS: NUTRITION, EXERCISE, AND SLEEP

1. Lynn Sonberg, *The Health Nutrient Bible* (New York: Simon & Schuster, 1995), 8.

2. "Female adolescents need calcium during 'window of opportunity,' " *Purdue News* (August 13, 1997), http://www.purdue.edu/UNS/html4ever/970808.Weaver.adoles.html, accessed May 22, 2001.

3. "Dietary Reference Intakes," Food and Nutrition Board of the National Academy of Sciences.

4. "A Guide to Eating for Sports," Nemours Foundation, Kidshealth.org/teen/ nutrition/menu/eatnrun_p6.html, accessed June 5, 2001.

5. "Do You Know How to Feed Your Child Athlete," Nemours Foundation, Kidshealth.org/parent/nutrition_fit/fitness/feed_child_athlete.html, accessed June 5, 2001.

6. "What Teens Should Know About Caffeine," Nemours Foundation, Kidshealth.org/teen/nutrition/menu/caffeine.html, accessed June 5, 2001.

7. Jane E. Brody, "For lifelong gains, just add water. Repeat," *New York Times*, 11 July 2000, F8.

8. Louise Hagler, *Tofu Quick and Easy* (Summertown, Tenn.: Book Publishing Company, 1986).

9. Amy Dacyczyn, *The Tightwad Gazette II* (New York: Villard Books, 1995), 74–75.

10. "School Breakfast and School Performance," *Am. J. Dis. Children* 143 (October 1989).

11. "The Relationship of School Breakfast to Psychosocial and Academic Functioning," *Archives of Pediatric and Adolescent Medicine* 152 (September 1998).

12. "Improving Reading and Math Scores: The School Breakfast Connection" (New York City: Community Food Resource Center, December 1999).

13. Nikki Goldbeck and David Goldbeck, *The Good Breakfast Book* (Woodstock, N.Y.: Ceres Press, 1992), i.

14. "Guidelines for School and Community Programs to Promote Lifelong Physical Activity Among Young People," supplement to *MMWR* 46 (March 7, 1997), no. RR-6, Centers for Disease Control and Prevention.

15. Ibid.

16. Operation Fit Kids, http://www.operationfitkids.org, accessed May 29, 2001.

17. "Physical Activity and Health: A Report of the Surgeon General," 1996, http://www.cdc.gov/nccdphp/sgr/adoles.htm, accessed May 29, 2001.

18. 1997 Youth Risk Behavior Surveillance System (YRBSS), Centers for Disease Control and Prevention, *MMWR* 45 (1998), no. SS-4.

19. Eric Jensen, "Moving with the Brain in Mind," *Educational Leadership* (November 2000), 34–37.

20. "Exercise Found Effective Against Depression," *New York Times*, 10 October 2000.

21. Bill McKibben, *Long Distance: A Year of Living Strenuously* (New York: Simon & Schuster, 2000), 14.

22. "Why Exercise Is Wise," Nemours Foundation, October 12, 1998, Kidshealth.org/teen/nutrition/move/exercise.html, accessed June 24, 2001.

23. "Strength Training, Weight and Power Lifting, and Body Building by Children and Adolescents (RE9196)," policy statement of the American Academy of Pediatrics, November 1990, http://www.aap.org/policy/03327.html, accessed May 30, 2001.

24. Mark Story and Dianne Neumark-Sztainer, "Promoting Healthy Eating and Physical Activity in Adolescents," *Adolescent Medicine: State of the Art Reviews* 10, no. 1 (1999).

25. *Adolescent Sleep Needs and Patterns: Research Report and Resource Guide* (Washington, D.C.: National Sleep Foundation, 2000), 3.

26. Ibid.

27. Ibid.

28. "Sleep Needs, Patterns and Difficulties of Adolescents: Summary of a Workshop," Commission on Behavioral and Social Sciences and Education, 2000, p. 13, http://zoo.nap.edu/nap-cgi@isbn=0309071771&page=R11, accessed May 22, 2001.

29. *Adolescent Sleep Needs and Patterns: Research Report and Resource Guide* (Washington, D.C.: National Sleep Foundation, 2000), 1.

30. "National Sleep Foundation Releases New Statistics on Sleep in America," National Sleep Foundation, Washington, D.C., http://www.sleepfoundation.org/pressarchives/new_stats.html, accessed July 15, 2001.

31. *Adolescent Sleep Needs and Patterns: Research Report and Resource Guide* (Washington, D.C.: National Sleep Foundation, 2000), 13.

32. Ibid.

CHAPTER 4: COMMON HEALTH PROBLEMS OF BOYS AND GIRLS

1. "An Ounce of Prevention Keeps the Germs Away . . . Wash Your Hands Often," National Center for Infectious Diseases, U.S. Centers for Disease Control and Prevention, http://www.cdc.gov/ncidod/op/handwashing.htm, accessed December 25, 2001.

2. National Institutes of Health, Department of Health and Human Services, National Institute of Arthritis and Musculoskeletal and Skin Diseases (NIAMS) Information Clearinghouse, NIH publication no. 01-4998, October 2001.

3. "On the Teen Scene: Dodging the Rays," *FDA Consumer*, Food and Drug Administration, http://www.fda.gov/fdac/reprints/ots_rays.html, accessed December 23, 2001.

4. Robert Brain, *The Decorated Body* (New York: Harper & Row, 1979), 7.

5. Beth Wilkinson, *Coping with the Dangers of Tattooing, Body Piercing, and Branding* (New York: Rosen Publishing Group, 1998), 62.

6. "Are Tattoos Safe?" Alliance of Professional Tattooists, http://www.imagesinink.net/safe.html, accessed September 15, 2001.

7. American Dental Association, http://www.ada.org/public/faq/piercing.html, accessed February 8, 2002.

8. Arlene L. Bronzaft, Ph.D., "It Takes a 'Silent Village' to Harm a Child," *Hearing Rehabilitation Quarterly* 24, no. 1 (1999), http://www.aafp.org/afp/981101ap/tips.htm/#8 9.

9. Mark N. Goldstein, "Otolaryngology," *Comprehensive Adolescent Health Care*, ed. Stanford B. Friedman (St. Louis: Quality Medical Publishing, 1992), 1075.

10. David Satcher, M.D., U.S. Surgeon General, *The Face of a Child*, Surgeon General's Workshop and Conference on Children and Oral Health, draft, May 2001.

11. Surgeon General's Report on Oral Health, May 25, 2000, http://www.nidr.nih.gov/sgr/sgr.html, accessed December 27, 2001.

12. Oral Health in America: A Report of the Surgeon General, May 2000, http://www.nidcr.nih.gov/sgr/sgr.htm, accessed December 27, 2001.

13. "Tips to Help Families Achieve Optimal Oral Health," American Academy of Periodontology, http://www.period.org/consumer/family_tips.htm, accessed December 30, 2001.

14. "Protecting Children's Oral Health," American Academy of Periodontology, http://www.perio.org/consumer/children.htm, accessed December 30, 2001.

15. American Dental Association, http://www.ada.org/public/faq/braces.html, accessed January 9, 2002.

16. American Association of Orthodontists, http://www.braces.org/dental-insc/index.cfm, accessed January 9, 2002.

17. American Dental Association, http://www.ada.org/public/faq/braces.html, accessed January 9, 2002.

18. Surgeon General's Report, executive summary, part two.

19. Jeffrey T. Kirchner, "Clinical Behavior Problems in Children with Nocturnal Enuresis," *American Family Physician*, November 1, 1998, http://www.aafp.org/afp/981101ap/tips.htm/#8, accessed July 20, 2001.

20. "Bed-Wetting: A Common Problem," National Kidney Foundation, http://www.kidney.org/general/news/bedwettaq.ctm, accessed July 10, 2001.

21. "Encopresis," *Child Health A to Z*, http://www.childrenshospital.org/cfapps/A2ZtopicDisplay.ctm?Topic=Encopresis, accessed July 22, 2001.

22. Judy Blume, *Deenie* (New York: Bradbury Press, 1973), 78.

CHAPTER 5: HEALTH ISSUES FOR YOUR DAUGHTER

1. Laurie Lisle, *Portrait of an Artist: A Biography of Georgia O'Keeffe* (New York: Washington Square Press, 1981), 170.

2. Lisle, 170.

3. "TSS Now Rare, but Women Still Should Take Care," FDA Consumer Magazine, March–April 2000, http://www.fda.gov/fdac/features/2000/200_tss.html, accessed February 2, 2002.

4. Turner's Syndrome Society, http://www.turner-syndrome-us.org/resource/faq.html, accessed January 16, 2002.

5. "American College of Sports Medicine Position Stand on the Female Athlete Triad," *Medicine and Science in Sports and Exercise* 29, no. 5 (1997), 2.

6. Planned Parenthood Federation of America, http://www.plannedparenthood.org/bc/WaysToChart.htm, accessed January 19, 2002.

7. National Institute of Diabetes and Digestive and Kidney Diseases (NIDDK), http://www.niddk.nih.gov/health/urolog/pubs/utiadult/utiadult.htm, accessed January 19, 2002.

8. Pearl S. Buck, *Dragon Seed* (New York: John Day Company, 1941), 221.

CHAPTER 6: HEALTH ISSUES FOR YOUR SON

1. "Now News: New Options for Wellness," newsletter of Stanford University Medical School, Stanford Linear Accelerator Center, January 1999, www.slac.stanford.edu/esh/medical/now/news0199.pdf, accessed December 11, 2001.

2. Lawrence S. Neinstein, *Adolescent Health Care*, 2d ed. (Baltimore: Urban & Schwarzenberg, 1991), 813.

3. Hypospadias Association of America, http://www.hypospadias.org/index.html, accessed September 25, 2001.

CHAPTER 7: COPING WITH CHRONIC HEALTH PROBLEMS

1. Nicole Johnson, *Living with Diabetes* (Washington, D.C.: LifeLine Press, 2001), 18.

2. Martin E. P. Seligman, *Learned Optimism* (New York: Alfred A. Knopf, 1990), 14.

3. Harriet Sirof, *The Road Back: Living with a Disability* (Lincoln, Nebr.: iUniverse.com, An Authors Guild Backinprint.com Edition, 2000).

CHAPTER 8: RISKS AND REALITIES OF TEEN SEXUALITY

1. David Satcher, M.D., Ph.D., "The Surgeon General's Call to Action to Promote Sexual Health and Responsible Sexual Behavior," June 2001, http://www.surgeon general.gov/library/sexualhealth/call.htm, accessed January 31, 2002.

2. U.S. Centers for Disease Control and Prevention, "Youth Risk Behavior Surveillance—United States, 1999," *Morbidity and Mortality Weekly Report* 49, no. SS-5 (June 9, 2000), 19–21.

3. Jenny Comita, "Not That Innocent," *Teen Vogue* (Spring 2001), 108.

4. Gary Webb, "Sex and the Internet: A Special Report," *Yahoo!* (May 2001), 84.

5. "Talking to Your Kids About Sex," American Academy of Child & Adolescent Psychiatry, http://www.aacap.org/publications/factsfam/62.htm, accessed June 23, 2001.

6. The National Campaign to Prevent Teen Pregnancy, www.teenpregnancy.org, accessed July 2, 2001.

7. Susan Philliber, Jackie Kaye, and Scott Herrling, "The National Evaluation of the Children's Aid Society Carrera-Model Program to Prevent Teen Pregnancy," May 2001, http://www.childrensaidsociety.org/cas/teen_preg/program_report.html, accessed January 30, 2002.

8. Donna Shalala, remarks made at the Children's Aid Society Annual Symposium, October 19, 2000, http://www.os.dhhs.gov/news/speeches/001019a.html, accessed January 30, 2002.

9. Ellen Rosenberg, *Growing Up Feeling Good*, 2d rev. ed. (New York: Puffin Books, 1995), 90–91.

10. Carolyn J. T. Halpern, "Adolescent Males' Willingness to Report Masturbation," *Journal of Sex Research* (November 2000), http://www.findarticles.com/cf_0/m2372/4_37/72272306/print.jhtml, accessed July 20, 2001.

11. James Lock, "Gay, Lesbian, and Bisexual Youth Risks for Emotional, Physical, and Social Problems: Results from a Community-Based Survey," *Journal of the American Academy of Child and Adolescent Psychiatry* (March 1999), http://www.find articles.com/cf_0/m2250/3_38/54171868/print.jhtml, accessed July 21, 2001.

12. "Gay and Lesbian Adolescents," American Academy of Child and Adolescent Psychiatry, April 1998.

13. "Parents, Families and Friends of Lesbian, Gay, Bisexual and Transgendered Persons," www.pflag.org, accessed October 20, 2001.

14. Gay, Lesbian and Straight Education Network, www.glsen.org, accessed October 20, 2001.

15. Ibid.

16. American Social Health Association, http://www.ashastd.org/stdfaqs/statistics.html, accessed August 6, 2001.

17. P. S. Rosenberg, R. J. Biggar, and J. J. Goedert, "Declining age at HIV infection in the United States," *New England Journal of Medicine* 330 (1994), 789–90.

18. "Condom Use by Adolescents," *Pediatrics* 107, no. 6 (2001), 1466.

19. Donald E. Greydanus, "Contraception in the Adolescent: An Update," *Pediatrics* (March 2001), http://www.findarticles.com/cf_0/m0950/3_107/71873829/print.jhtml, accessed July 21, 2001.

CHAPTER 9: NO TEEN IS IMMUNE: SUBSTANCE USE AND ABUSE

1. *Statistical Abstract of the United States*, 2000 ed., U.S. Department of Commerce, Economics, and Statistics, U.S. Census Bureau, Washington Printing Office, 2000.

2. "Teens: Alcohol and Other Drugs," American Academy of Child and Adolescent Psychiatry, "AACAP Facts for Families #3," http://www.aacap.org/publications/factsfam/teendrug.htm, accessed June 16, 2001.

3. Christopher Buckley, *Thank You for Smoking* (New York: Random House, 1994), 5.

4. "Youth Tobacco Surveillance—United States, 2000" (YTS 2000), *Morbidity and Mortality Weekly Report*, Centers for Disease Control and Prevention, November 2001.

5. Richard B. Heyman, "Tobacco, Alcohol, and Other Drugs," *Primary Care of Adolescent Girls*, edited by Susan Coupey (Philadelphia: Hanley & Belfus, 2000), 187.

6. "Youth Risk Behavior Surveillance (YRBS), 1999," *Morbidity and Mortality Weekly Report*, June 9, 2000, 11–12.

7. "Bidi Use Among Urban Youth—Massachusetts, March–April 1999," Department of Health and Human Services, www.cdc.gov/epo/mmwr/preview/mmwrhtml/ mm4836a2.htm, accessed November 10, 2001.

8. American Cancer Society, http://www.guidestar.org/partners/helping/ index_ext.jsp?npoId=108977, accessed December 12, 2001.

9. Ibid.

10. "Youth Risk Behavior Surveillance Survey, 1999," *MMWR*, 12.

11. Ibid.

12. C. Everett Koop, *The Memoirs of America's Family Doctor* (New York: Random House, 1991), 186.

13. "Youth Risk Behavior Surveillance Survey, 1999," *MMWR:* http://www. cdc.gov/mmwr/preview/mmwrhtml/ss4905a1.htm, accessed October 21, 2002.

14. Ibid.

15. Heyman, 196.

16. "Inhalants," *Infofax*, National Institute on Drug Abuse, National Institutes of Health, http://drugabuse.gov/Infofax/inhalants.html, accessed December 14, 2001.

17. "Crack and Cocaine," *Infofax*, National Institute on Drug Abuse, National Institutes of Health, http://drugabuse.gov/Infofax/cocaine.html, accessed December 14, 2001.

18. Glen R. Hanson, "Looking the Other Way: Rave Promoters and Club Drugs," testimony before the Senate Caucus on International Narcotics Control, December 4, 2001, http://www.drugabuse.gov/Testimony/12-4-01/Testimony.html, accessed December 12, 2001.

19. Alan I. Leshner, "Club Drugs Aren't 'Fun Drugs,' " National Institute on Drug Abuse, http://www.drugabuse.gov, accessed July 10, 2001.

20. Substance Abuse and Mental Health Services Administration, http://www. samhsa.gov/centers/csap/csap.html, accessed December 12, 2001.

21. Ibid.

22. Hanson.

23. Hanson.

24. "LSD," *Infofax*, National Institute on Drug Abuse, National Institutes of Health, http://drugabuse.gov/Infofax/lsd.html, accessed December 14, 2001.

CHAPTER 10: PANIC AT THE MIRROR: TEENS AND EATING DISORDERS

1. *Mental Health: A Report of the Surgeon General*, http://www.surgeongeneral. gov/library/mentalhealth/home.html, 1999.

2. Alison E. Field, Sc.D., et al., "Peer, Parent, and Media Influences on the Development of Weight Concerns and Frequent Dieting Among Preadolescent and Adolescent Girls and Boys," *Pediatrics* 107, no. 1 (2001).

3. Lawrence S. Neinstein, *Adolescent Health Care* (Baltimore: Urban & Schwarzenberg, 1991), 487.

4. Field.

5. *Diagnostic and Statistical Manual of Mental Disorders* (DSM IV) 4th ed. (Washington, D.C.: American Psychiatric Association, 1994).

6. Neinstein, 487–88.

7. Martin Fisher, M.D., "Medical Complications of Anorexia and Bulimia Nervosa," *Adolescent Medicine: State of the Art Reviews* 3, no. 3 (1992).

8. Richard E. Kreipe and Marguerite Uphoff, "Treatment and Outcome of Adolescents with Anorexia Nervosa," *Adolescent Medicine: State of the Art Reviews* 3, no. 3 (1992).

9. National Center for Health Statisics, Centers for Disease Control and Prevention, National Health and Nutrition Survey, *Prevalence of Overweight Among Children and Adolescents: United States, 1999*, www.cdc.gov/nchs/products/pubs/pubd/hestats/overwght99.html, accessed December 5, 2001.

10. Robert Lipsyte, *One Fat Summer* (New York: HarperCollins Children's Books, 1977), 180.

CHAPTER 11: YOUR TEEN'S MENTAL HEALTH

1. John Donne, *John Donne: Poetry and Prose*, ed. Frank J. Warnke (New York: Modern Library/Random House, 1967), 41.

2. Melba Colgrove, Harold H. Bloomfield, and Peter McWilliams, *How to Survive the Loss of a Love* (New York: Prelude Press, 1991).

3. The reference for this entire chapter is *Diagnostic and Statistical Manual of Mental Disorders* (DSM IV), 4th ed. (Washington, D.C.: American Psychiatric Association, 1994).

4. National Youth Violence Prevention Resource Center, http://www.safeyouth.org/topics/suicide.htm, accessed February 2, 2002.

5. National Center for Health Statistics, www.cdc.gov, accessed February 2, 2002.

6. American Association for Suicide Prevention, http://www.afsp.org/index-1.htm, accessed February 2, 2002.

CHAPTER 12: PREVENTING ACCIDENTS AND INJURIES

1. "Facts on Adolescent Injury," National Center for Injury Prevention and Control, U.S. Centers for Disease Control and Prevention, http://www.cdc.gov/ncipc/factsheets/adoles.htm, accessed September 16, 2001.

2. "Correct Quotes for DOS," WordStar International, 1991, http://www.bemorecreative.com, accessed February 6, 2002.

3. National Institute for Occupational Safety and Health (NIOSH), http://www.cdc.gov/niosh/adoldoc.html, accessed September 16, 2001.

4. National Consumers League, http://www.nclnet.org/childpr626.html, accessed February 4, 2002.

5. National Center for Health Statistics (NCHS), Vital Statistics Morbidity Data 1997, Multiple Causes of Death (MCOD) File, NCHS, Centers for Disease Control and Prevention, www.cdc.gov/nchs.

6. "Facts on Adolescent Injury."

7. "Child and Adolescent Violence Research," National Institute of Mental Health, http://www.ncadd.com/youth/parents.cfm, accessed February 6, 2002.

8. Elisa Hae-Jung Song, M.D., and Jane E. Anderson, M.D., "How Violent Video Games May Violate Children's Health," *Contemporary Pediatrics* (May 2001), 102.

9. "Child and Adolescent Violence Research."

10. Michael Klonsky, "How Smaller Schools Prevent School Violence," *Educational Leadership* (February 2002), 65.

11. Harriet Sirof, *The Road Back: Living with a Disability* (Lincoln, Nebr.: iUniverse.com, An Authors Guild Backinprint.com Edition, 2000).

Bibliography

Angier, Natalie. *Woman: An Intimate Geography*. Boston: Houghton Mifflin, 1999.

Apter, Terri. *Altered Loves, Mothers and Daughters During Adolescence*. New York: Fawcett Columbine, 1990.

Bartle, Nathalie, with Susan Lieberman. *Venus in Blue Jeans*. Boston: Houghton Mifflin, 1998.

Bauer, Joy. *The Complete Idiot's Guide to Total Nutrition*. 2nd ed. New York: Alpha Books, 1999.

Brownmiller, Susan. *Femininity*. New York: Fawcett Columbine, 1984.

Brumberg, Joan Jacobs. *The Body Project: An Intimate History of American Girls*. New York: Random House, 1997.

Colgrove, Melba; Harold H. Bloomfield; and Peter McWilliams. *How to Survive the Loss of a Love*. Prelude Press, New York, 1991.

Corr, Charles A., and David E. Balk, eds. *Handbook of Adolescent Death and Bereavement*. New York: Springer Publishing, 1996.

Coupey, Susan, ed. *Primary Care of Adolescent Girls*. Philadelphia: Hanley & Belfus, 2000.

Dudman, Martha T. *Augusta Gone*. New York: Simon & Schuster, 2001.

Dyment, Paul, ed. *Male Reproductive Health*. Adolescent Medicine, State of the Art Reviews, Vol. 7, No. 1, Philadelphia: Hanley & Belfus, 1996.

Edut, Ophira, ed. *Adios, Barbie: Young Women Write About Body Image and Identity*. Seattle: Seal Press, 1998.

Emans, S. Jean, Marc R. Laufer, and Donald P. Goldstein, eds. *Pediatric and Adolescent Gynecology*. Philadelphia: Lippincott-Raven, 1998.

Fassler, David G., and Lynne S. Dumas. *Help Me, I'm Sad: Recognizing, Treating, and Preventing Childhood and Adolescent Depression*. New York: Viking, 1997.

Feinberg, Linda Sones. *Teasing: Innocent Fun or Sadistic Malice?* Far Hills, N.J.: New Horizon Press, 1996.

Feldman, S. Shirley, and Glen R. Elliott. *At the Threshold: The Developing Adolescent*. Cambridge, Mass.: Harvard University Press, 1990.

Fontenelle, Don. *Keys to Parenting Your Teenager*. Hauppauge, N.Y.: Barron's Educational Series, 2000.

Friedman, Stanford B., ed. *Comprehensive Adolescent Health Care*. St. Louis: Quality Medical Publishing, 1992.

Gabriel, H. Paul, and Robert Wool. *Anticipating Adolescence: How to Cope with Your Child's Emotional Upheaval and Forge a New Relationship Together*. New York: Henry Holt and Company, 1995.

Gullo, Stephen. *Thin Tastes Better*. New York: Carol Southern Books, 1995.

Haffner, Debra W. *From Diapers to Dating*. New York: Newmarket Press, 1999.

Hancock, Emily. *The Girl Within: A Groundbreaking New Approach to Female Identity*. New York: Ballantine, 1989.

Herman, Judith. *Trauma and Recovery: The Aftermath of Violence—from Domestic Abuse to Political Terror*. New York: Basic Books, 1997.

Heyman, Richard. *How to Say It to Teens: Talking About the Most Important Topics of Their Lives*. Paramus, N.J.: Prentice-Hall Press, 2001.

Homan, William P., and Betty Rothbart. *The Hernia Book*. Yonkers, N.Y.: Consumer Reports Books, 1993.

Kastner, Laura S., and Jennifer F. Wyatt. *The Seven-Year Stretch: How Families Work Together to Grow Through Adolescence*. Boston: Houghton Mifflin, 1997.

Levy-Warren, Marsha. *The Adolescent Journey*. Northvale, N.J.: Jason Aronson, 1996.

Mann, Judy. *The Difference: Discovering the Hidden Ways We Silence Girls; Finding Alternatives That Can Give Them a Voice*. New York: Warner Books, 1994.

Neinstein, Lawrence S. *Adolescent Health Care*. 2d ed. Baltimore: Urban & Schwarzenberg, 1991.

Nelson, Miriam E., with Sarah Wernick. *Strong Women, Strong Bones*. New York: Perigee/Berkley Publishing Group, 2000.

Northrup, Christiane. *Women's Bodies, Women's Wisdom*. New York: Bantam, 1998.

Orenstein, Peggy, in association with the American Association of University Women. *Schoolgirls: Young Women, Self-Esteem, and the Confidence Gap*. New York: Anchor Books/Doubleday, 1994.

Pipher, Mary. *Reviving Ophelia: Saving the Selves of Adolescent Girls*. New York: Grosset/Putnam, 1994.

Pitman, Theresa, and Miriam Kaufman. *The Overweight Child*. Buffalo, N.Y.: Firefly Books, 2000.

Pollack, William S., with Todd Shuster. *Real Boys' Voices*. New York: Penguin Books, 2000.

Ponton, Lynn E. *The Romance of Risk: Why Teenagers Do the Things They Do*. New York: Basic Books/HarperCollins, 1997.

Pratt, Jane. *For Real: The Uncensored Truth About America's Teenagers*. New York: Hyperion, 1995.

Pruitt, D., ed. *Your Adolescent: Emotional, Behavioral, and Cognitive Development from Early Adolescence Through the Teen Years*. New York: HarperCollins, 2000.

Roan, Sharon L. *Our Daughters' Health*. New York: Hyperion, 2001.

Rosemond, John. *Teen-Proofing: Fostering Responsible Decision Making in Your Teenager*. Kansas City, Mo.: Andrews McMeel Publishing, 1998.

Rosenberg, Ellen. *Growing Up Feeling Good*. New York: Puffin Books, 1995.

Sanders, Summer, with Melinda Marshall. *Champions Are Raised, Not Born: How My Parents Made Me a Success.* New York: Dell Publishing, 1999.

Schydlower, Manuel, ed. *Substance Abuse: A Guide for Health Professionals.* Elk Grove Village, Ill.: American Academy of Pediatrics, 2002.

Shandler, Nina. *Ophelia's Mom: Women Speak Out About Loving and Letting Go of Their Adolescent Daughters.* New York: Crown Publishers, 2001.

Siegler, Ava L. *The Essential Guide to the New Adolescence.* New York: Dutton, 1997.

Silby, Caroline, with Shelley Smith. *Games Girls Play: Understanding and Guiding Young Female Athletes.* New York: St. Martin's Press, 2000.

Snyderman, Nancy, and Peg Streep. *Girl in the Mirror: Mothers and Daughters in the Years of Adolescence.* New York: Hyperion, 2002.

Sonberg, Lynn. *The Health Nutrient Bible.* New York: Fireside/Simon & Schuster, 1995.

Steinberg, Laurence, and Ann Levine. *You and Your Adolescent.* New York: Harper-Perennial, 1997.

Stepp, Laura S. *Our Last Best Shot: Guiding Our Children Through Adolescence.* New York: Riverhead Books, 2000.

Stern-LaRosa, Caryl, and Ellen Bettmann. *Hate Hurts: How Children Learn and Unlearn Prejudice.* New York: Anti-Defamation League/Scholastic, 2000.

Story, M.; K. Holt; and D. Sofka, eds. *Bright Futures in Practice: Nutrition (2000).* Washington, D.C.: National Center for Education in Maternal and Child Health, Georgetown University, 2000.

Swets, Paul W. *The Art of Talking with Your Teenager.* Holbrook, Mass.: Media Corporation, 1995.

Theodosakis, Jason, and David T. Feinberg. *Don't Let Your HMO Kill You: How to Wake Up Your Doctor, Take Control of Your Health, and Make Managed Care Work for You.* New York: Routledge, 2000.

Thompson, Michael. *Boys: Answers to the Most-Asked Questions About Raising Sons.* New York: Ballantine Books, 2000.

Wilens, T. E. *Straight Talk About Psychiatric Medications for Kids.* New York: Guilford Publications, 1998.

Wolf, Anthony E. *Get Out of My Life, but First Could You Drive Me and Cheryl to the Mall? A Parent's Guide to the New Teenager.* New York: Noonday Press/Farrar Straus Giroux, 1991.

Woody, Jane D. *How Can We Talk About That?* New York: Jossey-Bass, 2002.

Youngs, Bettie B. *Safeguarding Your Teenager from the Dragons of Life.* Deerfield Beach, Fla.: Health Communications, 1993.

Books for Teens (and Their Parents)

One effective way to help adolescents learn about health is by guiding them toward good books—not just reference books, but also memoirs and novels. It is a great idea for parents to read these books, too. Reading the same book gives you and your teen an enjoyable way to find common ground and initiate discussion.

- Use reference books to explain health issues, check out their advice, and identify questions to ask your doctor.
- Use memoirs to learn about other people's points of view, to spark recollections of your own teen years, and to encourage your adolescent to compare the writer's experience with that of your teen and his or her friends.
- Use novels to open discussions about the characters' personalities, challenges, and relationships with family, friends, and romantic partners. Talk about the choices the characters made, how they worked out, and what might have made things work out differently.

Books not only illuminate health issues your teen may be facing but also build knowledge and empathy for the experiences of others. It can be an eye-opener to read about an obese boy's difficulties in *One Fat Summer*, or an anorexic girl's fearful journey toward recovery in *Life-Size*, or how a girl's obsessive-compulsive disorder gets her into trouble in *Multiple Choice*. Books can take your adolescent into different cultures and into the mind of someone of the opposite sex. Reading about the problems (and problem solving) of others can show adolescents that they are not alone in sometimes feeling insecure, overwhelmed, sad, or confused. Through books adolescents can see how other people experience, express, and transcend life's challenges.

The following list only begins to hint at the great array of books that your adolescent (and you) can explore. You may also want to check out the American Library Association website, www.ala.org.parents. It lists recommended books, resources, and websites for parents, teens, and children.

GENERAL HEALTH REFERENCE BOOKS

Boston Women's Health Book Collective. *Our Bodies, Ourselves for the New Century*. New York: Simon & Schuster, 1998.

Fine, Judylaine. *A Book for Families to Share About Cancer*. New York: Lothrop, Lee & Shepard, 1984.

Gravelle, Karen, and Jennifer Gravelle. *The Period Book: Everything You Don't Want to Ask (But Need to Know)*. New York: Walker and Company, 1996.

Haffner, Debra. *Beyond the Big Talk: Every Parent's Guide to Raising Sexually*

Healthy Teens—from Middle School to High School and Beyond. New York: New-market Press, 2001.

Hipp, Earl. *Fighting Invisible Tigers: A Stress Management Guide for Teens.* Minneapolis: Free Spirit Publishing, 1985.

Madaras, Lynda. *The What's Happening to My Body? Book for Boys.* New York: Newmarket Press, 1988.

———. *The What's Happening to My Body? Book for Girls.* New York: Newmarket Press, 1988.

McCoy, Kathy, and Charles Wibbelsman. *The New Teenage Body Book.* Los Angeles: Body Press, 1987.

Metzl, Jordan D., with Carol Shookhoff. *The Young Athlete: A Sports Doctor's Complete Guide for Parents.* Boston: Little, Brown & Company, 2002.

Rosenberg, Ellen. *Growing Up Feeling Good.* Rev. ed. New York: Puffin Books, 1995.

Sirof, Harriet. *The Road Back.* New York: iUniverse.com, 2000. (How young people fight back after becoming injured.)

Slap, Gail, and Martha Jablow. *Teenage Health Care.* New York: Pocket Books, 1994.

Wilkinson, Beth. *Coping with the Dangers of Tattooing, Body Piercing, and Branding.* New York: Rosen Publishing Group, 1998.

NONFICTION BOOKS ABOUT THE ADOLESCENT EXPERIENCE

Carter-Scott, Cherie. *If High School Is a Game, Here's How to Break the Rules.* New York: Delacorte Press, 2001.

Fried, Scott M. *If I Grow Up: Talking with Teens about AIDS, Love, and Staying Alive.* New York: TALKAIDS, 1997.

Johnston, Andrea. *Girls Speak Out: Finding Your True Self.* New York: Scholastic, 1997.

Kirberger, Kim. *Teen Love: On Relationships.* Deerfield Beach, Fla.: Health Communications, 1999.

Weston, Carol. *All the Stuff Your Sister Never Told You.* New York: HarperPerennial, 1997.

COOKBOOKS

Bates, Dorothy R.; Bobbie Hinman; and Robert Oser. *Munchie Madness: Vegetarian Meals for Teens.* Summertown, Tenn.: Book Publishing Company, 2001.

Pierson, Stephanie. *Vegetables Rock: A Complete Guide for Teenage Vegetarians.* New York: Bantam Books, 1999.

Raab, Evelyn. *Clueless in the Kitchen: A Cookbook for Teens.* New York: Firefly Books, 1998.

———. *The Clueless Vegetarian: A Cookbook for the Aspiring Vegetarian.* New York: Firefly Books, 2000.

Winkler, Kathleen. *Vegetarianism and Teens: A Hot Issue.* Springfield, N.J.: Enslow Publishing, 2001.

POETRY

Glenn, Mel. *Class Dismissed: High School Poems.* New York: Clarion Books, 1986.

Harrison, David L. *Wild Country—Outdoor Poems for Young People.* Honesdale, Pa.: Wordsong/Boyd Mills Press, 1999.

Hearne, Betsy. *Love Lines: Poetry in Person.* New York: M. K. McElderry Books, 1987.

Mora, Pat. *My Own True Name: New and Selected Poems for Young Adults.* Houston: Piñata Books, 2000.

Watson, Esther P., and Mark Todd, eds. *The Pain Tree and other Teenage Angst-Ridden Poetry.* Boston: Houghton Mifflin, 2000.

MEMOIRS FOR ADOLESCENTS

Brimner, Larry Dane. *Being Different: Lambda Youths Speak Out.* New York: Franklin Watts, 1995. (About the teenage gay and lesbian experience.)

Burke, Chris, and Jo Beth McDaniel. *A Special Kind of Hero.* New York: Doubleday, 1991. (A boy with Down's syndrome becomes the star of a TV series and helps change America's image of the mentally handicapped.)

Cunneff, Tom. *Walk a Mile in My Shoes, the Casey Martin Story.* Nashville, Tenn.: Rutledge Hill Press, 1998. (Disabled at birth with a degenerative condition that makes walking difficult, the golfer sued the PGA tour for the right to ride a golf cart in tour competition.)

Domenick, Andie. *Needles: A Memoir of Growing Up with Diabetes.* New York: Scribner's, 1998. (The author and her sister take different paths in coping with the disease.)

Duffy, Karen. *Model Patient, My Life as an Incurable Wise-Ass.* New York: Harper-Collins, 2000. (A young model's tale of coping with sarcoidosis of the central nervous system.)

Edut, Ophira, ed. *Adios, Barbie: Young Women Write About Body Image and Identity.* Seattle: Seal Press, 1998. (Young women write about body image, self-esteem, and identity.)

Gordon, Jacquie. *Give Me One Wish.* New York: W. W. Norton, 1988. (Describes the author's relationship with her daughter, who is battling cystic fibrosis.)

Gravelli, Karen, and Bertram John. *Teenagers Face to Face with Cancer.* New York: Julian Messner, 1986. (Teenagers who have or had cancer talk about their experiences.)

Gutman, Bill. *Jim Eisenreich, Overcoming the Odds.* Austin, Tex.: Raintree Steck-Vaughn, 1996. (Story of a baseball player with Tourette's syndrome.)

Heppner, Cheryl. *Seeds of Disquiet.* Washington, D.C.: Gallaudet University Press,

1992. (After losing most of her hearing at age six from spinal meningitis, a young woman has two strokes, becomes profoundly deaf, and learns sign language.)

Hornbacher, Marya. *Wasted: A Memoir of Anorexia and Bulimia*. New York: Harper-Flamingo, 1998. (The author states: "I fell for the great American dream, female version . . . once I just lost a few pounds . . . I would become rich and famous and glamorous.")

Johnson, Nicole. *Living with Diabetes*. Washington, D.C.: Lifeline Press, 2001. (Miss America 1999 reveals how she has coped with diabetes and advocated for research to find a cure.)

Krementz, Jill. *How It Feels to Live with a Physical Disability*. New York: Simon & Schuster, 1992. (Stories of twelve children whose physical disabilities include blindness, dwarfism, paralysis, birth anomalies, spasticity, and cerebral palsy.)

Krumme, Cynthia. *Having Leukemia Isn't So Bad. Of Course It Wouldn't Be My First Choice*. Winchester, Mass.: Sargasso Enterprises, 1993. (The author describes her fight against this life-threatening illness.)

Laborit, Emmanuelle. *Cry of the Gull*. Washington, D.C.: Gallaudet University Press, 1998. (A deaf French girl pursues an acting career.)

Macht, Norman. *Roy Campanella, Baseball Star*. New York: Chelsea House, 1996. (Roy Campanella was one of the first black baseball players in the major leagues. After a car accident left him paralyzed from the shoulders down, he returned to the Brooklyn Dodgers to become a successful coach.)

———. *Jim Abbott: Major League Pitcher*. New York: Chelsea House, 1994. (Born without a hand, Jim Abbott went on to become a famous pitcher for the Yankees.)

Musgrave, Susan, ed. *Nerves Out Loud: Critical Moments in the Lives of Seven Teen Girls*. Toronto: Annick Press, 2001. (Seven writers describe events that changed their lives.)

Pendergrass, Teddy, and Patricia Romanowski. *Truly Blessed*. New York: G. P. Putnam's Sons, 1998. (At the age of thirty-one, at the height of his success as a singer, a car accident left him a quadriplegic, yet he made a successful comeback.)

Schrader, Steven. *Silent Alarm: On the Edge with a Deaf EMT*. Washington, D.C.: Gallaudet University Press, 1995. (The account of a firefighter and emergency medical technician who copes with a severe hearing loss.)

Shandler, Sara., ed. *Ophelia Speaks: Adolescent Girls Write About Their Search for Self*. New York: HarperPerennial, 1999.

Steele, Danielle. *His Bright Life*. New York: Delacorte Press, 1998. (Portrait of this best-selling author's son and his struggles with manic depression.)

Vizzini, Ned. *Teen Angst? NAA. . . .* Minneapolis: Free Spirit Publishing, 2000. (". . . taking my boring, scary, embarrassing high school moments and turning them into something people could read about.")

Wilensky, Amy. *Passing for Normal*. New York: Broadway Books, 1999. (A young woman struggles to come to terms with her irrational behavior.)

Zazove, Philip. *When the Phone Rings My Bed Shakes: Memoirs of a Deaf Doctor.* Washington, D.C.: Gallaudet University Press, 1993. (A deaf child grows up to become a respected family practitioner.)

NOVELS ABOUT ABUSE, DOMESTIC VIOLENCE, AND SEXUAL ASSAULT

Anderson, Laurie H. *Speak.* New York: Farrar Straus Giroux, 1999. (Melinda was raped at a party and finds herself unable to speak during her freshman year in high school.)

NOVELS ABOUT EATING DISORDERS

Frank, Lucy. *I Am an Artichoke.* New York: Holiday House, 1995. (A writer clashes with her anorexic daughter.)

Lipsyte, Robert. *One Fat Summer.* New York: HarperCollins Children's Books, 1977. (An obese boy manages to lose weight when he gets a summer job.)

Shute, Jenefer. *Life-Size.* Boston: Houghton Mifflin, 1992. (A young woman with anorexia gradually comes to understand her disease and accept help.)

NOVELS ABOUT COPING WITH CRISIS, MENTAL HEALTH, AND SUICIDE PREVENTION

Blume, Judy. *It's Not the End of the World.* New York: Macmillan Books for Young Readers, 1972. (An adolescent comes to terms with her parents' divorce.)

Foon, Dennis. *Double or Nothing.* Toronto: Annick Press, 2000. (A high school boy has a gambling problem and must cope with increasing debts.)

Greenberg, Joanne. *I Never Promised You a Rose Garden.* New York: New American Library, 1964. (A young girl battles mental illness.)

Hesser, Terry S. *Kissing Doorknobs.* New York: Bantam Doubleday Dell Books for Young Readers, 1998. (A vivid story of a girl with obsessive-compulsive disorder.)

Konigsburg, E. L. *Silent to the Bone.* New York: Atheneum Books for Young Readers, 2000. (A thirteen-year-old is wrongly accused of injuring his baby half sister and loses his power of speech.)

Sirof, Harriet. *Bring Back Yesterday.* iUniverse.com reprint. New York: Atheneum/ Simon & Schuster, 1996. (After her parents die in a plane crash, a teenage girl copes with crisis in both present-day New York and Elizabethan England.)

Tashjian, Janet. *Multiple Choice.* New York: Henry Holt, 1999. (Monica, a compulsive perfectionist, creates a dangerous game to help her control her behavior and comes close to causing a tragedy before she obtains the help she needs.)

NOVELS ABOUT CHRONIC HEALTH PROBLEMS

Anderson, Rachel. *Bus People.* New York: Henry Holt, 1992. (Stories about mentally handicapped teenagers.)

Baer, Judy. *Silent Thief.* Minneapolis: Bethany House, 1995. (A family must face a mother's multiple sclerosis.)

Betancourt, Jeanne. *My Name Is Brain Brian.* New York: Scholastic, 1993. (For Brian, who has dyslexia, writing his name as Brain is only one of the problems he has in school.)

Bloor, Edward. *Tangerine.* New York and San Diego: Harcourt Brace, 1997. (A visually impaired boy battles with his older brother when they move to an ominous Florida town.)

Blume, Judy. *Deenie.* New York: Bradbury Press, 1973. (Scoliosis puts a teen's modeling career on hold.)

Bowler, Margaret K. *Midget.* New York: McElderry Books, 1994. (A fifteen-year-old boy is called Midget by his seventeen-year-old brother because of his small stature and physical handicaps.)

Corcoran, Barbara. *May I Cross Your Golden River?* New York: Atheneum, 1975. (An eighteen-year-old boy is diagnosed with the fatal disease ALS, Lou Gehrig's disease.

Helfman, Elizabeth. *On Being Sarah.* Morton Grove, Ill.: Albert Whitman & Co., 1992. (Twelve-year-old Sarah, born with cerebral palsy, gets around in a wheelchair and uses a symbol board because she cannot speak.)

Hill, David. *See Ya, Simon.* New York: Dutton Children's Books, 1992. (Simon has muscular dystrophy.)

Hurwin, Davida W. *A Time for Dancing.* New York: Puffin Books, 1995. (A sixteen-year-old girl dancer is stricken with cancer.)

Janover, Caroline. *The Worst Speller in Junior High.* Minneapolis: Free Spirit Publishing, 1995. (A girl with dyslexia yearns for romance and copes with a learning disability.)

Jordan, Sheryl. *Raging Quiet.* New York: Simon & Schuster, 1999. (In this historical novel a young woman invents a way to communicate with a deaf boy.)

Keith, Lois. *A Different Life.* London: Livewire Books/Women's Press, 1997. (A fifteen-year-old becomes disabled after a swim in the ocean, and fights to be able to continue her education.)

McElfresh, Lynn. *Can You Feel the Thunder?* New York: Atheneum Books for Young Readers, 1999. (A thirteen-year-old boy struggles with his feelings about his deaf and blind sister.)

Philbrick, W. R. *Freak the Mighty.* New York: Blue Sky Press, 1993. (A learning-disabled boy and a brilliant boy with a birth defect team up in the eighth grade.)

Rubin, Susan G. *Emily in Love.* San Diego, Calif.: Harcourt Brace, 1997. (A developmentally disabled fourteen-year-old enters a "regular" high school and finds her first romance.)

Scott, Virginia M. *Finding Abby.* Hillsboro, Oreg.: Butte Publications, 2000. (Many challenges confront a teenager with diminishing hearing.)

Shreve, Susan. *The Gift of the Girl Who Couldn't Hear*. New York: Tambourine Books, 1991. ("I've thought what it must be like not to hear music, or the sound of your mother's voice or your own.")

Strachan, Ian. *Flawed Glass*. Boston: Little, Brown, 1989. (A relationship with a boy changes the life of an isolated and disabled teenage girl.)

NOVELS ABOUT ACCIDENTS AND INJURIES

Calvert, Patricia. *Picking Up the Pieces*. New York: Scribners, 1993. (A young woman must overcome physical and emotional trauma when she suffers a spinal cord injury.)

DeLaCroix, Alice. *Mattie's Whisper*. Honesdale, Pa.: Caroline House, 1992. (After an automobile accident, a girl whose skill in riding horses won her many awards must learn to walk with crutches.)

Feuer, Elizabeth. *Paper Doll*. New York: Farrar Straus Giroux, 1990. (After an accident leaves his daughter an amputee, a father encourages her to play the violin.)

Orr, Wendy. *Peeling the Onion*. New York: Holiday House, 1996. (A girl faces the uneven road of recovery after a terrible accident.)

Sirof, Harriet. *Because She's My Friend*. iUniverse.com reprint. New York: Atheneum, 1993. (Two very different girls become friends when one is seriously injured in an accident and is cared for in the hospital where the other volunteers.)

Slate, Joseph. *Crossing the Trestle*. New York: Marshall Cavendish, 1999. (After a fourteen-year-old girl loses her eye in a car accident, her relationships with family and friends change.)

ANTHOLOGY

Rochman, Hazel, and Darlene Z. McCampbell, eds. *Leaving Home: 15 Distinguished Authors Explore Personal Journeys*. New York: HarperCollins, 1997.

Resources

NUTRITION

American Dietetic Association's Nationwide Nutrition Network—Resource for easy-to-understand nutrition information.
   www.eatright.org

American School Food Service Association—Resource for research on the newest legislation and regulations; provided by child nutrition professionals covering a wide range of information.
   700 S. Washington Street, Suite 300, Alexandria, VA 22314, 703-739-3900
   www.asfsa.org

Child Nutrition Programs, the U.S. Department of Agriculture Food, Nutrition, and Consumer Services—Provides food assistance and nutrition education for consumers.
   www.usda.gov/fcs/cnp

Dietary Guidelines for Americans—Provides a joint publication of the Departments of Health and Human Services and Agriculture.
   Available by phone at 1-888-878-3256.
   Available on-line at www.health.gov/dietaryguidelines.

Dole Company's Nutrition and Health Program—Provides nutrition education to promote consumption of fruits and vegetables.
   www.dole5aday.com

5-A-Day for Better Health—Provides programming to educate consumers about the need to eat more fruits and vegetables.
   Eat 5 A Day for Better Health, 5301 Limestone Road, Suite 101, Wilmington, DE 19808-1249, 309-235-ADAY
   www.5aday.com

Fresh Starts—Provides resources that can help students maintain proper nutrition, student activities, and a great deal of information about vitamins.
   www.freshstarts.com

National Center for Nutrition and Dietetics, Consumer Nutrition Hotline—Part of the American Dietetic Association. Provides links to nutrition resources, a nutrition fact sheet, healthy lifestyle tips, and a food and nutrition guide.
   1-800-366-1655
   www.eatright.org

National Dairy Council—Provides current scientific research supporting the health benefits of dairy foods.

> 10255 West Higgins Road, Suite 900, Rosemont, IL 60018
>
> www.nationaldairycouncil.org

Tufts University Nutrition Navigator—A rating and review guide for on-line nutrition information.

> http://navigator.tufts.edu/about

U.S. Department of Agriculture: Nutrition Explorations, Guide to Nutrition and Health Information on Federal Government Web Sites—Makes available "Teenagers' Guide for Better Living."

> www.usda.gov

EXERCISE

American Fitness Alliance—Provides information teachers can use in implementing health-related physical education programs and information for parents about their children's exercise programs.

> www.americanfitness.net

Operation Fit Kids—Provides information about improving the health and fitness of American youth.

> www.operationfitkids.org

PECentral—Exercise site for health and physical education teachers, parents, and students. Provides information about developmentally appropriate physical education programs for children and youth.

> www.pecentral.org

PELinks4U—Provides health, fitness, and sports information for students of all ages.

> www.pelinks4u.org

President's Council on Physical Fitness and Sports—Encourages Americans of all ages to become physically active and participate in sports.

> PCPFS, 200 Independence Avenue SW, Room 738H, Washington, D.C., 20201-0004, 206-690-9000
>
> www.fitness.gov

Sports Media—Platform where coaches, teachers, and students exchange ideas about physical education and sports.

> www.sports-media.org

HEALTH CARE

American Academy of Dermatology—Provides access to a wide variety of information about dermatology.
> 884-462-DERM
> www.aad.org

American Academy of Pediatrics—Provides general information for parents of children from birth through age twenty-one.
> Department of Federal Affairs, 601 13th Street NW, Suite 400N, Washington, D.C. 20005, 202-347-8600
> www.aap.org

American Cancer Society—Provides information on cancer types, and information for patients, families, and friends on coping with cancer and its effects.
> 1-800-227-2345
> www.cancer.org

American Dental Association—Information about dental hygiene and oral health. Free brochures about dental care are available.
> www.ada.org

American Diabetes Association—Provides basic information and other services to people with diabetes and their families; community resources, information about Types 1 and 2 diabetes, research information, and information about advocacy efforts.
> www.diabetes.org

American Medical Association Adolescent Health Resources—The American Medical Association has developed materials on adolescent health related issues to be provided to physicians working with adolescents. These may be viewed and printed.
> American Medical Association, 515 N. State Street, Chicago, IL 60610, 312-464-5000
> www.ama-assn.org/ama/pub/category/1981/

American Medical Women's Association—Provides information about a variety of different medical issues of interest to women.
> 801 N. Fairfax Street, Suite 400, Alexandria, VA 22314, 703-549-3864
> www.amwa-doc.org

American Podiatric Medical Association—Provides foot health information and foot facts, with the aim of increasing awareness of the importance of foot health among the general public and other health professionals.
> 1-800-FOOT-CARE, 1-800-366-8227
> www.apma.org

Arthritis Foundation—The American Juvenile Arthritis Organization focuses on the needs of children, teens, and adults. This site provides fact sheets, information about contacting local support groups, and the opportunity to ask questions via E-mail.
   www.arthritis.org

Asian and Pacific Islander American Health Forum—An advocacy organization that promotes policy, programs, and research efforts for the improvement of the health status of Asian American and Pacific Islander communities.
   942 Market Street, Suite 200, San Francisco, CA 94102, 415-954-9988
   www.apiahf.org

Band-Aides and Blackboards When Chronic Illness . . . Or Some Other Medical Problem Goes to School—A site offering content on chronic illness for parents, teens, and children about health and illness, medical conditions, physical differences, and serious medical problems. Many stories about teens with serious chronic medical problems are presented.
   www.faculty.fairfield.edu/fleitas/sitemap.html

Bright Futures—From the Maternal and Child Health Bureau, this organization provides guidelines for the health care of infants, children, and adolescents.
   www.brightfutures.org/index

Children's Health Links—A project of Harvard University's Center for Children's Health. It provides a list of related web links to advocacy groups, policy organizations, research and statistics sites, and other child health organizations.
   www.hsph.harvard.edu/children/links/newslinks5

Family Doctor—Provides health information for the entire family from the American Academy of Family Physicians, the national association of physicians who specialize in family practice.
   www.familydoctor.org

Family Voices—A national organization that addresses the common problems of children with special health needs.
   3411 Candelaria NE, Suite M, Albuquerque, NM 87107, 1-888-835-5669
   www.familyvoices.org

Health Finder—A website developed by the U.S. Department of Health and Human Services. Provides health information "from A to Z," medical dictionaries, an encyclopedia, journals, information on health care, and a directory of other health information sites.
   www.healthfinder.gov

Joslin Diabetes Center—This center is dedicated solely to diabetes treatment, research, and cure. It provides free information packets, free on-line classes on the treatment of diabetes, and access to professionals who will answer questions about diabetes.

www.joslin.harvard.edu

Just for Teens, American Diabetes Association—Provides diabetic teens with information about how to work with their health care team, confidentiality, and telling friends about their disease.

www.diabetes.org/ada/c50g.asp

Juvenile Diabetes Research Foundation International—Its focus is entirely on research. It provides information on clinical trials, research, links, and answers to questions about juvenile diabetes.

120 Wall Street, NY 10005-4001, 1-800-533-CURE

www.jdrf.org

Mayo Clinic—Provides information on diseases and conditions, drugs, first aid and self-care, and a section called "Answers from Mayo Experts."

200 First Street SW, Rochester, MN 55905

www.mayoclinic.com

Medem—The medical library site of the American College of Obstetrics and Gynecology. Provides information about women's health derived from leading medical societies.

www.medem.com

MedicAlert—Source for purchasing the MedicAlert emblem, which may be worn on a bracelet or neck chain, and is used for providing information in a medical emergency.

1-888-633-4298

www.medicalert.org

Medscape Pediatrics—A collection of the latest medical news and information on a wide range of conditions and health issues.

www.medscape.com

National Eye Institute—Through its National Eye Health Education Program (NEHEP), this organization conducts large-scale public and professional education programs. Obtain information here about its programs and free materials.

2020 Vision Place, Bethesda, MD 20892-3655, 301-496-5248

www.nei.nih.gov

National Health Information Center—Search the database for answers to any health-related issues.

1-800-336-4797

www.health.gov/nhic

National Heart, Lung, and Blood Institute Information Center—Provides information on prevention and treatment of heart, lung, and blood diseases. Free publications are available.

> NHLBI Health Information Center, Attention Web Site, P.O. Box 30105, Bethesda, MD 20824-0105
> www.nhlbi.nih.gov/health/infoctr

National Institute for Diabetes, Digestive, and Kidney Disease—Provides health information on diabetes; kidneys; nutrition; urologic problems; hematologic, endocrine, and metabolic disorders; clinical trials; and other information.

> Office of Community and Public Liaison, NIDDK, NIH Building 31, Room 9A04, Center Drive MSC 2560, Bethesda, MD 20892-2560
> www.niddk.nih.gov

National Institutes of Health—Provides publications and fact sheets, information on clinical trials, A–Z topic index, MEDLINEplus, and other resources.

> 6001 Executive Boulevard, Bethesda, MD 20892-9561
> www.nih.gov

National Oral Health Information Clearinghouse—Provides information about special care in oral health, and information on an approach to oral health management designed to meet the needs of people with a variety of medical conditions or limitations that require more than routine delivery of oral care.

> 1 NOHIC Way, Bethesda, MD 20892-3500, 301-402-7364
> www.nidr.nih.gov

National Organization for Rare Disorders—Provides a rare disease database, information about rare diseases, support groups, and information about new drugs.

> P.O. Box 8923, New Fairfield, CT 06812-8923
> www.rarediseases.org

National Women's Health Network—Advocates for improved women's health policies in legislative, research, and regulatory areas. Acts as a clearinghouse for information on women's health.

> 514 10th Street NW, Suite 400, Washington, D.C. 20004, 202-347-1140
> www.womenshealthnetwork.org

Ortho Dermatological Company—Website for teens that offers personal care information and includes an "Ask the Dermatologist" section.

> www.pimpleportal.com

Society for Adolescent Medicine—Promotes the development and dissemination of scientific knowledge unique to the health needs of adolescents.

> 1916 NW Copper Oaks Circle, Blue Sprints, MO 64015, 816-224-8010
> www.adolescenthealth.org

Testicular Cancer Resource Center—Information about testicular self-exam, cancer, and treatment.

>   http://tcrc.acor.org

SEXUALITY

Advocates for Youth—Program built around the "3 R's—Rights, Respect, Responsibility." Provides information to help organizations assist youth in making responsible decisions about their sexual and reproductive health.

>   www.advocatesforyouth.org

American College of Obstetricians and Gynecologists—Provides information on women's issues, government affairs, and the latest news releases on women's health.

>   409 12th Street SW, P.O. Box 96920, Washington, D.C., 20090-6920
>   www.acog.org

American Social Health Association—Its stated mission: to stop sexually transmitted diseases and their consequences to individuals, families, and the community. Provides an interactive website for teens, education, and information.

>   www.ashastd.org

Chromosome Deletion Outreach—An international support group for families with chromosome deletions, additions, inversions, translocations, and rings.

>   P.O. Box 724, Boca Raton, FL 33429-0724, 1-888-CDO-6880
>   www.chromodisorder.org/index

Dignity/USA—Organization of gay, lesbian, bisexual, and transgendered Catholics, and their families and friends. Works to promote educational outreach, social reform, and the advocacy of feminist issues.

>   1500 Massachusetts Avenue NW, Suite 11, Washington, D.C. 20005,
>   202-861-0017
>   www.dignityusa.org

Gay and Lesbian Medical Association—An organization of lesbian, gay, bisexual, and transgendered physicians, medical students, and supporters. Its stated purpose: to combat homophobia in the health community.

>   459 Fulton Street, Suite 107, San Francisco, CA 94102
>   www.glma.org

Gay, Lesbian and Straight Education Network—Offers a resource center and information about making schools safe for gays, lesbians, bisexual, and transgendered people.

>   www.glsen.org

If Plan A Fails, Go to Plan B—Website intended to give women, men, and health care providers more information about levonorgestrel, a new contraceptive method.
    www.gotoplanb.com

International Gay and Lesbian Human Rights Commission—The commission states that it addresses the need to protect the human rights of all people and communities subject to discrimination or abuse on the basis of sexual orientation, gender identity, or HIV status.
    1360 Mission Street, Suite 200, San Francisco, CA 94103, 415-255-8680
    www.iglhrc.org

Making Schools Safe—This ACLU site supports lesbian, gay, bisexual, transgendered, and questioning teens who are being harassed at school because of their sexuality.
    125 Broad Street, 18th floor, New York, NY 10004, 212-549-2627
    www.aclu.org/safeschools

National Campaign to Prevent Teen Pregnancy—Website for teens on how to avoid pregnancy.
    1776 Massachusetts Avenue, #200, Washington, D.C. 20036, 202-478-8500
    www.teenpregnancy.org/teen

National Women's Health Information Center—Features women's health information from the Office on Women's Health. Phone for free health information.
    The Office on Women's Health, Department of Health and Human Services,
    1-800-994-WOMAN
    www.4women.gov

Planned Parenthood Federation of America—A site for teens in which are discussed teens' changing bodies and the topics of choosing whether or not to have sex, how to protect yourself from sexually transmitted diseases, and the prevention of pregnancy.
    Call 1-800-230-PLAN to find the nearest Planned Parenthood Center.
    www.teenwire.com

Sexuality Information and Education Council of the United States (SIECUS)—Develops, collects, and disseminates information on sex, advocating the right of the individual to make responsible sexual choices.
    130 West 42nd Street, Suite 350, New York, NY 10036-7802, 212-819-9770
    www.siecus.org

Surgeon General's Call to Action to Promote Sexual Health and Responsible Sexual Behavior—This site lists strategies that focus on increasing awareness, implementing interventions, and expanding the research base related to sexual matters.
    www.bchumanservices.net/news/satcher1

Unique—A rare chromosome disorder support group. Source of information, support, and self-help for families of children with any rare chromosome disorders.

  www.rarechromo.org

SEXUALLY TRANSMITTED DISEASES, HIV/AIDS

AIDS Alliance for Children, Youth, and Families—Trains youth and HIV prevention leaders through the Youth Corps Leadership Project; provides technical assistance to community-based organizations; serves as a national policy forum to exchange ideas on HIV prevention for youth.

  1600 K Street NW, Suite 300, Washington, D.C. 20006, 202-785-3564
  www.aids-alliance.org

Balm in Gilead—Works through black churches to support those infected with, and affected by, HIV/AIDS; works to stop the spread of HIV in the African American community.

  130 West 42nd Street, Suite 450, New York, NY 10036, 212-730-7381
  www.balmingilead.org

Centers for Disease Control and Prevention—The national center for reference, referral, and distribution of information about STDs and HIV/AIDS.

  P.O. Box 6003, Rockville, MD 20849-6003
  www.cdcnpin.org

Children's AIDS Fund—Provides care, services, resources, referrals, and education.

  P.O. Box 16433, Washington, D.C. 20041, 703-433-1560
  www.childrensaidsfund.org

Gay Men's Health Crisis—Provides AIDS service; includes education about HIV prevention and treatment; and serves men, women, and children with HIV and AIDS.

  Tisch Building, 119 West 24th Street, New York, NY 10011, 1-800-AIDS-NYC
  www.gmhc.org

HIV/AIDS and Adolescents—Provides materials from the Centers for Disease Control and Prevention, information on HIV/AIDS for young people, journals, newsletters, and web resources.

  http://hivpositive.com/f-Resources/f-17-NewslettersInfo/f-teenagers/
  Organizations

Metro TeenAIDS (Youth HIV/AIDS Prevention Service Organization)—Focuses its efforts on the prevention, education, and treatment needs of youth. Provides services to advance the overall health of at-risk and HIV-positive adolescents.

  651 Pennsylvania Avenue SE, Washington, D.C. 20003, 202-543-9355
  www.metroteenAIDS.org

Mothers' Voices—Mobilizes parents and other concerned individuals as educators and advocates for HIV prevention, expanded research, and better medical treatments.
165 West 46th Street, Suite 701, New York, NY 10036, 212-730-2777
www.mvoices.org

National Alliance for Hispanic Health—Provides HIV/AIDS prevention education to large populations of high-risk Hispanic youth using theater.
1501 16th Street NW, Washington, D.C. 20036, 202-387-5000
www.hispanichealth.org

National Hemophilia Foundation—Provides information on hemophilia and HIV/AIDS.
116 West 32nd Street, 11th Floor, New York, NY 10001, 1-800-42-HANDI
www.hemophilia.org

National Latina Health Network—Addresses the disease prevention needs of youth sixteen to twenty-four years of age. Its stated mission is to enhance the quality of life of Latinas and their families.
1680 Wisconsin Avenue, 2nd Floor, Washington, D.C. 20007, 202-965-9633

National Native American AIDS Prevention Center—Works to establish collaborative agreements with local service providers that ensure access to services by HIV-infected Native Americans.
436 14th Street, Suite 1020, Oakland, CA 94612, 510-444-2051
www.nnaapc.org

Project Inform—Provides information on the diagnosis and treatment of HIV; advocates for strengthened regulatory, research, and funding policies.
205 13th Street, Suite 2001, San Francisco, CA 94103, 415-558-8660
www.projectinform.org

Teen Health—Provides links to many websites covering a wide spectrum of health education for teens and youth for prevention of HIV and other sexually transmitted diseases.
www.mihivnews.com/teenweb

SUBSTANCE ABUSE

Alateen—Assistance for families and friends of alcoholics in recovering from the effects of living with the problem drinking of a relative or friend.
Al-Anon Family Group Headquarters., Inc., 1600 Corporate Landing Parkway, Virginia Beach, VA 23454-5617, 1-888-4AL-ANON
www.al-anon-alateen.org

Alcoholics Anonymous—Support for those combating the disease of alcoholism.
475 Riverside Drive., 11th Floor, New York, NY 10115, NY, 212-870-3400
www.alcoholics-anonymous.org

American Council on Alcoholism—Provides publicity dedicated to educating the public about the adverse effects of alcohol, alcoholism, and alcohol abuse.
1-800-527-5344
www.aca-usa.org

American Lung Association—Its mission is to fight lung disease and promote lung health. Provides in-school programs.
1740 Broadway, New York, NY 10019, 212-315-8700
www.lungusa.org

Centers for Disease Control and Prevention—Provides a catalog of available publications, research, and data, and reports on tobacco information and prevention tips for teens.
www.cdc.gov/tobacco

Center for Substance Abuse Treatment—Provides assistance in finding the right drug abuse or alcohol abuse treatment program.
U.S. Department of Health and Human Services, 1-800-662-HELP
http://findtreatment.samhsa.gov

Children of Substance Abusers Initiative—The National Youth Anti-Drug Media Campaign offers help to teens and preteens who live with a chemically dependent parent; provides life-coping skills and preventive resources.
www.mediacampaign.org/newsroom/factsheets/children.html

Club Drugs—A service of the National Institute on Drug Abuse. Provides information on club drugs.
www.clubdrugs.org

Dance Safe—Promotes health and safety within the rave and nightclub communities.
www.dancesafe.org

Foundation for a Smokefree America—Provides antismoking live assembly programs for middle and high schools.
The Foundation for a Smokefree America, P.O. Box 492028, Los Angeles, CA 90049-8028
www.tobaccofree.org/children

Freevibe—Statistics on teen drug and alcohol abuse. Teens can post messages, read stories about teens with drug problems, and share their own stories.
www.freevibe.com

Join Together Online—Resource for communities working to reduce substance abuse and gun violence. Offers information on current issues, ways to make positive changes in the community, and support services for families and friends.
>441 Stuart Street, 7th Floor, Boston, MA 02116, 617-437-1500
>www.jointogether.org

MADD, Mothers Against Drunk Driving—Promotes legislation relating to alcohol and traffic safety laws. Coordinates efforts to prevent drunk driving in communities across the nation.
>1-800-GET-MADD
>www.madd.org

Narcotics Anonymous—Provides a forum for "recovery from the disease of addiction."
>P.O. Box 9999, Van Nuys, CA 91409 USA, 818-773-9999
>www.na.org

National Asian-Pacific American Families Against Substance Abuse—Organization devoted to addressing alcohol, tobacco, and other drug issues of the Asian and Pacific Islander populations.
>340 East 2nd Street., Suite 409, Los Angeles, CA 90012, 213-625-5975
>www.napafasa.org

National Clearinghouse for Alcohol and Drug Information—A service of the Substance Abuse and Mental Health Administration. Clearinghouse for alcohol and drug information.
>P.O. Box 2345, Rockville, MD 20847-2345, 1-800-729-6686
>www.health.org

National Council on Alcoholism and Drug Dependence—Information on substance abuse. Call to get resources and referrals to local support groups.
>20 Exchange Place, Suite 2902, New York, NY 10005, 1-800-NCA-CALL
>www.ncadd.org

National Institute on Drug Abuse—Provides information on drugs of abuse, and information for researchers and health programmers.
>National Institute of Health, 6001 Executive Boulevard, #5213, Bethesda, MD 20892-9561, 1-800-662-HELP
>www.drugabuse.gov

Nicotine Anonymous—Support for those trying to gain freedom from nicotine.
>419 Main Street, PMB #370, Huntington Beach, CA 92648, 415-750-0328
>www.nicotine-anonymous.org

No Tobacco.org—Website for teens that focuses on motivating them to quit or remain tobacco free.

> Foundation for a Smokefree America, P.O. Box 492028, Los Angeles,
> CA 90049-8028
> www.notobacco.org

Parents Resource Institute for Drug Education (PRIDE)—Provides programming devoted to reaching parents and youth at home, school, and work.

> 1-800-279-6361
> www.prideusa.org

Quitnet.org—An on-line program providing support to smokers trying to quit, and a guide to smoking cessation programs throughout the United States.

> www.quitnet.org

SADD, Students Against Driving Drunk (also, Students Against Destructive Decisions)—School-based organization dedicated to addressing the issues of underage drinking, impaired driving, and drug use.

> SADD, Inc., P.O. Box 800, Marlborough, MA 01752, Fax 508-481-5759
> www.saddonline.com

STAT, Stop Teenage Addiction to Tobacco—Describes strategies for building successful prevention programs.

> www.open.org/~westcapt/bp96.htm

Substance Abuse Facility Locator—Searchable directory of drug and alcohol treatment programs, shows the locations around the country that treat alcoholism, alcohol abuse, and drug abuse problems.

> Substance Abuse & Mental Health Services Administration, U.S. Department of
> Health and Human Services
> http://findtreatment.samhsa.gov

Tips 4 Youth—Provides resources for adolescents and young adults about smoking and tobacco. Also provides order forms for free posters and publications.

> www.cdc.gov.tobacco/tips4youth

EATING DISORDERS

About-Face—Site designed to combat negative and distorted images of women. Provides information on eating disorders, body image, and other issues. Provides many resources for study.

> P.O. Box 77665, San Francisco, CA 94107, 415-436-0212
> www.about-face.org

Academy of Eating Disorders—This site focuses on anorexia nervosa, bulimia nervosa, binge eating disorder, and related disorders, and includes downloadable newsletters, information, and links to other eating disorder sites.

    6728 Old McLean Village Drive, McLean, VA 22101, 703-556-9222

    www.aedweb.org

Anorexia Nervosa and Related Eating Disorders, Inc.—Provides detailed consumer information about anorexia nervosa, bulimia nervosa, binge eating disorder, compulsive exercising, and other less-well-known food and weight disorders.

    www.anred.com

Eating Disorder Referral and Information Center—Provides a wide range of general information about the treatment and prevention of eating disorders, and referrals to practitioners, treatment facilities, and support groups.

    www.edreferral.com

Eating Disorders Awareness and Prevention, Inc.—A national organization promoting the awareness and prevention of eating disorders by encouraging positive self-esteem and size acceptance. The site describes programs and activities, and gives information about prevention, diagnosis, and treatment; lists publications.

    603 Stewart Street, Suite 803, Seattle, WA 98101, 1-800-931-2237

    www.edap.org

National Association of Anorexia Nervosa and Associated Disorders—Free hot line counseling; operates network of support groups for sufferers and their families, and offers referrals to health care professionals.

    ANAD, P.O. Box 7, Highland Park, IL 60035; hot line: 847-831-3438

    www.anad.org

National Eating Disorders Association—Provides prevention efforts, education, referral, support services, advocacy, training, and research.

    603 Stewart Street, Suite 803, Seattle, WA 98101, 1-800-931-2237

    www.edap.org

Weight Control Information Network—Provides health professionals and consumers with information on obesity, weight control, and nutrition.

    1 WIN Way, Bethesda, MD 20892-3665, 1-877-946-4627

    www.niddk.nih.gov/health/nutrit/nutrit.htm

CRISIS COUNSELING AND MENTAL HEALTH

American Academy of Child and Adolescent Psychiatry—Provides general information for parents and families on development, behavioral, emotional, and mental disorders affecting children and adolescents.
> 3615 Wisconsin Avenue NW, Washington, D.C. 20016-3007, 202-996-7300
> www.aacap.org

American Psychiatric Association—This site is primarily for mental health professionals, but it offers some general information and several links on mental health and public policy.
> 1400 K Street NW, Washington, D.C. 20005, 1-888-357-7924
> www.psych.org

American Psychological Association—Provides general information for patients and families on mental health, when and how to seek help.
> 750 First Street NE, Washington, D.C. 20002-4242, 1-800-374-2721
> www.helping.apa.org

Children and Adults with Attention Deficit–Hyperactivity Disorder—Activities include education, advocacy, and support. Obtain fact sheets on diagnosis and treatment of AD/HD, legal rights, parenting, and education.
> 8181 Professional Place, Suite 201, Landover, MD 20785, 1-800-233-4050
> www.chadd.org

Mental Health: A Report of the Surgeon General—The first report on mental illness by the surgeon general states: "Mental Illness is a critical public health problem that must be addressed by the nation." The report contains a separate section on children.
> For a copy of the report, write to: Mental Health, Pueblo, CO 81009,
> or call 1-800-789-2647.
> Access the report on-line at www.surgeongeneral.gov.

National Alliance for the Mentally Ill—Information for families of the mentally ill on support, education, advocacy, and research.
> Colonial Place Three, 2107 Wilson Boulevard, Suite 300, Arlington, VA 22201,
> 703-524-7600
> www.nami.org

National Institute of Mental Health—General information on mental health, including current research.
> 6001 Executive Boulevard, Room 8184, Bethesda, MD 20892-9663,
> 301-443-4513
> www.nimh.nih.gov

National Mental Health Association—General information on mental health for patients and families.

    1021 Prince Street, Alexandria, VA 22314-2971, 1-800-969-NMHA

    www.nmha.org

Toughlove—Provides ongoing and active support to families, empowering parents and helping young people to take responsibility for their actions.

    P.O. Box 1069, Doylestown, PA 18901, 215-348-7090

    www.toughlove.com

CHRONIC HEALTH PROBLEMS AND DISABILITIES

Commission of the Mental and Physical Disability Law—Site of the American Bar Association. Serves people who have been discriminated against because of a disability.

    www.abanet.org

Disability Rights Education and Defense Fund—National law and policy center that advocates for the rights of people with disabilities through litigation, technical assistance, and training of attorneys, advocates, persons with disabilities, and parents of children with disabilities.

    2212 6th Street, Berkeley, CA 94710, 510-644-2555

    www.dredf.org

Exceptional Parent *Magazine*—Provides information, support, and outreach for parents of children with disabilities or special care needs and the professionals who work with them.

    65 East Route 4, River Edge, NJ 07661, 201-489-4111

    www.eparent.com

Parent to Parent—Provides support and information to parents of children with special needs. This is a New York site, but it provides links to a national directory of Parent to Parent sites.

    www.parenttoparentnys.org

ADDITIONAL RESOURCES

American Association of University Women—Use this site as a guide to research that the studies organization has completed about the problems girls face in school. Included are the following: "Shortchanging Girls: Shortchanging America," "Hostile Hallways," "Beyond the Gender Wars," and many others.

    www.aauw.org/2000/research

Congress of National Black Churches—Addresses a variety of health issues that cause premature death and illness in the black community: HIV/AIDS, diabetes, substance abuse, etc.

www.cnbc.org

Henry J. Kaiser Family Foundation—Provides tips for parents about talking to their children about drugs, alcohol, AIDS, sex, and other issues.

Call 1-800-CHILD-44 to get the book *Talking with Kids About Tough Issues*.
www.talkingwithkids.org

National Campaign Against Youth Violence—Offers tips for preventing violence, and information about starting antiviolence programs in your community.

2115 Wisconsin Avenue NW, 6th Floor, Washington, D.C. 20007, 202-687-1660
www.ncayv.org

National Network for Youth—Represents many community-based youth services. It is engaged in public education efforts promoting youth-adult partnerships.

1319 F Street NW, Suite 401, Washington, D.C. 20004, 202-783-7949
www.NN4Youth.org

Nemours Foundation Center for Children's Health Media—Has separate areas for kids, teens, and parents, with hundreds of articles for teens on a variety of subjects.

www.kidshealth.org

Parent Dex—Sponsored by the National Children's Coalition and Streetcats Foundation. This site provides links to a wide range of subjects for and about children, including health, disabilities, behavioral risk issues, education, juvenile justice, runaways, and national hot lines.

www.child.net/childco

Hot Lines and Related Websites

Use these numbers to get help for yourself, your adolescent, a friend, or another loved one.

ABUSE, DOMESTIC VIOLENCE, SEXUAL ASSAULT

Child Abuse Hotline—Receives calls from children in the midst of abuse, troubled parents, individuals concerned that abuse is occurring, and others requesting child abuse information.

> 1-800-540-4000
>
> www.thechildabusehotline.com

Childhelp USA—Provides assistance if child abuse is suspected or immediate help is required.

> 1-800-422-4453
>
> www.childhelpusa.org

National Child Abuse Hotline—Provides information for reporting child abuse to appropriate agencies for immediate action.

> 1-800-422-4453
>
> www.childhelpusa.org

National Domestic Violence Hotline—Provides crisis intervention, information about domestic violence, and referrals to local service providers.

> 1-800-799-SAFE
>
> www.ndvh.org

National Sexual Assault Hotline—Counseling for victims of rape and assault, advice for friends and families.

> 1-800-656-HOPE
>
> www.rainn.org

Rape, Abuse & Incest National Network—Call if you or your adolescent has been sexually assaulted, or for information on how to reduce the risk of sexual assault.

> 1-800-656-HOPE
>
> www.rainn.org

CRISIS COUNSELING, MENTAL HEALTH, SUICIDE PREVENTION, SUBSTANCE ABUSE

Al-Anon/Al-Ateen—Call for assistance with the problem drinking of a relative or friend. Referrals provided throughout the country.
  1-800-356-9996
  www.al-anon-alateen.org

American Foundation for Suicide Prevention—If you or someone you know is contemplating suicide, use this hot line. Immediate counseling and referral to local assistance.
  1-800-SUICIDE

Covenant House Nineline/Crisis Intervention Center—Volunteers available to speak with adolescents and their parents about all types of crises. Referrals provided if requested.
  1-800-999-9999
  www.covenanthouse.org

Girls and Boys Town—Adolescents and parents can call with any problem.
  1-800-448-3000

Kids Peace—Crisis Intervention. Counseling provided by clinicians.
  1-800-8KID-123
  www.kidspeace.org

National Alliance for the Mentally Ill—Provides information on family support and self-help groups.
  1-800-950-6264

National Depressive and Manic-Depressive Association (NDMDA)—Provides information about local patient and support groups.
  1-800-826-3632

National Institute of Mental Health (NIMH)—Provides information on depression and other mental health issues.
  1-800-421-4211

National Mental Health Association—Provides information about depression and referrals to local screening sites.
  1-800-969-6642

National Suicide Hotline—Provides directive counseling and referrals to local numbers, and special hot lines for teens, parents, and counselors.
  1-800-784-2433

Yellow Ribbon Project—Provides counseling and referrals for suicide prevention.
   303-429-3330
   www.yellowribbon.org

Youth Crisis Hotline—For youth under eighteen in crisis situations, if a runaway, or if struggling with drugs, physical abuse, rape, suicide, pregnancy, or any other crisis. Provides options and referral services.
   P.O. Box 178408, San Diego, CA 92177-7480, 1-800-448-4663
   www.icfs.org/bluebook/bb000658

EATING DISORDERS

Bulimia/Anorexia Self-Help Hotline—Provides resources on how to deal with these life-threatening eating disorders.
   1-800-227-4785

Eating Disorder Awareness and Prevention (EDAP)—Provides counseling and resources for those suffering from eating disorders.
   1-800-931-2237
   www.edap.org

National Association of Anorexia Nervosa and Associated Disorders—Counseling services and referrals to support groups for people with eating disorders and their families.
   847-831-3438
   www.anad.org

RUNAWAYS, PROSTITUTION

Children of the Night—Provides assistance for runaway youth ages eleven to seventeen who have been forced into prostitution.
   1-800-551-1300
   www.childrenofthenight.org

HIPS Hotline—For adolescent prostitutes. Provides counseling and referrals.
   1-800-676-4477

National Runaway Switchboard—An adolescent crisis line for teens thinking about running away; also provides services for those who have run away, counseling for parents, and information for teachers.
   1-800-621-4000
   www.nrcrisisline.org

SEXUALITY

National Gay and Lesbian Hotline—Referrals, peer counseling, and information for people who are gay, lesbian, bisexual, or transgender.
   1-888-843-4564
   www.ginh.org

Teen Pregnancy Hotline—Gives referrals to places of prenatal and related care, and local referrals for testing. Also offers, through an Adolescent Pregnancy Providers Program outreach, referrals to health, vocational, educational, and social care centers to pregnant and parenting adolescents.
   1-800-522-5006
   www.ccy.org/teenp

SEXUALLY TRANSMITTED DISEASES, HIV/AIDS

AIDS Clinical Trials Information Service—all to obtain information about participating in research studies and obtaining information about current clinical trials.
   1-800-TRIALS-A
   www.actis.org

CDC Hearing Impaired AIDS Hotline
   1-800-243-7889

CDC National Prevention Information Network—Provides revised guidelines for HIV counseling and testing.
   1-800-458-5231
   www.cdcnpin.org

CDC National STD Hotline—Provides information on STDs and HIV to the general public, and referrals to free or low-cost clinics. Free educational literature is available.
   1-800-227-8922
   www.ashastd.org/NTSD

CDC Spanish HIV/AIDS Hotline
   1-800-344-7432

Hepatitis and Liver Disease Hotline
   1-800-223-0179

National AIDS Hotline—Call with questions on HIV, AIDS, and latest U.S. trends.
   1-800-342-2437
   www.ashastd.org/nah/tty

National Herpes Hotline—Provides information and appropriate referrals to anyone concerned about herpes.
   919-653-4325
   www.ashastd.org/hotlines/herphotline

Project Inform—Provides information on the diagnosis and treatment of HIV. Is an advocate for research and funding policies.
   1-800-822-7422
   www.projinf.org

STD and AIDS Hotline—Find answers to frequently asked questions about sexually transmitted infections and obtain referral to a local support group.
   1-800-227-8922
   www.ashastd.org

Teen AIDS Hotline—Teens provide AIDS prevention education under the supervision of adult mentors.
   1-800-440-TEEN
   www.volunteersolutions.org/volunteerway/volunteer/opp/one_170386.html

TEENS TAP—Call to find information about teens teaching AIDS prevention.
   1-800-234-TEEN

Index

obesity, 50–51, 255–62
  or "baby fat," 256–57
  causes of overeating, 258
  changing habits, 259
  and diets, 257–58
  getting help with, 260–61
  and menstrual cycle, 122
  setting realistic goals in, 261
  as social hardship, 256
  weight-loss coach, 259
obsessive-compulsive disorder (OCD), 286–87
obstructive sleep apnea, 62
oils and fats, 36, 43
opiates, 236–37
oppositional defiant disorder (ODD), 284
oral care, 87–88
oral contraceptives, 119, 203, 211, 212–13
oral health, 84–88, 225
oral sex, 198, 203
orchitis, 154
Ortho Evra patch, 214
osteopenia, 126
osteoporosis, 126
otitis media, 89–90
outercourse, 198
ovaries, 112
  and PCOS, 124–25
overeating, see obesity
ovo-lacto vegetarians, 43
ovulation, 113–14

paint thinner sniffing, 232
panic attacks, 285–86
panic disorder, 285–86
Pap tests, 141, 206
papules, 72
paraphimosis, 159
parents:
  abusive, 265–66
  conflict between, 266
  cooperation among networks of, 240
  and discussions about sex, 189
  and doctors, 18, 31–32
  health-partnering tips for, see health-partnering
    tips
  as role models, 56, 239, 298
  as school advocates, 53, 277
  separation or divorce of, 266
  substance-abusing, 265–66
  values of, 194
  as volunteers, 57
Paxil (paroxetine), 280, 285
PCOS (polycystic ovary syndrome), 124–25
pediatricians, 19
peer pressure:
  and dating abuse, 272–73
  and eating disorders, 244–45
  and mental health, 268–73
  sexual, 218
  in substance abuse, 222, 241
pelvic exam, first, 108
penile disorders, 160–62

penile hygiene, 159–60
penile meatus, 148
petting, 198
pharyngitis, 92–93
phimosis, 159
physical education classes, 52, 53–54
physical examinations, 26, 291–92
physicians, see doctors
piercing, 79–81
pimples, see acne
pink pearly papules, 160
PMS (premenstrual syndrome), 118–19
pneumococcal vaccine, 28
pneumonia, 90–91
polycystic ovary syndrome (PCOS), 124–25
polythelia, 138
post-traumatic stress disorder (PTSD), 286
power naps, 63
precum, 151
pregnancy, 190–91, 216–17
  abortion, 217
  adoption, 217
  contraceptive failure rates, 211
  keeping the baby, 217
  and menstruation, 115, 123–24
  protection from, see contraception
premenstrual syndrome (PMS), 118–19
preseminal fluid, 151
priapism, 161
privacy, 241
progestin-only pill (POP), 213
prostate gland, 148
prostatitis, 150
proteins, 36, 44
Prozac (fluoxetine), 119, 254, 281, 286
psychiatrists, 274
psychologists, 274
psychotherapists, 274
psychotherapy, 273–75
PTSD (post-traumatic stress disorder), 286
puberty:
  for boys, 144–46
  communication during, 9
  for girls, 105–7, 122
pubic area, 148
pubic hair, 106–7, 146
pubic lice, 205, 208
pyelonephritis, 133
pyridium, 134

rape, and post-traumatic stress disorder, 286
rebellion, in chronic health problems, 169
recurrent abdominal pain (RAP), 94–95
relationships, healthy, 194, 218
relaxation techniques, 119
reproductive system:
  of boys, 146–51
  of girls, 107–12
respiratory problems, 88–91
retrograde ejaculation, 150
ring contraception, 214
risky situations, avoiding, 198, 291

Permissions

About the Authors

ANDREA MARKS, M.D., a specialist in adolescent medicine, directed academic programs for sixteen years before opening a private practice in 1990 for patients ages 9 to 30. She is on the faculty of The Mount Sinai School of Medicine and has published widely in the field of adolescent health for both health professionals and the general public (her monthly column, "Ask Dr. Marks," appears in *Cosmo Girl* magazine). An advocate for adolescents as a speaker and in the media, she was recently selected to be President of the Society for Adolescent Medicine in 2004.

BETTY ROTHBART, M.S.W., a psychiatric social worker, educator, and speaker, is the author of several books about parenting and health. She creates health and literacy education programs for the New York City Department of Education and conducts parent/adolescent workshops. She taught at Bank Street College of Education and Hunter College, and has been a consultant to such organizations as Planned Parenthood Federation of America and SIECUS. She has served on the Board of Directors of the American Society of Journalists and Authors.

Both authors have adolescent children and live in New York City.